A FROG UNDER THE TONGUE

T0385557

# THE LITTMAN LIBRARY OF JEWISH CIVILIZATION

*Life Patron*
COLETTE LITTMAN

*Dedicated to the memory of*
LOUIS THOMAS SIDNEY LITTMAN
*who founded the Littman Library for the love of God*
*and as an act of charity in memory of his father*
JOSEPH AARON LITTMAN
*and to the memory of*
ROBERT JOSEPH LITTMAN
*who continued what his father Louis had begun*
יהא זכרם ברוך

'*Get wisdom, get understanding:*
*Forsake her not and she shall preserve thee*'
PROV. 4: 5

*The Littman Library of Jewish Civilization is a registered UK charity*
*Registered charity no.* 1000784

# A FROG UNDER THE TONGUE

## *Jewish Folk Medicine in Eastern Europe*

MAREK TUSZEWICKI

*Translated by*
JESSICA TAYLOR-KUCIA

London
**The Littman Library of Jewish Civilization**
in association with Liverpool University Press

The Littman Library of Jewish Civilization
Registered office: 14th floor, 33 Cavendish Square, London W1G 0PW

in association with Liverpool University Press
4 Cambridge Street, Liverpool L69 7ZU, UK
www.liverpooluniversitypress.co.uk/littman

Managing Editor: Connie Webber

Distributed in North America by Longleaf Services
116 S Boundary St, Chapel Hill, NC 27514, USA

First published in Polish © 2015 Wydawnictwo Austeria, Kraków
First published in English 2021
First published in paperback 2024

English translation of this abridged edition
© The Littman Library of Jewish Civilization 2021

Catalogue records for this book are available from the
British Library and the Library of Congress

ISBN 978–1–802075–83–0

Publishing co-ordinator: Janet Moth
Copy-editing: Agnes Erdos
Proof-reading: Bonnie Blackburn
Indexes: Marek Tuszewicki
Designed and typeset by Pete Russell, Faringdon, Oxon.

Printed and bound in Great Britain by
CPI Group (UK) Ltd., Croydon, CR0 4YY

*To Monika, my only medicine*

# ACKNOWLEDGEMENTS

I WISH to express gratitude to all those who supported the idea of trans-
lating *A Frog under the Tongue*. This book would not have come into
being without the involvement of Connie Webber (the Littman Library of
Jewish Civilization) and Michał Galas (Jagiellonian University of Kraków),
whose enthusiasm for my vision greatly contributed to its realization. My
special thanks are also extended to Wojciech Ornat of the publishing house
Austeria for making this translation a natural consequence of our previous
collaboration. The book has profited enormously from critical insights
and advice from Leszek Hońdo, Zbigniew Libera (Jagiellonian University of Kraków), and Monika Adamczyk-Garbowska (Catholic University
of Lublin), who supervised and reviewed the original dissertation, devoted
to the beliefs and healing practices of the Jewish people, long before it
received its current form. Collecting the scattered and patchy source
material and its evaluation would have been difficult without the help of
Anna Jakimyszyn-Gadocha, Alicja Maślak-Maciejewska, Monika Biesaga,
Zuzanna Kołodziejska, Magdalena Kozłowska, Jolanta Kruszniewska,
Monika Szabłowska-Zaremba, Karolina Szymaniak, Sylwia Szymańska-
Smolkin, Ewa Węgrzyn, Piotr Grącikowski, and Yaad Biran. Certainly, my
work on the project would have taken longer, and perhaps not even led
to the goal at all, had it not been for the presence of my spouse, Monika
Tuszewicka. Last, but not least, I owe a debt of gratitude to my outstanding
translator Jessica Taylor-Kucia, as well as to the editorial team, especially
Agi Erdos and Janet Moth, for their help and assistance in making this
'peculiar' topic available to international readers.

# NOTE ON
# THE ENGLISH EDITION

THIS work differs from the original Polish edition in a number of ways. Long passages about Jewish holidays and liturgies have been deleted, on the grounds that they will be familiar to Littman readers; on the other hand, information needed to understand the Slavic–Jewish interface has been added. Some passages have been abridged, on the recommendation of reviewers of the Polish edition. In particular, I have pruned the tangle of concepts rooted in Polish literature and ethnographic studies that might cloud the picture for a modern English readership.

# CONTENTS

**PART IV**

UNCLEAN FORCES

# NOTE ON
# TRANSLITERATION

## Hebrew

The transliteration of Hebrew in this book reflects consideration of the type of book it is, in terms of its content, purpose, and readership. The system adopted therefore reflects a broad approach to transcription, rather than the narrower approaches found in the *Encyclopaedia Judaica* or other systems developed for text-based or linguistic studies. The aim has been to reflect the pronunciation prescribed for modern Hebrew, rather than the spelling or Hebrew word structure, and to do so using conventions that are generally familiar to the English-speaking reader.

In accordance with this approach, no attempt is made to indicate the distinctions between *alef* and *ayin*, *tet* and *taf*, *kaf* and *kuf*, *sin* and *samekh*, since these are not relevant to pronunciation; likewise, the *dagesh* is not indicated except where it affects pronunciation. Following the principle of using conventions familiar to the majority of readers, however, transcriptions that are well established have been retained even when they are not fully consistent with the transliteration system adopted. On similar grounds, the *tsadi* is rendered by 'tz' in such Anglicized words as barmitzvah. Likewise, the distinction between *ḥet* and *khaf* has been retained, using *ḥ* for the former and *kh* for the latter; the associated forms are generally familiar to readers, even if the distinction is not actually borne out in pronunciation, and for the same reason the final *heh* is indicated too. As in Hebrew, no capital letters are used, except that an initial capital has been retained in transliterating titles of published works (for example, *Shulḥan arukh*).

Since no distinction is made between *alef* and *ayin*, they are indicated by an apostrophe only in intervocalic positions where a failure to do so could lead an English-speaking reader to pronounce the vowel-cluster as a diphthong—as, for example, in *ha'ir*—or otherwise mispronounce the word. An apostrophe is also used, for the same reason, to disambiguate the pronunciation of other English vowel clusters, as for example in *mizbe'aḥ*.

The *sheva na* is indicated by an *e*—*perikat ol, reshut*—except, again, when established convention dictates otherwise.

The *yod* is represented by *i* when it occurs as a vowel (*bereshit*), by *y* when it occurs as a consonant (*yesodot*), and by *yi* when it occurs as both (*yisra'el*).

## Yiddish

Names have generally been left in their familiar forms, even when this is inconsistent with the overall system.

# INTRODUCTION

IT IS WRITTEN: 'Happy is he who is thoughtful of the wretched. And there are none more wretched than the sick.'[1] It is with these words from Psalm 41 that Rabbi Yehudah Yudl Rosenberg, the tsadik of Tarłów and Łódź in the late nineteenth century, began his medical manual *Rafa'el hamalakh*.[2] The Tarler Rebbe was a fascinating figure: an energetic Orthodox leader and writer, alternative medical practitioner steeped in the hasidic tradition and practising homeopathy, and in later years rabbi to the Jewish community in Montreal. He was a man who, like many of his contemporaries, still breathed the spirit of tradition, but with time became increasingly influenced by modern life. The book written by Rabbi Rosenberg around 1910 superbly reflects the multiplicity of health-related views, beliefs, and practices that held sway in the world of which he was a representative. It is an anthology of advice and wisdom sourced from medical, religious, and folk literature, and is highly conservative in its literary and linguistic form. The opening words of the work, whose title contains the name of the angel Raphael (Heb. 'God will heal'), highlight the fundamental significance of such concepts as health and sickness to the east European Jewish community, and particularly to that traditional stratum of the Ashkenazi world which in the collective memory is often reduced to a single generic image: that of the devout scholar versed in the sacred books and kabbalah, and who exists almost outside the corporeal dimension.

My fundamental aim in writing this book was to bring to light the wealth of notions connected with the folk medicine of Ashkenazi Jews living in eastern Europe around 1900. In order better to describe the scope of this subject, the first step must be to define what exactly folk medicine is. Of course,

---

[1] Ps. 41: 2. Unless otherwise stated, biblical quotations are taken from Berlin and Brettler (eds.), *The Jewish Study Bible* (Jewish Publication Society Tanakh Translation).

[2] Rosenberg, *Rafa'el hamalakh*, 3. For more on the work and writings of Rabbi Rosenberg, see Robinson, 'The Tarler Rebbe of Łódź', 53–61, and id., 'Literary Forgery and Hasidic Judaism', 61–78.

it is a somewhat ambiguous concept, long tarred by the derogatory description 'superstition'. In common parlance the term 'folk medicine' is usually used to describe remedies and treatment methods specific to traditional culture and which do not fall within the contemporary dominant biomedical model.[3] Magic practices are one area of activity often categorized as 'folklore'. Largely incomprehensible to the majority of the uninitiated, they tend to be perceived as bizarre and mysterious, and are commonly associated with bats, garlic, and arcane incantations, though some do cherish the hope of experiencing the powerful healing they promise. Elsewhere this descriptor is used to refer to medications drawn from the broad canon of natural medicine, sanctified by generations of experience. Passed down over centuries, such knowledge has been considered an important element of the heritage of a given community, whether village, town, or nation, and testimony to the development of material and spiritual culture in the *longue durée*. An equivalent assumption regarding the curative therapies accumulated over generations among Ashkenazi Jews would be overly simplistic, however, as is revealed by the image which emerges from research into the sources available to us.

In the ethnological literature that covers the Slavic lands, the question of the scope of the term 'folk culture' has been the subject of extensive discussion. This has rarely extended to matters closely connected to the Jewish populace, however, since the main focus of debate has tended to be the ethnic Slavic peasantry. Nonetheless, since this region essentially corresponds to the lands inhabited by the eastern Ashkenazim, and since the subject of this book—health and healing—is by definition universal in character, it is worth pausing to look at two interpretations of the folk medicine of the Slavs inspired by the theories of structuralism and cultural semiotics. Some scholars, among them Ludwik Stomma in his work *Antropologia kultury wsi polskiej XIX w.* (The Anthropology of the Culture of Rural Poland in the Nineteenth Century), claim that 'traditional folk culture' never existed in any pure form, and that cultural types are mutually permeable. In this discourse, it would be more accurate to speak of a 'folk-type' culture dominated by mythical thinking, of its visible expressions, and of its subsequent decline in the sphere of peasant culture. 'Folk medicine' (of necessity in inverted commas) would thus be based on myth rather

---

[3] In accordance with contemporary medical anthropological convention I use the term 'biomedicine' to refer to Western medicine founded on the paradigm of the biological sciences.

than rational analysis and experience, and any efficacy of its various manifestations would have to be attributed to chance.[4] For the purposes of this
book, I shall refer to this as the narrow definition. One of those who dis-
agree with Stomma's views is Zbigniew Libera, who, in his book *Medycyna
ludowa. Chłopski rozsądek czy gminna fantazja?* (Folk Medicine: Peasant Sense
or Communal Fantasy?), attributes fundamental significance to myth in
the shaping of popular views on health, but at the same time emphasizes
the complexity of these views and the rational element inherent in them.
In his opinion,

only by taking account of convictions and practices . . . in the fullness of their
mutual relations and by taking into consideration the mythological imaginings
which are at their roots is it possible to define the medical system within the traditional image of the world, to express it in terms of therapeutic magic and other
cultural texts, to treat medicine as one form of interpretation of the world and of
humanity, and to discern the sense behind various forms of treatment.[5]

I am far more convinced by Libera's 'broad' definition of the concept of
folk medicine. The primary reason for this is that, as scholars including the
North American ethnologist Don Yoder have noted, folk medicine should
not be confused with primitive or 'native' medicine, which is essentially
devoid of links to other systems of medicine. Folk medicine is not a collection of views enclosed within the embrace of a single social stratum (the
common people, the peasantry, country folk); it is an aspect of life that was
perceptible and recognizable in the culture of every level of society and of
every community living in eastern Europe in the period that interests us
here.[6] Secondly—and this is particularly important from the perspective of
research into Jewish culture—as recently as the early twentieth century,
traditional health-related practices still held considerable sway in urban
environments. Although the proportion of the populace that employed
them had shrunk discernibly, and the practices themselves had succumbed
to the influences of modernity, they had not become invisible even to the
most dedicated proponents of biomedicine. As such, then, folk medicine
was a complex system which comprised both natural and magic elements of
highly diverse provenance. On the one hand it remained dependent upon

---

   [4] Stomma, *Antropologia kultury wsi polskiej*, 126.
   [5] Libera, *Medycyna ludowa*, 12. 'Other cultural texts' refers to songs, stories, and proverbs,
which provide a more general insight into the traditional world-view.
   [6] Yoder, 'Folk Medicine', 192–3.

the conception of the construction of the world that was dominant within a given community, as one of the manifestations of folk cosmology and of the rationality and logic specific to that system. On the other it was shaped by official policies on health-related matters, whether these happened to be anachronistic or thoroughly modern, as well as by other systems of medicine, including the beliefs and practices of neighbouring ethnic groups.

Broadening the conceptual scope of folk medicine enables us to solve certain methodological problems. It is true that the Jewish community stood somewhat apart from the other ethnic groups inhabiting eastern Europe, in particular from the peasant classes. The Israeli ethnographer Haya Bar-Itzhak lists the following as unique features of Jewish folklore: multiculturalism, due to the scattering of the Jews in the diaspora; multilingualism; and the presence of written sources.[7] These attributes lent the Jews' customs distinctiveness, though they were not exclusive in character. They might cause obstacles, but they could also create new interfaces for intercultural relations. Multilingualism, when it appeared in non-Jewish sources, was one of the attributes of magic in therapeutics. In the context of a multi-ethnic society, where many and varied dialects were in use, contact with a healer or physician necessitated negotiation of a shared platform of communication. As Stomma demonstrates, in folk culture the fact of speaking a different language was rarely a barrier in itself. It was more a marker of 'outsiderdom', which functioned primarily at the level of myth, that is, as a means of ordering otherness in the collective consciousness.[8] The question of handwritten and printed collections of wisdom regarding therapies was similar. Written sources—in various forms and in a range of ways—also influenced the medical practices of the Christian populace, though to a lesser extent than among the Jews. Any group that has even the most limited contact with books and letters will ultimately be influenced by them in some way. This is also true of illiterate communities insofar as they have regular contact with individuals or groups in possession of libraries or other collections of books. The oral transmission of tradition in the field of folk medicine should not be treated as the only form of its dissemination. It certainly does not preclude—on the contrary, it is far more likely to promote—the popularization of views which may have originated in books.[9]

---

[7] Bar-Itzhak, 'Introduction: Folklore and Jewish Folklore', pp. xiii–xiv.

[8] Stomma, *Antropologia kultury wsi polskiej*, 40–1.

[9] See e.g. Hufford, 'Medicine, Folk', 849; Libera, *Znachor*, 42–5.

The question of Jewish folklore, as a phenomenon at once local and quasi-global, however, is somewhat more complex. It forces the scholar to define precisely the group of Jews about which he or she undertakes to write. While keeping sight of the ties that bound the Ashkenazi diaspora to geographically distant centres of Jewish culture, I nonetheless consider the primary subject of my interest to be its east European branch, along with its Christian environment. More specifically still, I focus on that part of this society which remained faithful to its traditional Ashkenazi Jewishness (*yidishkayt*) and retained its attachment to aspects of that tradition such as time-honoured forms of religiosity, social institutions, values, and language. It is the views and beliefs of this group, the customs it observed, and the procedures it followed in the field of healthcare and medicine that are the focus of this book.

The research perspective outlined above represents a strongly comparative approach to relations between the Jewish community and other groups inhabiting the same geographical region. Readers will undoubtedly notice how many of the footnotes in this book cite publications which discuss the therapeutic beliefs and practices of rural residents: Poles, Ukrainians, and Belarusians,[10] and also early modern medical manuals, mostly in Polish.[11] This is a deliberate and very important decision in view of the relatively short history of comparative research and of the obstacles that have to date prevented comparison of similar documents with testimonies in Yiddish and Hebrew. Including reference to Slavonic and German sources in the analysis of Jewish folk medicine enables us to note differences, but also provides broad scope for the discussion of similarities, shared traditions, influences, and cultural diffusion. At this point it is worth skipping ahead of the narrative somewhat to emphasize that the Jews constituted an integral element of the mosaic of east European medical practices and healthcare. Representatives of the Jewish community played an active part in the medical culture of eastern Europe on many levels, as practitioners of biomedicine, as paramedics of various sorts, as healers, and as patients. This participation was not confined to the sphere of symbolic

[10] e.g. Udziela, *Medycyna i przesądy lecznicze ludu polskiego*; Talko-Hryncewicz, *Zarys lecznictwa ludowego na Rusi Południowej*; Wereńko, 'Przyczynek do lecznictwa ludowego'; Biegeleisen, *Lecznictwo ludu polskiego*; Moszyński, *Kultura ludowa Słowian*.

[11] e.g. *Vade mecum medicum*; Haur, *Ekonomika lekarska albo domowe lekarstwa*; *Apteka domowa i podróżna doznawana lekarzami*.

connotations which, in the Slavic imagination, linked adherents of Judaism with otherness and witchcraft; neither was it restricted to the Jewish court physicians or Jews studying medicine when the universities were opened up to them. And it most certainly was not expressed in the exclusivism that was purported to be the ever-present issue keeping the Ashkenazi community and the non-Jewish world apart.

This book preserves a distinction between the natural and the magical,[12] both in terms of the aetiology of disease and in respect of the remedies used. Nonetheless, given the blurred boundaries between these two aspects of folk medicine and healthcare, and the limited availability of historical sources, this does not form the main axis of my analysis. Neither is there any attempt to verify popular health-related beliefs and practices against the biomedical paradigm, or to pass judgement on the validity of views on the nature of illnesses or the efficacy of remedies applied. This would do little to increase our knowledge of the basis on which a given remedy was used, and would therefore be of limited use in recreating the folk world-view.[13]

The history of research shows that little work has been done in the field of Jewish folk medicine in eastern Europe. There have, to date, been no monographs on the subject, which may come as something of a surprise given the rich traditions of German, Polish, and Russian ethnography, and the considerable achievements of YIVO centres and Israeli scholars. Many of the works of ethnographic literature written in Polish in the 1880s and 1890s include information on the characteristics and way of life of the Jewish population. Key contributors to this research were the pioneers who wrote for the periodicals and book series *Wisła*, *Lud*, and *Zbiór Wiadomości do Antropologii Krajowej*, foremost among them Regina Lilientalowa, Benjamin Wolf Segel, and Samuel Adalberg. Others wrote in the Polish-language Jewish press, including Henryk Lew (in the Warsaw paper *Izraelita*), Izrael Fels (in the Lwów-based *Wschód*), and Giza Frenklowa (in *Chwila*, also published in Lwów), and to a certain extent also Henryk Biegel-

---

[12] Although Judaism expressly prohibited the use of spells, and the ethical literature of Ashkenazi Jews exhorted people to shun magic in any and all of its manifestations (see e.g. T. H. Koydanover, *Kav hayashar*, 88), Jewish culture, in particular its therapeutic practices, was steeped in magical lore.      [13] Moszyński, *Kultura ludowa Słowian*, 216.

eisen. Their studies, supplemented by numerous press articles on the living circumstances of Ashkenazi Jews around 1900, proved sufficiently modern and of such breadth as to make a lasting contribution to the specialist literature. They served Polish, Russian, and Ukrainian ethnologists as comparative material that provided a basis from which to draw wider conclusions. However, they remained almost entirely undiscovered, and therefore absent from contemporary Jewish studies, in other parts of the world. The research of Olga Goldberg-Mulkiewicz, a professor at the Hebrew University who strove to make the bibliography of Polish ethnographic sources accessible to scholars working in English, did little to improve this state of affairs.[14]

In the same period a lot of material amassed by Jewish collectors of folklore was also published in other languages. 'Superstitions' (*abergloybns*) and 'old wives' tales' (*zabobones*) were matters of interest to Jewish ethnography from its birth as a discipline, when its development was significantly influenced by the German *Volkskunde*. Although its proponents (such as Julius Preuss) evinced a strong bias towards research into the mores of the biblical and talmudic age,[15] they rapidly branched out into the field of the traditions of east European Jews. Descriptions of beliefs and practices from the realm of healthcare were printed in papers published in Germany by Rabbi Max Grunwald[16] and Friedrich Salomon Krauss.[17] A few articles by authors including Samuel Weissenberg, Demeter Dan, Raimund Friedrich Keindl, and the aforementioned Biegeleisen were published in other German and Austrian ethnographic journals, such as *Globus*. Matters relating to Jewish folklore, and in some cases specifically folk medicine, surfaced in Russian- and Ukrainian-language publications in both tsarist and Soviet Russia. Folk medicine was also one of the significant areas of interest on the pioneering research expedition to the towns of Volhynia organized by the St Petersburg-based Jewish Historical and Ethnographic Society and led by S. An-sky (Salomon Zaynvl Rapoport) in 1912–14. This expedition bore fruit in a series of articles published in the journal *Yevreiskaya Starina* and in the fifteenth volume of An-sky's *Collected Writings*, and in a short though interesting study by one of its participants, Avrom Rechtman.[18]

[14] The publication intimated here is her slim volume *Ethnographic Topics Relating to Jews in Polish Studies*. [15] Preuss, *Biblisch-talmudische Medizin*.
[16] *Mitteilungen der Gesellschaft für Jüdische Volkskunde*, 1898–1904; *Mitteilungen zur Jüdischen Volkskunde*, 1905–22, 1926–9; *Jahrbuch für Jüdische Volkskunde*, 1923–5.
[17] *Am Ur-Quell*, 1890–6; *Der Urquell*, 1897–8.  [18] *Jewish Ethnography and Folklore* (Yid.).

Health-related issues were also of interest to the Jewish intelligentsia, for whom ethnography held a particular fascination. Mordkhe Spektor recognized this trend, and had Avrom Yitshok Buchbinder's article 'Jewish Omens (Zabobones)' printed in *Hoyz-fraynd* in 1909. Many collectors of folk medicine 'curios' were themselves doctors, and it was this group that initiated the compilation and publication of a survey questionnaire in the popular Yiddish science journal *Folksgezunt* (1923) and called for a collection of 'folk superstitions' to be compiled. But in fact it was the Ethnographic Committee of the Jewish Scientific Institute (YIVO) in Vilna (now Vilnius, Lithuania) that in the 1920s and 1930s played the most important role in amassing such material. Its scholars in both Vilna and Warsaw published a number of documents and articles (their own and others submitted to them by collectors of folklore such as Regina Lilientalowa) on the subject of beliefs and practices connected with health and medicine,[19] both in periodicals and in book series.[20] These publications were followed by three slim pamphlets released by the Yehudah Leyb Cahan Folklore Club in New York between 1954 and 1962 and entitled *Yidisher folklor*. Similar material was also published in Zionist journals, above all in *Reshumot*, founded by the Hebrew poet Hayim Nahman Bialik, Alter Druyanov, and Yehoshua Chone Ravnitzki, and from the late 1940s in *Yeda am* and *Edot*. Barbara Kirshenblatt-Gimblett has written an extensive article on many aspects of the history of Jewish folklore and ethnography studies,[21] while Itzik N. Gottesman, in his book *Defining the Yiddish Nation*, takes a broader angle on the history of Jewish ethnography as a project to 'invent' the tradition of the Ashkenazi diaspora in eastern Europe.

Most authors of articles and studies written in the early twentieth century made no attempt to interpret or analyse their observations in this field. As Kazimierz Moszyński noted, such texts tended to take the form of more or less systematized collections of information in which there was no attempt to apply a 'point of comparison on any wider scale'.[22] At best (as in the work of Max Weinreich, for instance) they concentrated on philological analysis, shifting their focus to explaining the genesis of the cultural facts

[19] e.g. Bastomski, *At the Source: Jewish Proverbs* (Yid.); Lilientalowa, 'Additions: The "Evil Eye"' (Yid.).

[20] Periodicals included *Yidishe filologye*, 1924, *Filologishe shriftn*, 1926–9, and *Pinkes*, 1927–9, as well as other titles published in the series Shriftn fun yidishn visnshaftlekhn institut between 1926 and 1939.          [21] 'Folklore, Ethnography and Anthropology'.

[22] Moszyński, *Kultura ludowa Słowian*, 174.

they discussed. While doing little to explicate the intricacies of folk culture, however, they nonetheless undeniably created repositories of ethnographic notes. Among the exceptions to this rule were the mature analyses of practices observed in the context of a cholera epidemic published in the 1930s in *Sotsyale meditsin* by Naftole Veynig.[23] Any continuation of this research from a sociological and functional perspective was prevented by the annihilation of the Jewish population in the Holocaust.

It was some time before a more comprehensive approach to the subject was forthcoming. The first harbinger of this development was *Jewish Magic and Superstition* by Joshua Trachtenberg, which marked the beginning of a period dominated by works written in English. Issues related to health and sickness were touched on by Elizabeth Herzog and Mark Zborowski in their groundbreaking though now outdated book *Life Is with People: The Jewish Little-Town of Eastern Europe*, written under the supervision of Margaret Mead. Thereafter, interest in the medical practices of the European branch of the Ashkenazi diaspora (as opposed to the Americas and Israel) faded rapidly. Only customs and rituals surrounding childbirth seemed still to attract some modest attention from scholars. These practices had been a major area of interest for Lilientalowa in the early twentieth century; her extensive essay 'Dziecko żydowskie' (The Jewish Child) has recently been reissued in book form.[24] The field of pregnancy and childbirth was also the subject of Raphael Patai, who published a number of scientific articles on related matters, including aids to conception, and also wrote an entire chapter on this area in the volume *On Jewish Folklore*.[25] Finally, the work of Michele Klein must be mentioned; this tackles the subject of childbirth in an accessible, if not particularly revelatory, form.[26] In parallel to these works, since the mid-1940s there have been many publications deepening our insight into Jewish folk culture in general. Chaim Schwarzbaum's *Studies in Jewish and World Folklore*, the anthologies *Yiddish Folktales* by Beatrice Silverman-Weinreich and *Folktales of the Jews* by Dan Ben-Amos and Dov Noy (in particular its second volume), and the multi-volume series *Sefer hamo'adim* edited by Yom-Tov Levinski are just a few works of immense value which shed light on the cultural background to beliefs and practices connected with health.

[23] Veynig, '*Mageyfe* Weddings' (Yid.); id., 'Medicaments and Remedies among the Jews' (Yid.).    [24] Lilientalowa, *Dziecko żydowskie*, based on the 1927 edition of the essay.
[25] Patai, 'Jewish Folk-Cures for Barrenness' and 'Jewish Folk-Cures for Barrenness. II'; id., *On Jewish Folklore*.    [26] Klein, *A Time To Be Born*.

Post-war studies of folk medicine launched in Israel initially followed trends that had been typical of pre-Holocaust folkloristic research. A few of those who published collections of folk curios with analytical comments and explanations were themselves immigrants from eastern Europe, among them talented writers and ethnographers such as Akiva Ben-Ezra (Kostrometski), Yehudah Avida (Złotnik), and Yitshak Ganuz (Ganuzowicz). In successive decades research at Israeli universities switched its focus to communities that, unlike the east European diaspora, were still in existence. Thenceforth it emphasized the unity of the nation's culture regardless of obvious differences; the drive to build a new society based on immigrants arriving from a range of cultural spaces provided the perfect context for this. In the 1990s Hagit Matras defined Jewish folk medicine in terms of its unique characteristics, writing: 'This distinctiveness is rooted in the Hebrew language, in the Written and Oral Law, and in Jewish symbolism.'[27] This was the line also taken by Gideon Bohak, author of *Ancient Jewish Magic*. In his endeavour to concentrate on magic as a kind of learned art of influencing the world and people, he decided to exclude the realm of medicine and health from his sphere of attention, but included a detailed analysis of the outside influences that were present in Jewish folk culture. In recent decades interest in the ethnography of contemporary Ashkenazi collectivities, particularly hasidic communities, has increased in both Israel and the USA. Unfortunately, this has not translated into a significant contribution in terms of the historical view. There are, however, a number of promising studies in the form of unpublished dissertations, which enhance our knowledge of various aspects of Jewish medical practices and healthcare. Of particular note in this group are Lisa Epstein's study of the history of Jewish medicine in tsarist Russia[28] and a survey of amulets by Daniela Schmid.[29] Interesting work has also been produced in the form of analyses of hasidic writings, such as the studies of Ira Robinson on Yehudah Yudl Rosenberg[30] and of Daniel Reiser on the writings of the tsadik Kalman Shapiro of Piaseczno.[31] My own essay on Abraham Abele Kanarvogel, a hasid of the Rymanów community, focuses on health-related strands in his

[27]  Matras, 'Jewish Folk Medicine in the 19th and 20th Centuries', 118.
[28]  Epstein, 'Caring for the Soul's House'.
[29]  Schmid, 'Jüdische Amulette aus Osteuropa'.
[30]  Robinson, 'The Tarler Rebbe of Łódź'.
[31]  Reiser, 'Idea nieuświadomionego (the unconscious) a chasydyzm'.

book *Be'erot hamayim*.[32] Most of these analyses place the medical practices
of the traditional Jewish community within the context of medical currents
contemporary to them.

Recently this area of study has seen limited interest from historians and
cultural studies scholars. Historical narrations usually relegate the ethno-
medical aspect of Ashkenazi Jewish culture to the margins of broader
research, though in some cases they do afford it somewhat more attention.
Among the scholars who have addressed this aspect of Ashkenazi life are
Marcin Wodziński; Hanna Węgrzynek, who has written on 'black weddings'; Yohanan Petrovsky-Shtern, the author of a number of studies on
early modern medicine; and Glenn Dynner, who has written a book on the
hasidic movement in the Kingdom of Poland.[33] Excerpts of previously
unpublished material from Lilientalowa's archives were published in 2010
in an essay by Piotr Grącikowski, who plans to release the archives in full at
some point.[34] The subject of Jewish medical practices has been taken up to
a lesser extent by ethnologists, however, since it entails looking back into
the past instead of focusing on living and thriving cultures. Their limited
knowledge of Yiddish and Hebrew sources has been a further barrier to
accessing the relevant ethnographic material.[35] Maria Barthel de Wyden-
thal, in her interesting work *Uroczne oczy* (Evil Eyes), drew almost exclusively on Polish texts by Lilientalowa. For the same reason the undeniably
fascinating snippets of Jewish folklore published in 1897 in the journal
*Wisła* by Ignacja Piątkowska—all of them verifiable in the original
sources—read bizarrely. The number of distortions and inaccuracies—testimony to her lack of comprehension of fundamental terms in Jewish culture—must today elicit profound consternation. Perhaps the most valuable
attempts at exploring the sources relating to Jewish folk medicine were
undertaken by scholars associated with the Sefer Center in Moscow in the
series edited by a team under Olga Belova. None of these publications,

[32] Tuszewicki, 'Chasydzi w Galicji wobec współczesnej farmacji'.
[33] Wodziński, 'Dybuk'; Węgrzynek, '"Shvartze khasene": Black Wedding among Polish
Jews'; Petrovsky-Shtern, '"You Will Find It in the Pharmacy": Practical Kabbalah and Natural
Medicine'; id., 'The Master of an Evil Name'; id., 'Magic and Folk Remedy' (Heb.); id., *The
Golden Age Shtetl*; Dynner, *Men of Silk*.
[34] Grącikowski, 'Kobieta żydowska w badaniach Reginy Lilientalowej'.
[35] Among the articles which address the subject of Jewish therapeutic practices we
might mention the following: Wasilewski, 'Tabu, zakaz magiczny, nieczystość'; Banasiewicz-
Ossowska, 'Warunki życia i stan zdrowia Żydów polskich'.

however, address more than isolated, fragmentary aspects of what is a much larger issue.

This study thus aims to fill the sizeable gap in the research into Jewish folk medicine in eastern Europe, and into Ashkenazi Jewish culture in general.

The period under scrutiny begins in the late nineteenth century and is linked to the birth of the ethnic studies movement and the awakening of interest among the Jewish intelligentsia in the medical customs of the community which they referred to as 'the folk', or 'the people'. It ends with the first decades of the twentieth century, specifically with the First World War and the conflicts played out on Polish territory shortly after its conclusion (fighting in the Ukraine and the Polish–Bolshevik War). Narrowing the perspective to a time frame defined in this way facilitates the detailed analysis of a cohesive body of material without having to address the consequences of the events that changed the face of eastern Europe. Nonetheless, in view of the need to delineate the broader historical background and demonstrate the continuity of certain phenomena characteristic of the turn of the century, it has proved necessary to make reference to some much earlier sources.

The territorial scope, in turn, is the region known in the terminology of contemporary Yiddish studies as eastern Ashkenaz (or Ashkenaz II).[36] Thus the primary focus of interest will be the lands of the former Polish Commonwealth within the Austrian and Russian partitions, in their boundaries as on the eve of the outbreak of the First World War, while the lands lying within the German empire, in view of the considerable degree of acculturation of the Jews there, are marginal to this work. The collectivity whose views on medical issues are the subject of this book also existed in pockets scattered beyond the historical borders of Poland and Lithuania. It will thus be expedient to take into account a considerable body of sources originating from northern Hungary (chiefly Slovakia and Transylvania), Bukovina, Romania, Bessarabia, the south of Ukraine, and Odessa, as well as material gathered or published by émigrés to western Europe, the USA, Argentina, and Israel. In view of the character of the study, however, and the paucity of comparative material, it seems neither justifiable nor even

---

[36]  See e.g. M. Weinreich, *History of the Yiddish Language*, 1–44.

possible to undertake an in-depth analysis of local variations on particular beliefs. For, as Lilientalowa noted, 'the customs . . . of the Jewish populace . . . are so internally similar that the non-existence of a superstition in one place and its existence in another should rather be considered a question of insufficiently systematic questioning on my part'.[37]

I have mainly drawn on sources in Yiddish and Hebrew, and also in Polish, English, German, Russian, and Ukrainian. The source base comprises selected manuscripts and printed publications dating from around 1900 and featuring therapeutic advice, recipes, magical incantations, and descriptions of kabbalistic methods, all used by the traditional Jewish community in the Polish lands. In addition to manuscripts, which have hitherto rarely been of interest to students of therapeutic practices, notable vademecums include: the anonymous *Sefer harefuot* (Lwów?, 1864/5; Vienna, 1926/7), *Sefer lakhashim usegulot vegoralot umazalot* by Israel Yudl Goldberg and Abraham Aba Eisenberg (Jerusalem, 1880/1), *Imrot shelomoh* by Solomon Wilff (Lwów, 1883/4), the above-mentioned *Rafa'el hamalakh* by Yehudah Yudl Rosenberg (Łódź, 1907), *Sefer haḥayim hanikra segulot yisra'el* by Shabetai Lifshits (Munkacs, 1905), and *Zikhron ya'akov yosef* by Yehoshua Yonatan Rubinstein (Jerusalem, *c*.1930), some of which were bilingual publications in Hebrew and Yiddish. Most of them may be classified as books of *segulot urefuot* (*segulot* are practical methods of a magical nature, while *refuot* are natural remedies). Among the sources of particular significance for the present study there were also a certain number of earlier—even medieval—titles, which were reprinted repeatedly up to the First World War and which continued to influence the character of popular medical views. These examples of ethical literature aspired not only to the moral improvement of their readers, but also to enlighten them on phenomena both visible and invisible. They included *Sefer ḥasidim*, *Shevilei emunah*, *Shenei luḥot haberit*, *Kav hayashar*, *Tsene urene*, *Ma'aseh tuvyah*, and *Sefer haberit*, as well as a number of manuals addressed to people performing circumcisions. Another point of reference was the pamphlets penned by *ba'alei shem* (healer kabbalists), such as the eighteenth-century *Sefer zekhirah*, *Mifalot elokim*, *Toledot adam*, and several other compilations of practical kabbalah, early apothecary arts, and folklore. Alongside these, books of customs also played an important role in my research, above all *Ta'amei haminhagim umekorei hadinim* by Abraham Isaac Sperling (Lwów, 1896), *Sefer*

---

[37] Lilientalowa, 'Przesądy żydowskie', 277.

*matamim* by Isaac Lipiets (Warsaw, 1890), and *Minhagei yeshurun* by Abraham Eliezer Hirshovitsh (Vilnius, 1899).

My research brought to light a considerable volume of material never previously exploited by scholars of folk medicine. The manuscripts on which I draw were sourced largely from the Library of the Jewish Theological Seminary (New York), the Bibliotheca Rosenthaliana (Amsterdam), the Archive of the Emanuel Ringelblum Jewish Historical Institute in Warsaw, and the bequest of Regina Lilientalowa held in the Public Library of the Capital City of Warsaw at Koszykowa Street.[38] The printed sources came from the collections of the Society for Preservation of Hebrew Books (New York), the New York Public Library (New York), the YIVO Institute for Jewish Research (New York), the National Library of Israel (Jerusalem), the Austrian National Library (Vienna), the Lithuanian National Library (Vilnius), the Library of the Jewish Historical Institute (Warsaw), and the National Library (Warsaw), as well as from the collection of Hebrew printed matter in the Institute of Jewish Studies at the Jagiellonian University and the Jagiellonian Library (Kraków). Some of these documents have been digitized, and access to them was facilitated by the websites of the respective archives and libraries.

The second main type of source used in this book is ethnographic material published from the late nineteenth century on, both in periodicals and as autonomous volumes. Among these items are systematized collections of descriptions of folk remedies and other documents of assistance in reconstructing commonly held views on health, illness, or the functioning of the human body (such as collections of omens, proverbs, songs, and folk tales). Aside from strictly ethnographic publications, this group of sources includes lexicons, encyclopedias, and popular scientific titles dating from the early twentieth century. The vast majority of the documentation on which these publications are based is deposited in the archives of the YIVO Institute for Scientific Research, whose main branches today are in Vilnius and New York, in the Israel Folktale Archives (Haifa), and in the State Museum in St Petersburg (in the S. An-sky collection). In view of both the immense volume of resources and the repetitive nature of the content, it proved necessary to narrow the field of interest to a representative portion of the previously published material. Use was also made of material gathered among Jewish émigrés from eastern Europe and accessible in the

---

[38] These are listed under the Archival Sources heading of the Bibliography.

Online Archive of American Folk Medicine (now the Archive of Healing, Ritual, and Transformation).[39] In addition to enabling the reconstruction of the overall picture of health-related beliefs and medical practices among the Jewish populace, the ethnographic sources also serve comparative analysis. This is true in particular of publications that merely make mention of the beliefs of Jews, or make no reference to them at all, focusing on other ethnic groups in eastern Europe.

The picture is supplemented by information discovered in Jewish memoiristic literature. This is a very broad category, encompassing autobiographies, diaries, memoirs, and a genre of literature unique to the Ashkenazi diaspora: the *izker-bikher*, or books of memory, commemorating the communities annihilated in the Holocaust. These sources were written primarily in Yiddish and Hebrew, though there is also interesting and extremely useful information in those that were published in Polish, German, English, and Russian. It is important to bear in mind, however, that these writings contain many errors and inaccuracies, the result of both the passage of time and the adoption by their authors of a more contemporary (or even biomedical) perspective, which skewed their attitude towards folk medicine. A similar caveat should be added in respect of sources from the genre of belles-lettres, which, notwithstanding the nature of this type of writing, are considered in contemporary ethnology to have undeniable value.

This book is divided into four parts, each of which examines a different issue within the wider theme.

Part I offers an overview of the levels on which such notions as health and sickness were uniquely understood within Jewish folk culture; these meanings differed markedly from contemporary mainstream interpretations, which were founded on the biological sciences. Among the first questions addressed are the ways of speaking about illness, including its concealment using euphemism and other linguistic devices due to religious

---

[39] University of California Los Angeles, <https://humtech.ucla.edu/project/archive-of-ritual-healing-and-transformation/> (accessed 3 Jan. 2020). The idea of this project formerly devoted to gathering examples of folk medical practices changed around 2015. Today the archive is used mostly as a platform for studying and teaching the ethics of digital publication of cultural information 'deriving from indigenous, dispossessed, or disenfranchised populations'.

and superstitious taboo, and the multiplicity and significance of available treatment options. The Ashkenazi community, which is ordinarily viewed in terms of its close attachment to religion, was influenced in health-related matters by many systems and models, few of which may be considered exceptional and specific to this segment of society. All of these are discussed, taking into consideration the successive steps followed in seeking medical assistance, starting with the Jewish tradition and the immediate family, through official and unofficial therapeutic practitioners without medical training, to the two ultimate platforms on which the battle against disease was fought, and which were only seemingly conflicted and mutually exclusive: the hasidic court and the doctor's consulting room.

Part II examines the far-reaching consequences of the persistent conviction in folk culture of the close bonds between the human body (the microcosm) and the world (the macrocosm). This conviction was not only the ground from which 'folk-type medicine' grew, but also key evidence that ancient theories surrounding the origins and functioning of the world, the anatomy and workings of the human body, and even astrology were very much alive in the medicine-related beliefs and practices of the residents of eastern Europe at the turn of the nineteenth century. This section therefore contains examples of treatments employing methods inspired by folk mythology and expressed in a language that used an anthropomorphic and cosmological code, and of the consequences of the perception of humans as a reflection of the world around them. In Chapters 7 and 8 I describe health-related convictions and recommendations based on the principles of humoral pathology and astrology, which had been a constant in Jewish culture down the ages, and were no less so in east European folk medicine around 1900.

In Part III more space is devoted to matters outside the remit of medical speculation and related to the theory of humours and the philosophy of nature. Rabbinical ethics, and in particular the concepts of sin, judgement, and evil decrees, played a major role in interpreting human fate. Popular ideas regarding the consequences for one's health of disobedience to the Creator and his commandments are discussed, as are traditional methods of reversing or annulling them. Chapter 10 covers that dimension of Jewish therapeutic practices which encompassed daily and annual rites, rituals, and customs. On the one hand, it looks at the health-related justifications for the rituals that God-fearing Jews were required to perform, and on the other it emphasizes the ubiquity in Jewish folk medicine of elements of the sabbath and festival liturgy, and of objects used in religious rites.

The fourth and final part of the book looks at Jewish conceptions of the world of demons, both those which in popular interpretations took the form of diseases operating within the human body, and forces of evil existing outside the body and doing their mischief by means of spells, incantations, dangerous tricks, and villainy. In addition to the aetiology, prevention, and treatment of complaints caused by the work of demonic beings, I also describe instances of interaction with evil forces which could, on occasion, promise benefits for both parties.

This book is essentially a historical work. The traditional Jewish community fell victim to incomprehensible crimes during the Second World War and no longer exists in the form that emerges from the sources accessible to us today. For this reason I often deliberately depart from the use of the 'ethnographic present tense' in favour of the past tense, especially in sections addressing issues related to Judaism. The diverse character of the subject of this study, and the aims I set myself, nonetheless also demanded recourse to methods used in a range of fields of the humanities. I could not have written this book without the possibilities presented by contemporary interdisciplinary studies, above all the tools supplied by linguistics, anthropology, and cultural studies.

Jewish folk medicine is a veritable tangle of meanings, and becomes ever harder to unravel the further we move from the Holocaust and the tragic end met by the traditional Jewish society of eastern Europe. My aim here is to provide a detailed explanation of issues that the student of Ashkenazi health-related beliefs and practices might encounter. I thus explore how traditional Jewish medicine in this region related to its historical, geographical, and social contexts, as well as to other traditions, and what aspects of it were elements of a wider, common heritage. The scale of this challenge is far beyond the capacity of a single volume. But despite the complexity of the phenomena under study here, and the various obstacles and limitations posed by the subject, I hope I have succeeded in contributing to the expansion of knowledge about Ashkenazi Jewish culture. History shows us that attempts to clear up the confusion caused by ethno-medical sources and their seemingly incomprehensible tangles of meaning need not invariably be doomed to irrelevance. Moses Maimonides (1135–1204), in his *Guide of the Perplexed*, remarks upon the similarity between the biblical concepts of life, convalescence, and good fortune on the one hand, and death, sickness, and misfortune on the other.[40] This brief disquisition, in which philological analysis combined with the philosopher's genius to produce a thoroughly modern interpretation of culture, was a source of inexhaustible inspiration to me as I wrote this book.

[40] *Guide of the Perplexed*, i. 42.

# PART I

# HEALTH AND SICKNESS
# IN THE CULTURE OF
# ASHKENAZI JEWS

# CHAPTER ONE

# HEALTH AS A VALUE

CONTEMPORARY medical anthropology differentiates between several distinct meanings of the notion of sickness and, following the example of Anglo-Saxon scholars including Horatio Fabrega, Arthur Kleinman, and Alan Young, employs separate terms for each one, thereby emphasizing the various different dimensions of the generic concept. In the first place, in referring to the body as a system and to the afflictions affecting it, the word 'disease' is used. These afflictions may be organic or functional in character; they also exist outside the consciousness of the sufferer until such time as he or she begins to experience problems or is informed of the disease by a specialist. Although the taxonomy of ailments is culturally conditioned, to simplify slightly, disease can be said to comprise afflictions known to contemporary biomedicine. From this perspective, 'healthy' means 'free from pathological states'. In the second meaning, the subjective experience of health and sickness is emphasized, and the phenomenon is labelled 'illness'. This covers a wealth of cultural aspects of the issue: convictions surrounding the aetiology and nature of diseases, ways of explaining their symptoms, actions taken when faced with health-related indisposition, and assessments of treatment outcomes. Different individuals set the limits of their reactions to their afflictions differently, though in this respect we are in thrall not only to our own character, but above all to the symbolic system in which we were brought up and in which we live. It is also on the basis of subjective feelings translated into the language of our culture that we define our state as 'good', and thus structure the boundaries of our concept of health.[1]

The use of biomedical terminology as the basis for interpretation of culturally conditioned conceptions and behaviours inevitably causes misunderstandings. The reason for this is that the phenomena referred to

---

[1] See e.g. Penkala-Gawęcka, 'Antropologia medyczna dzisiaj', 219–42; Kleinman, *The Illness Narratives*, 3–8. Kleinman also introduces a third concept: 'sickness', which he uses in relation to macrosocial (economic, political, institutional) forces.

colloquially as 'health', 'illness', or 'medicine' do not form a coherent, finite system delineated by the well-being of the human body but are understood variously by different human collectivities. In fact, in folk culture the minimal degree of differentiation of a range of fields precludes the precise definition of that encompassing the complete set of facts associated with 'medicine'.[2] It is impossible to disentangle ideas relating to medicine from views on the structure and functioning of the world, ethics and the role of humanity, imaginings of the extra-sensory world, and historical or social circumstances. Because folk medicine is multiplanar, it is difficult to examine its medical content. At the same time, however, it presents a broad spectrum of possibilities for exploring a culture—in this case the culture of Ashkenazi Jews—in all its dimensions, including its historical aspect and its links with the surrounding culture.

Popular views within the Jewish community on matters of health fell into three main categories of complaint: general (problems that might afflict anyone in the adult population, irrespective of age or sex), female (those connected with fertility, birth, nursing, etc.), and childhood (those specific to infants and children up to the age of religious maturity). This division, familiar from works focusing on other ethnic groups,[3] is very simplistic, however, and lends only the most basic degree of order to this immensely complex area of life. While it offers a point of reference for further considerations, it reduces the matter to but one of its many aspects and reveals relatively little about either the unique characteristics of Jewish folk medicine or the overall medical landscape of Ashkenazi culture. In any examination of cultural representations of health and related issues it is worth going a few steps further and exploring what mechanisms caused certain thought constructs to be elevated to the status of treatment-related beliefs and convictions, what types of aetiology were attributed to diseases, what characteristics were attributed to them, and, consequently, why certain actions and not others were taken. These representations differed in their genealogy and were shaped and altered by their users in different periods; therefore their comprehension requires an approach that takes account of the multifaceted character of this research subject. In order to be able to analyse it in any depth, however, we must, in the first place, turn

[2] Libera, *Medycyna ludowa*, 12–13.
[3] It is in evidence not only in older studies (e.g. by Julian Talko-Hryncewicz), but also more recent ones; see Robotycki and Babik (eds.), *Układ gniazdowy terminów*.

our attention to the matter of health as a significant value for the community of east European Jews, a collectivity culturally immersed in the biblical and talmudic tradition, but in possession of a range of therapeutic alternatives.

It would be something of a truism to point out that the vast majority of the Jews who lived in Galicia, the Congress Kingdom of Poland, and the Russian Pale of Settlement were an urban populace engaged in crafts and trade. It is nonetheless important to remember that until the twentieth century most towns, whether large or small, were relatively poorly developed. In parallel with their other occupations, residents cultivated gardens and fields, raised livestock, and performed basic crop-processing work. They also maintained close economic relations with the surrounding rural areas, supplying them with crafts and services, and in some cases lived outside towns as innkeepers or managers of mills or other properties belonging to the nobility. Their culture was not bound up with agriculture by such a dense mesh of symbols as that of the peasant populace, who lived off the land and held their relationship with it to be the essence of their fate. Only a tiny minority could afford to eschew physical labour entirely, however, and as such the Ashkenazi view of health incorporates a considerable body of references to the world of nature.

In east European folk culture, including its Jewish variant, the term 'health' (Yid. *gezunt, gezunthayt*) was colloquially understood as the state of full vitality. Attributes that fell within the scope of this concept included vigour, energy, ruddiness, and even the broader quality of longevity. The epithet *a gezunter yid* (a healthy Jew) designated not so much a person free of illnesses, but rather someone strong and fit, even in some contexts exuberant. People tended not to use the terms 'recover' or 'cure', preferring to speak of regaining vital forces or gaining new strength (*krign naye koykhes*). In Jewish eyes, the social stratum closest to the paragon of vigour was the peasantry. Although the legal position of peasant farmers in most of the Polish lands was unenviable until as recently as the second half of the nineteenth century, the idea of physical work in the sun and fresh air created a positive image of the peasant's body, particularly in contrast with the rather 'anti-physical' bodily image of the scholar bent over the pages of the Talmud day in, day out. As such, Yiddish developed the expressions *gezunt vi a poyer/a goy/ivan/yura* (as healthy as a peasant/a goy/Ivan/Yura), and *shtarke poyerishe/goyishe hent* (strong peasant/goy hands). One resident of Poczajów in the Podolye region (now Pochaiv, Ukraine) encapsulated the paradox of the ideal of health in Jewish culture in this passage from his memoirs:

The Russians [*katsapes*] brought in to work—healthy, stockily built, and with fine, full faces—bore little resemblance to the people of Poczajów. Mountains of *sunitsi* [wild strawberries] grew in the forests where they lived. Their young girls gathered them by the basketful and brought them to town to sell. These ruddy-faced goy maidens were exquisite. Barefooted, and dressed in short skirts to the knee, they caught everyone's eye. Many a devout Jewish youth sinned in thought at the sight of these beautiful, full-blooded *katsap* girls.[4]

The symbolic sphere of health drew to a similar extent on the animal world, above all on livestock, which was an everyday sight, hard at work. It might be said, then, that someone was as healthy as an ox or a horse, especially if they 'laboured like a horse' (*horeven vi a ferd*). And someone who had recovered after a serious illness was said to have 'grown a new coat', just like animals regaining their healthy appearance after the winter.[5] Another noteworthy point is the shared Hebrew root *ḥai* (alive, living) in the Yiddish words *khaye* (animal, pl. *khayes*) and *khayes* (life, vitality). Indeed, the kabbalistic number eighteen, which recurred in many curative rituals, owed its popularity to the fact that its letters formed the same root.

Aside from vitality, another constituent element in the state of full health in Jewish folk phraseology was one's aesthetic appearance. Only someone who was resilient enough to fight off illness could look 'well' (*frish*, lit. 'fresh'). A healthy person 'blossomed' or exuded other qualities characteristic of the plant world—they might be *frish vi a royz* (as fresh as a rose), *gezunt vi a rib/demb/kirbes* (as healthy as a turnip/oak/pumpkin). A corpulent, 'healthy' woman would be described as 'firm' (*zaftik*, lit. 'juicy'), an adjective used to describe fruits and vegetables. A fundamental indication of illness was the loss of 'colour', a pale physiognomy, which gave rise to the saying, regarding uncertain prospects: *oder toyt oder royt*, 'either dead or ruddy'.[6] Another visible symptom of illness was a dull gaze,

[4] Salz, 'My Town Pochayiv' (Yid.), 222–3.

[5] Stutshkov, *Thesaurus of the Yiddish Language* (Yid.), 419.

[6] Esterzon, *500 Rhyming Proverbs and Sayings* (Yid.), 14; Lew, 'O lecznictwie i przesądach', *Izraelita*, 40, p. 382; Lilientalowa, 'Dziecko żydowskie', 149. Perhaps this was why children were frequently pinched on the cheeks, and, alongside water, sugar, and breast milk, camomile was a staple element of the infant diet. In the Slavonic languages the name of the camomile plant—*rumianek* (Pol.), *rumianok* (Ukr.), *romashka* (Rus.)—is cognate with the adjective 'ruddy'

while conversely it would be said of someone returning to health that their 'eyes were brightening'.[7]

For the traditional Jewish population, health was one of the most significant factors in everyday life. *Vos tut men nit tsulib dem gezunt?* (What doesn't one do for one's health?), the saying went. And this conviction was echoed in everyday greetings. *Zay gezunt!* (Be healthy!) or *For gezunt!* (Go in good health!) were popular valedictions, especially when someone was embarking on a long journey. Customers buying new clothes were commended to health with *Tiskhadesh* (May you be renewed) or *Tserayst gezunterhayt* (May you tear off your clothes in good health).[8] Blessings of vitality and resilience to illness were standard elements of the lullabies sung by Jewish mothers.[9] In traditional communities thanks were also expressed in the form of a blessing; instead of saying *A dank*, a Galician hasid would likely use the phrase *Shkoyekh!*, meaning 'May you go from strength to strength'.[10]

Diseases were at the opposite end of this continuum of meaning. Poverty was spoken of as a fever (*kadokhes*),[11] and in general physical ailments were used as synonyms for all misfortunes, regardless of whether these 'plagues' were material in character or not (*Yak khvore to tsore*, If sick then worried;[12] *a brokh*, hernia or break, *a plog*, plague). The exclamation *Oy vey!*, so often on the lips of the Jews, and most simply translated as 'Woe!', was at its root a cry of pain. Of cumulated troubles it would often be said, *Oyf a bloter a prishtsh, un oyf der make a bloter* (A pimple on an abscess, and an abscess on an ulcer),[13] and talking about them was almost like a visit to the doctor. Problems were characterized as 'burning' (*gebrente*) or 'swollen' (*ongeshvolene*), and had to be fought (*plogn zikh*) like physical weaknesses; someone might be 'sitting in wounds' (*zitsn in gehakte vundn*)[14] and 'eating illness' (*esn krenk*)—often referring to long-lasting poverty without

---

(e.g. Pol. 'rumiany'); in Yiddish this plant from the genus Matricaria was also called by a name borrowed from these languages, usually the local variant. Presumably, in addition to the name, Jews also shared their neighbours' convictions as to the curative properties of camomile.

[7] Stutshkov, *Thesaurus of the Yiddish Language* (Yid.), 419.

[8] Ibid. 635. See *Shulḥan arukh*, 'Oraḥ ḥayim', 223: 6.

[9] Ginzburg and Marek (eds.), *Yevrieyskaya narodnaya piesni*, 67; Wiener, 'Aus der Russisch-Jüdischen Kinderstube', 49.     [10] Heb. *yasher ko'aḥ*; see Rothstein, *Tsanzer khsides*, 180.

[11] Hurvits, 'My Mother's Sayings' (Yid.), 92; Ginzburg and Marek (eds.), *Yevrieyskaya narodnaya piesni*, 278.     [12] Rabokh, 'Another Handful of Jewish Cares' (Yid.), 61.

[13] I. Bernstein, *Jewish Proverbs and Sayings* (Yid.), 45.

[14] Stutshkov, *Thesaurus of the Yiddish Language* (Yid.), 432.

prospects for the future.[15] The sense that everyday troubles were reminiscent of physical afflictions was reflected most vividly in the saying that
regular employment or some other source of income was 'the cure for all
ills' (*a refue tsu ale krenk*).[16] The connection between weakness and troubles
was bidirectional. On the one hand failing health was a source of worry,
while on the other excessive troubles took their toll on one's physical
health. *A kharote iz a sukhote* (Sadness is consumption),[17] it was said, and
*Tsores leygn zikh nit in di kleyder nor in di beyner* (Cares build up not in the
clothes but in the bones).[18] Plenty and calm, by contrast, were seen as salutary: *Gute tsaytn makhn sheyn di haytn* (Good times make the skin beautiful).[19] Everyday worries were nonetheless nothing compared to bodily
ailments, and this was best expressed in the thought: *Beser a fule zorg eyder
eyn zorg* (Better many worries than one worry [serious illness]).[20]

   Jewish curses frequently invoked illness and death, and were graphically
expressed. Among the mildest and least convoluted was the wish that a
miser be forced to spend his money on doctors. More incisive ones expressed the vindictive desire for an enemy to succumb to misfortunes such as
'rheumatism in the heels';[21] to break his leg on a flat road; or to be struck
down by cramp in the guts, an attack of apoplexy, the 'seventh fever', convulsions, or other similar afflictions.[22] There were also curses with a sting in
the tail, such as *Zolst zayn shtark un gezunt vi an ayzn, un zolst dikh nit kenen
aynbeygn* (May you be as strong and healthy as iron, and may you never be
able to bend).[23] Read literally, of course, and seeming, perhaps, unneces-
sarily cruel, they might lead one to suspect Jews of an inordinate fondness
for wishing the misfortune of ill health upon others; this was naturally not
the case. Driven to distraction by noisy neighbours or recalcitrant servants,
spouse, or children, they might be somewhat free with their malevolent

   [15] Y. Tsherniak, 'Linguistic Folklore in Yiddish' (Heb.), 100.
   [16] Stutshkov, *Thesaurus of the Yiddish Language* (Yid.), 525.
   [17] Esterzon, *500 Rhyming Proverbs and Sayings* (Yid.), 66; Stutshkov, *Thesaurus of the Yiddish
Language* (Yid.), 381.        [18] I. Bernstein, *Jewish Proverbs and Sayings* (Yid.), 224.
   [19] Einhorn, 'Folk Proverbs' (Heb.), 344.
   [20] Beilin, 'Jüdische Sprichwörter und Redensarten aus Russland', 133; Golenpol, *Lexicon of
Hebrew Folklore* (Heb.), 38, 70.        [21] Bastomski, *At the Source: Jewish Proverbs* (Yid.), 100.
   [22] Interesting ethnographic collections which list curses wishing ill health upon an enemy
include: Grunwald, 'Aus unseren Sammlungen. Teil I', 34–41; Bastomski, *At the Source: Jewish
Proverbs* (Yid.), 96–100; 'Minor Collections of Folklore' (Yid.), 201–4; 'From the Folklore of
Parysów' (Yid.), 396–7. According to some sources, cursing an orphan could prove dangerous,
because of the protection extended to the child by its dead mother in heaven; see Yoffie, 'Popular Beliefs and Customs', 390.        [23] Kaindl, 'Die Juden in der Bukowina', 161.

words even towards those closest to them. But the availability of such a rich tapestry of curses did not mean that they were bandied around without any fear of the consequences. Jewish women would hang up onions in their home to offset the results of thoughtless use of impure words towards their children. They might also 'bite their tongue', and, instead of shouting more literal curses at their mischievous offspring, mitigate them appropriately: *Krep . . . lekh zolstu esn!* (May you . . . eat *kreplakh*!).[24] Curses cast after dark, when demonic *mazikim* (destructive forces), quick to latch on to conjurations spoken in anger, were abroad, were thought to be particularly dangerous.[25] In certain circumstances individuals thought to possess the power to cause harm using words were cosseted and humoured. The sick, and pregnant women, whom the folk imagination considered to be teetering on the brink between life and death, ought never to be refused anything; curses pronounced by them were perceived to be especially powerful.[26]

*Aby ja zdrów* (That I [might be] healthy), Jews might say in the language of their Slavic neighbours.[27] Health was paramount among the values perceived by the Jewish community as important. One might forget about it for a brief while; caught up in the humdrum of daily life, one might fall into the trap of thinking it was one's right. But sooner or later sickness would catch up with anyone so frivolous, and remind them of the respect with which they should treat their body. Health was considered more important than anything the material world could offer. A number of Yiddish sayings provide excellent illustration of this sentiment: 'better a healthy pauper than a sick rich man';[28] 'he who is healthy is rich';[29] 'when one is healthy one will be happy anywhere';[30] 'better to sleep with a sound head on a broken bed than with a broken head in a sound bed';[31] and 'better sauerkraut in happiness than beef in suffering'.[32] Seeking help in sickness might entail the sacrifice of significant material assets or financial outlay. As the popular

---

[24] Yoffie, 'Popular Beliefs and Customs', 390. It is possible that some role in the popularity of this curse was played by the phonological similarity of the words *kreplekh* and *krep/krop* (croup).

[25] Segel, 'Wierzenia i lecznictwo', 51; Bastomski, *At the Source: Jewish Proverbs* (Yid.), 102.

[26] Lilientalowa, *Dziecko żydowskie*, 24–5; Bastomski, *At the Source: Jewish Proverbs* (Yid.), 109.

[27] Bastomski, *At the Source: Jewish Proverbs* (Yid.), 40.

[28] Stutshkov, *Thesaurus of the Yiddish Language* (Yid.), 414.

[29] I. Bernstein, *Jewish Proverbs and Sayings* (Yid.), 59.

[30] Beilin, 'Jüdische Sprichwörter', 134.

[31] Stutshkov, *Thesaurus of the Yiddish Language* (Yid.), 414.

[32] Frumkin, *Eternal Sources* (Yid.), 79.

maxim went, a poor man would slaughter his only chicken (i.e. a consider-able portion of his assets) when sick; it was either him or the chicken.[33] A recurring strand in Jewish folk tales is the motif of being forced to make a choice between wealth and a cure for infertility. The miracle that was the birth of a child might be heralded by an encounter with an angel or one of the holy men of old; it was often also a reward for a good deed or a devout life.[34]

Fear of illnesses, above all the most serious and incurable sort, made its mark on the Yiddish language also in terms of what was better left unsaid. In view of the belief that the spoken word could attract evil or cause misfor-tune (or, conversely, bring well-being), one popular precautionary measure was desisting from garrulity. A number of popular commentaries evolved around the talmudic phrase 'One should not open one's mouth unto Satan':[35] *In a guter sho tsu redn, in a shlekhter sho tsu shvaygn* (Speak in a good hour, be silent in an ill hour),[36] and *Nit rir on di tsore ven zi shloft* (Rouse not evil when it sleeps).[37] When the need to pass on news of a misfortune nonetheless made silence impossible, the names of diseases would be fol-lowed, for prudence' sake, by the words 'May the merciful God protect us' (*Rakhmone litslan*). This would be accompanied by a protective ritual, which involved spitting and the adjuration *Nit oyf mir/oyf mayne kinder gedakht/gezogt* (May it not be thought/said of me/my children).[38] Rather than saying outright that someone felt ill, it was considered better to say *lo-aleykhemdik* (from Heb. *lo aleikhem*, 'not on you').[39] When asked how he felt, the patient might answer 'better', and the questioner would then add: 'May you be better.' Repetition throughout a brief conversation of the con-viction that things were 'better' and would yet be better still was considered a method of actually improving the sufferer's health.[40] According to some testimonies, such dogged denial of misfortune was considered a truly Jew-ish trait. Anyone mentioning their own death and not adding the words 'God forbid' was perceived as a heathen and a boor. Such a person would be

---

[33] See e.g. I. Bernstein, *Jewish Proverbs and Sayings* (Yid.), 22; Golenpol, *Lexicon of Hebrew Folklore* (Heb.), 272; Kazdan, 'Imagery in Jewish Folk Language' (Yid.), 44.

[34] See e.g. Wiener, 'Märchen und Schwänke in Amerika aus dem Munde russischer Juden aufgezeichnet', 104; Silverman-Weinreich (ed.), *Yiddish Folktales*, 73; Krausz, *The Life of the Ba'al Shem Tov* (Yid.), 114.      [35] *Ber.* 19*a* and 60*a*; *Ket.* 8*b*.

[36] Stutshkov, *Thesaurus of the Yiddish Language* (Yid.), 361.

[37] Hurvits, 'My Mother's Sayings' (Yid.), 91.      [38] Lilientalowa, *Dziecko żydowskie*, 66–7.

[39] Also *Lo aleinu!* (Not on us!); Stutshkov, *Thesaurus of the Yiddish Language* (Yid.), 634.

[40] Lilientalowa, *Choroby, lecznictwo*, fo. 196.

said—perhaps with the addition of a formula to protect them from actual misfortune—to 'talk like our cat in the attic'.[41]

A range of methods for neutralizing potential threats was also used. The first was to hire an outsider (usually a non-Jew) or a child to be the bearer of bad news. The popular logic in this was that misfortune, once expressed verbally, lost its inauspicious power and could cause no further harm. It was either nullified by the innocence of the intermediary or transferred to the outsider.[42] The second method was to avoid speaking about illnesses overtly and use instead language purged of any obvious reference to them. As in other cultures, this preference for evasive turns of phrase, inverted meanings, and euphemisms broadened the vocabulary connected with health. Hunches, swellings, and mange were all 'painful sites'.[43] Epilepsy and convulsions were referred to as 'the serious sickness',[44] 'the saintly sickness',[45] or 'the bad thing',[46] or it might even be said that a child suffered from 'may the pure Shekhinah rest'.[47] Tuberculosis was 'the good sickness'.[48] The evil eye (*ayn hore*) would be called the 'good eye';[49] demons were known as *yene layt*, 'those people', and the word *shed* (demon), rather than being pronounced normally, would be spelled out (*shin-dalet*).[50] Cholera was termed *kholi-ra*—'the evil sickness'[51]—or 'the misfortune which will not come, may [God] have mercy on us'.[52] In official community documents likewise, the records do not specify 'in the time of the cholera epidemic', but 'when by the will of God it is lifted'.[53]

This juggling of euphemisms has a tradition in Jewish literature reaching back at least as far as the talmudic era. In the musings of the rabbis we come across the expression 'enemies of Israel' in contexts which leave no doubt that it is Israel itself that is meant, and leprosy is referred to as 'another thing' (*davar aḥer*, BT *Pes.* 76*b*). Hasidim believed that it was possible to combat a disease by calling it by a different name. This claim was

---

[41] Lew, 'Z ludoznawstwa', *Izraelita*, 17, p. 186.

[42] Khayes, 'Death-Related Beliefs and Customs' (Yid.), 311.

[43] Mark (ed.), *Great Dictionary of the Yiddish Language* (Yid.), iv. 2213.

[44] Rosenberg, *Der malekh refoel*, 62–3.

[45] Wolf, *Yarum mosheh*, 5*b*.                    [46] Schneersohn, *Sefer refuot*, 4.

[47] Khayes, 'Death-Related Beliefs and Customs' (Yid.), 284. The Shekhinah, an aspect of God's presence among the people of Israel, emanates holiness capable of overcoming illness perceived as a demonic being.        [48] Stutshkov, *Thesaurus of the Yiddish Language* (Yid.), 408.

[49] Ibid. 717.                    [50] Lilientalowa, *Złe duchy*, 51.

[51] Perets, *One Does Not Die of Cholera if One Does Not Want To* (Yid.).

[52] *Shemirot usegulot nifla'ot*, 2.

[53] Orinski, 'A Document about Cholera in Pruzhana' (Yid.), 39–42.

made by Yehudah Tsevi Brandwein, the tsadik of Stratin, on the basis of a
passage from the Torah: 'I will drive out before you the Amorites, the
Canaanites, the Hittites, the Perizzites, the Hivites, and the Jebusites'
(Exod. 34: 11). The grounds for his statement lay in the kabbalistic theory
that diseases came from the 'husks of impurity' which characterized the
nations mentioned in the verse.[54] The taboo surrounding words overtly
describing ailments might also have been connected with the belief that
it was unwise to talk about or even mention one's enemies, in order not to
give them extra strength.[55] Such precautions notwithstanding, we must remember that folk culture was fond of exceptions. Where some people feared
to verbalize the names of diseases, others went to the opposite extreme,
actually employing those names for instrumental purposes (for example
to exorcise Lilith, or when treating erysipelas. In incantations for driving
out parasites, for instance, or reversing enchantments, all the possible variants of such misfortunes that came to mind would be enumerated.[56]

Health was identified with life; sickness was tantamount to death. In
order to convince someone that a statement was true, one would swear:
'May I live as I do now, may I be as healthy as this.' Where their Slavic
neighbours drank 'to health', the Jews preferred *Leḥayim!* (To life!). Death,
which was never far away and visited all too frequently in an age of epidemics and high infant mortality, was something to be marginalized in any
way possible. Close encounters with it, such as the sight of a funeral
cortège, required extra safety measures. The deceased should not be mentioned, and on no account spoken ill of, unless a caveat was added, such as
*Er zol zayn an opkhaver fun undz* (May he not accompany us).[57] If someone
sneezed or yawned in the presence of the body of the deceased, they should
pull their left earlobe (an uninitiated child should be protected in this way
by a parent). The significance of this action was that the human soul was
believed to leave the body via the nose, and tugging on the ear was believed
to keep the soul inside the body (either by physically preventing its exit in
twisting the nasal passages, or by symbolically keeping hold of it in holding
on to the earlobe).

In order to maintain a clear and unequivocal separation between the
spheres of life and death, and between the worlds of the living and the dead,

---

[54] Berger, *Imrei yisra'el*, 13*a*–*b*.
[55] Ibid. 14*a*.                          [56] Cf. Moszyński, *Kultura ludowa Słowian*, 300.
[57] Khayes, 'Death-Related Beliefs and Customs' (Yid.), 284.

the rituals connected with serving the dying, burial, and mourning, and likewise any of the individual elements of those rituals, were not to be imitated in any way without good reason. In the popular consciousness, performing such actions in trivial circumstances, whether or not deliberately, would bring bad luck to the offender, such as a difficult birth for women, dwarfism in children, and dull-wittedness in children and adult men. In extreme cases it could also bring about the death of the offender or of a member of their family. Thus children would be forbidden to climb out of a window (and would never be passed out of the house through the window), for fear that they would stop growing or would grow a hump.[58] This was related to the custom of passing the body of the deceased through the window. The rooms would never be cleaned just after someone had left the house,[59] or just before someone was due to depart on a long journey, again in response to these actions being performed after the removal of a corpse from a house.[60] Chipped or otherwise damaged vessels would not be kept in the house, as clay pots were typically smashed when someone died, and the shards were placed on the eyelids of the deceased.[61] An empty cradle should not be rocked,[62] nor a child be dressed by two people at once, as this is how the dead were usually dressed.[63] It was considered risky to sleep in one's shoes, as shoes were put on the feet of the dead before burial; moreover, sleep was said to be a foretaste of death from which one might not wake up again.[64] Similarly, one was not to walk around the house in one's socks, which was a mourning custom,[65] or place a candle on the floor[66] or at the head of a cradle.[67] The buttons on the pillow on which one slept should be on the underside,[68] and mirrors should not be covered up, as this was done

[58] Lilientalowa, 'Dziecko żydowskie', 150; Bastomski, *At the Source: Jewish Proverbs* (Yid.), 105; Pulner, 'Obryadi i povirya', 112; Khayes, 'Death-Related Beliefs and Customs' (Yid.), 311; Fayvushinski, 'The Folklore of Pruzhana' (Yid.), 200.

[59] Segel, 'Wierzenia i lecznictwo', 51.       [60] Ibid. 52.       [61] Ibid. 53.

[62] Lilientalowa, *Dziecko żydowskie*, 39. Boys at school (and when sitting on a chair or bench anywhere) should not swing their legs, as this was tantamount to cursing their parents; Lilientalowa, 'Dziecko żydowskie', 158; 'Aus unseren Sammlungen. II', 8; Weissenberg, 'Kinderfreud und -leid bei den südrussischen Juden', 317; Ben-Ezra, 'Customs' (Yid.), 175.

[63] Fayvushinski, 'The Folklore of Pruzhana' (Yid.), 199.

[64] Lilientalowa, 'Wierzenia, przesądy i praktyki', 152; Bastomski, *At the Source: Jewish Proverbs* (Yid.), 107.

[65] Khayes, 'Death-Related Beliefs and Customs' (Yid.), 323; Fayvushinski, 'The Folklore of Pruzhana' (Yid.), 200.

[66] Khayes, 'Death-Related Beliefs and Customs' (Yid.), 301; Fayvushinski, 'The Folklore of Pruzhana' (Yid.), 201.       [67] Lew, 'O lecznictwie', *Izraelita*, 40, p. 381.

[68] Bastomski, *At the Source: Jewish Proverbs* (Yid.), 112.

in a house of mourning.[69] Water should never be boiled unless for a specific purpose,[70] and one should never sleep on the table top because both these actions were among the preparations for washing a corpse.[71] Customs connected with the memory of the dead should likewise not be imitated or echoed in dealings with the living. For this reason people avoided marrying off a child to someone who had the name of a living father- or mother-in-law, or calling a baby after any living relative—in a community where being named after deceased forebears was an important symbol of the unbroken 'golden chain' of generations, this could be perceived as wishing for the death of the living relative. Wherever possible, on Saturday evening, the traditional time for burying those whom it had not been possible to bury before the sabbath, one would not put on a clean shirt as this might be interpreted as a harbinger of imminent misfortune.[72]

According to Jewish folklore, people fighting illness did not need to be reminded of the ephemerality of life. Thus, as sewing clothes might be reminiscent of the preparation of a shroud, such work should be put away until the patient was restored to full health.[73] Digging a grave for someone who was not yet dead was seen as sealing the verdict of heaven. Death was never referred to as such, but as 'resting', 'falling asleep', 'closing one's eyes', or sometimes by ironically tinged euphemisms such as 'laying out one's legs', 'going to meet one's ancestors', or 'going to the boards'. If the word itself was uttered, however, every attempt would be made to deflect the impression that it had any connection with a particular person by adding phrases such as: *Nisht im meyn ikh, di vant meyn ikh* (I don't mean him, I mean the wall) or *Vi di erd shvaygt, azoy zol al dos beyz shvaygn* (As the earth is silent, so may all mischief be silent).[74] Likewise, it was customary to avoid speaking of a funeral (which was coyly alluded to as 'moving to the apartment' or 'taking refuge beneath seven locks'), of the deceased ('the one lying in the ground'), and even of the cemetery (a 'bare field', an 'empty field', or the 'house of life').[75] There was also a broad palette of euphemisms

[69] Fayvushinski, 'The Folklore of Pruzhana' (Yid.), 205.

[70] Lilientalowa, 'Kult wody u starożytnych Hebrajczyków i szczątki tego kultu u współczesnego ludu żydowskiego', 7; Fayvushinski, 'The Folklore of Pruzhana' (Yid.), 200.

[71] Khayes, 'Death-Related Beliefs and Customs' (Yid.), 323.

[72] Lilientalowa, 'Przesądy żydowskie', 277; Fayvushinski, 'The Folklore of Pruzhana' (Yid.), 204.            [73] Khayes, 'Death-Related Beliefs and Customs' (Yid.), 296.

[74] Buchbinder, 'Jewish Omens' (Yid.), 255.

[75] Zelkovitsh, 'Death and Its Accompanying Moments' (Yid.), 150–2.

available to convey the fact that someone was dying, for 'When one speaks of death one cannot be sure of life.'[76] A dying person would be said to be 'hanging on narrowly' (*haltn shmol*), or be 'making ready for the road' (*greyt zikh in veg*).[77]

In colloquial speech, words from the Bible and the Talmud were often used to 'neutralize' expressions associated with uncleanliness and disease. Similarly, words derived from Hebrew were used to denote embarrassing or shameful parts of the body, for example *tokhes* (the behind), *eyver* (the 'member'), *beytsim* ('balls'), *oyse-mokem* ('that place'), and for all manner of health complaints (for example *segi-noher*, literally 'full of light', to refer to a blind person). According to one Jewish saying, Hebrew was used to refer to things one was too embarrassed to say in Yiddish, such as *beys-hakise* (toilet) or *mashtin zayn* (to urinate).[78] It was often also the case that Yiddish words or phrases would be replaced with Hebrew ones in the context of death (*mes*—the deceased; *bar-minyen*—corpse; *brengen tsu kvure*—bury; *beys-oylem*, *beys-hakhayim*, *beys-kvores*—cemetery). At the same time, words derived from the sacred language were believed to have greater power. As Avrom Rechtman noted, a sick Jew should be said to be *krank*, while the word *khoyle* (from the Hebrew *ḥoleh*) might be used only in respect of a non-Jew, because, like all Hebrew words, it was seen as an expression of the Creator's power and hence as having the potential to 'create' illness.[79]

Nonetheless, it is important to remember that there were values to which greater worth was attached—if not by society at large, then certainly by the intellectual elites—than health. Foremost among these was the idea of a reward in heaven, which prompted mystics to promote fasting and bodily privations. This idea originated in the thinking of the rabbis of the talmudic era, and in the culture of Ashkenazi Jews it grew to remarkable proportions via the agency of the medieval Ashkenazi Pietist movement (Hasidei Ashkenaz). The ethical literature of the early modern age upheld the conviction of the superiority of the World to Come over this world, devoting considerable space to asceticism and interventions affecting the body. At the same time, the hasidism that emerged in the lands of the

---

[76] Khayes, 'Death-Related Beliefs and Customs' (Yid.), 284.
[77] Zelkovitsh, 'Death and Its Accompanying Moments' (Yid.), 164.
[78] Cahan, *The Jew on Himself and Others* (Yid.), 7.
[79] Rechtman, 'Some Customs and Their Folk Explanations' (Yid.), 253. According to another interpretation, a sick person should be said to be not *khoyle* but unhealthy (*er iz nisht bekav-habriyes*); Yelin, *Derekh tsadikim*, 10.

Commonwealth of the Two Nations in the mid-eighteenth century drew attention to the negative consequences of such practices, arguing that they weakened people's vital forces and distracted them from joyful service of God. In place of these it advocated procedures such as ritual bathing in the *mikveh*.[80] Nonetheless, many charismatic hasidic leaders (tsadikim) practised self-mortification, at least in secret—and irrespective of whether their names went down in hasidic history as a result of their poverty or by virtue of their palatine grandeur. Rebbe David Biderman of Lelów, an extremely modest man, practised *gilgul sheleg*: in the winter he would climb a hill just outside the town and roll down it dozens of times in rapid succession, doused each time with hot water.[81] Rebbe Israel of Ruzhyn, known for living in the splendour befitting an aristocrat (and said to be descended from the royal line of David), would wear shoes without soles in the winter, and at feasts would swallow such large mouthfuls of the fine foods as not to be able to taste them.[82] The hasidic literature, and to some extent also kabbalistic and rabbinic writings, abounded in descriptions of similar privations.

Saintliness underscored by self-mortification was something that ordinary people accepted and respected. Devout practices that honed the soul at the cost of its material hull were considered proper for rare individuals. They testified to the saintliness and exceptionality of those figures. In the form of fasts and less onerous privations, they also found a permanent place in the Jewish liturgical calendar, though they certainly did not dominate everyday life. What is more, in spite of the general approval of such actions, Jewish society as a whole remained aware of their negative impact on one's health. Evidence of this is not only the hasidic recommendation to practise regular ablutions in place of fasts, but also the numerous exemptions from the duty to observe the fast days enshrined in Jewish religious law, which applied to pregnant and nursing women and to the sick. Taking advantage of these exemptions was recommended even if the illness was not life-threatening.[83]

[80] *Keter shem tov hashalem*, 125.　　　[81] Weinstock, *Kodesh hilulim*, 82.
[82] Rothstein [Nisnzohn], *Dos malkhesdike khsides*, 47.
[83] Ganzfried, *Kitsur shulḥan arukh*, 121: 9.

CHAPTER TWO

# BIBLICAL AND TALMUDIC
# TRADITION

IT WAS IN THE SPHERE of religious belief that the difference of the
Jewish population from their east European neighbours became most
clearly manifest. At the centre of this sphere was, for the Jews, the Penta-
teuch, also known as the Written Torah, which comprised the first five
books of the Bible and was considered to be the Law given to Israel by God.
Together with the books of the Prophets (Nevi'im) and the Writings (Ketu-
vim), it made up the Hebrew Bible (the Tanakh). The rabbinic exegesis and
interpretation of the Holy Scriptures, which was known as the Oral Torah,
was not initially codified. It was only recorded in writing between the
third and sixth centuries CE, in the two parts of the Talmud: the Mishnah
and the Gemara. In the succeeding centuries this body of law did not wane
in importance; on the contrary, it took on new dimensions, for instance in
the collections of rabbinic responsa and in legal codes. The biblical and talmudic tradition formed the framework of everyday life for Jews and determined their ritual duties. It ordained what was fitting, what was permissible
in certain circumstances, and what, as a Jew, one should eschew at all costs.
Every action performed, whether on a festival, on the sabbath, or on an
ordinary day, was to a greater or lesser extent imbued with religious significance, and actions connected with health and sickness were no exception;
in the premodern era they in particular were subject to interpretations
inspired by motifs and stories familiar from religious texts.

The treatment of medical matters in the Bible and the Talmud is a subject for separate research. A vast and fascinating body of literature has
developed around this topic, including the works of specialists in a range of
areas—from historians of medicine, through scholars of ethics, to rabbis.[1]

---

[1] There are publications on this subject in many languages. Titles released even before the
outbreak of the Second World War include Preuss, *Biblisch-talmudische Medizin*; Perlman, *The
Midrash of Medicine* (Heb.); Katsenelson, *The Talmud and Medical Knowledge* (Heb.); and Lewin,

This literature cannot be ignored in any exploration of the folk medicine of east European Jews. The discussion below, however, will be limited to the main issues regarding the way in which the holy books, as well as the midrashic, ethical, and kabbalistic literature based on them, influenced curative practices in Jewish society. What I am interested in here is the many aspects of the popular perception of the sacred texts of Judaism, which often produced creative interpretations of their content.

For many centuries Jewish culture in eastern Europe developed along the line where orality met literacy. To a considerable extent its form was dependent not so much on the text itself as on its oral interpretation. Only the educated had the privilege of communing directly with the content of the canonical books. For the most part, this excluded women, as well as the many men who were forced to devote their time not to study but to feeding their families. Tradition rationed access to public readings of the Torah in the synagogue. In the *ḥeder*, too, more time was spent studying religious law than reading its biblical source; indeed, on occasion this latter was treated as the root of potential heresies. A strict taboo had grown up around touching the Torah scrolls with one's bare hands. Sacred books were likewise greatly venerated: they were kept in covers to protect them from dirt and damage, and were kissed as they were replaced on the shelf. Religious texts recorded in Hebrew script were denoted by the collective term *sheymes*, or 'divine names', and when too worn out to be of further use, they were stored in a special repository called a *genizah*.

Written form had the power of preserving words. The skill of encapsulating utterances in visible characters not only did not destroy the potency of the sacred message, but actually lent it entirely new dimensions. Words, which were considered to have practical impact on reality, could be poured out onto the parchment, thus becoming material objects. They might be manipulated even by those unable to decipher them correctly. For societies immersed in oral culture, books have always been important instruments in view of the holiness emanating from them, their connection with the priesthood, and their potential as a means of communication with the other world.[2] They could be used independently of their content, and the in-

*Ochrona zdrowia i eugenika w Biblii i Talmudzie.* At present some of the seminal works include those by the ethics scholar and historian of medicine Fred Rosner (e.g. *Medicine in the Bible and the Talmud*), who was also the author of the English translation of Preuss's book, *Biblical and Talmudic Medicine.*

[2] Goody, 'Restricted Literacy in Northern Ghana', 206.

ability to read them constituted no hindrance in this respect. Although a considerable proportion of Jewish society was literate, among its customs there are many examples of instrumental treatment of books, in particular the five books of Moses. Anyone wishing to be cured of infertility, for instance, would be advised to finance the copying of a Torah scroll.[3] For a woman in childbirth to have physical contact with the Torah, whether directly or by means of surrogate actions—wrapping the band used to bind the scrolls around her belly, or laying the Torah mantle or curtain from the ark on it; or running a thread from the Torah ark in the synagogue to her bed—was said to assuage labour pains and accelerate a birth free of complications.[4] Some of these procedures violated tradition and rabbinic lore, but, while they might be criticized by figures of authority for their sacrilegious character, they were treated with understanding in view of the circumstances surrounding them—situations of threat to human life and health.

The influence of religious tradition on the curative beliefs and practices of a society which, in the late nineteenth century, still recognized the supreme authority of that tradition was perceptible on a number of levels. At the most basic, it shaped the general normative expectations surrounding the life of members of the community. The Bible and Talmud created a system of laws regulating all aspects of a Jew's life, and contained many detailed pronouncements on health-related issues, including physical cleanliness, procedures designed to help maintain physical health, and the correct diet. Rabbis living in the modern era could not ignore the subject of treating sickness. They addressed issues such as the optimum times for bloodletting and attitudes towards physicians, quacks, and purveyors of magic. The collectivity gave considerable weight to their suggestions for provision of medical care and aid to the poor by the community and its organizations. So many and such varied matters were regulated in various places scattered throughout the extensive treatises and chapters that it seemed impossible to know them all fully. Even those with the talent and the time would have had to devote a considerable part of their life to them.

[3] Rosenberg, *Rafa'el hamalakh*, 17. The Torah joins the beginning with the end: the first commandment, 'multiply', and the last, 'write a Torah'. In fulfilling the latter, the former is at once fulfilled. For if a man had children, they would study for him; if he did not, however, someone else must study from his Torah (Lipiets, *Sefer matamim*, 85).

[4] Wilff, *Imrot shelomoh*, 103; Pulner, 'Obryadi i poviryà', 103; Lilientalowa, *Dziecko żydowskie*, 26.

Assistance was at hand in the form of the halakhic codes, the most important of which was the *Shulḥan arukh*. This was a four-part collection of religious laws and prescriptions published in the sixteenth century by the Sephardi rabbi Joseph Karo (1488–1575) and expanded shortly thereafter by Moses Isserles of Kraków (1520–72) to include Ashkenazi practice. Since for most people, on account of their rather poor command of Hebrew, the contents of this code remained hermetic, it too was abridged and updated several times. In the nineteenth century a number of publications came out which expressed religious law in yet more condensed and accessible form. Among the most important of these were Abraham Danzig's books *Ḥayei adam* (Vilnius, 1810) and *Ḥokhmat adam* (Vilnius, 1814), which discussed issues in Karo's code taking into account more recent halakhic rulings. Danzig's code, in turn, provided the inspiration for Solomon Ganzfried's popular book *Kitsur shulḥan arukh* (Ungvár, 1864). Among the many other legal issues, separate chapters in these works addressed questions of significance for health and well-being—from natural ways of maintaining vitality, through general prophylaxis, the blessings to be recited on evading danger and during therapy (for example bloodletting), taking medication on the sabbath and from a non-Jew, birth, and contact with a physician, to the rules for visiting the sick and handling a dying patient. Some of these prescriptions (such as those regarding vaccinations) betray attempts to reconcile current biomedical knowledge with the constraints of rabbinical Judaism. Aside from countless Hebrew-language editions, before long there were also translations of Danzig's and Ganzfried's codes into Yiddish.[5]

Thanks to the ubiquity of printing across Europe in the period under scrutiny, it was possible to reach a wide circle of readers and to pass on tradition in a reliable manner. However, this often required acceptance of the necessity to translate writings from the original Hebrew or Aramaic into vernacular languages. Attitudes among the rabbinic authorities of Ashkenaz regarding such translations had long been ambivalent. They recognized the potential for reinforcing religious attitudes among the Jewish

---

[5] The *Kitsur shulḥan arukh*, though extremely widely read, was not considered grounds on which to take a halakhic stand. In rabbinic law, greater significance was attached to the books of Danzig, and later to the *Mishnah berurah*, a commentary on the *Shulḥan arukh* compiled by Israel Meir Kagan of Raduń (also known as Hafets Hayim, 1838–1933). The first volume of his work was published in 1884, and the sixth and final volume in 1907.

populace, but at the same time feared the strengthening of heterodox stances and the undermining of the key role of the rabbinate as authoritative interpreter of the Law and as arbiter. Neither did they entirely trust these translations, and for this reason they unequivocally discouraged study of halakhic matters from sources other than those written in Hebrew, and treated Yiddish-language versions exclusively as serving to reinforce and refresh previously acquired knowledge. At the same time, they accepted the existence of a vast body of ethical literature, which was intended not so much to take the place of the sacred texts as to offer an alternative to non-Jewish secular literature.

Ethical literature in Yiddish had emerged at the beginning of the sixteenth century, and before long titles began to appear which can confidently be termed bestsellers. These books did not contribute any fundamentally new content, but drew on the reservoir of talmudic, rabbinical, and ethical literature in Hebrew. One such compilation was the immensely popular *Tsene urene*, a homiletic adaptation of the text of the Torah supplemented with stories from later traditions.[6] Works whose didactic value had been recognized in the Hebrew version were often published in Yiddish in abridged form. These editions made it possible for many women and men without an education in Hebrew and Talmud to access rabbinic culture and thus satisfy their aspiration to partake of the spirituality of the Jewish elites. Literature of this type remained in circulation for a remarkably long time, gracing the shelves of devout households and study halls in eastern Europe until the Holocaust.

Aside from the above, around 1900 there was a return to the use of *sifrei minhagim*—books of customs, which explained the meaning of the commandments and juxtaposed the halakhah with the standard custom (Heb. *minhag*) in a given region. This literature, which had its roots in the talmudic era, had first blossomed among Ashkenazi Jews in the late Middle Ages.[7] In their heyday, the Jewish communities in Poland and Lithuania adopted a unique model, developed in medieval Germany, in which local custom was considered equally authoritative as the deliberations of the ancients. In the late nineteenth century several new collections of *minhagim* were published in major centres of Jewish life in the Polish lands,

---

[6] Baumgarten, *Introduction to Old Yiddish Literature*, 113–22.

[7] See Ta-Shma, 'Minhagim Books', 278–9; Kosofsky, *The Book of Customs*, pp. xv–xxx; Baumgarten, *Introduction to Old Yiddish Literature*, 250–9.

including *Ta'amei haminhagim umekorei hadinim*, *Sefer matamim*, and *Minhagei yeshurun*. The explications of the rituals contained in them varied from traditional readings of the scriptures to demonology and contemporary science. They contain a considerable number of instructions on the proper fulfilment of the commandments, supplemented by health warnings and information on the curative properties of ritual objects and amulets. The *Ta'amei haminhagim* also includes a whole collection of health-related advice and prescriptions, some of them given weight by the authority of professors of medicine. Nineteenth-century books of customs were released as popular, widely available publications and ran into numerous editions, usually translated from Hebrew into Yiddish shortly after their initial launch.

The legal and moral interpretations of the biblical and talmudic literature were only two of many types of exegesis. The spectrum of issues that the holy writings addressed was so broad that the religious tradition could be treated as a treasure trove of health-related advice, among other things. This instrumentalization of the classical texts raised objections from rabbis and physicians long before the era of biomedicine. Both Moses Maimonides and Joseph Karo warned against the direct implementation of such ancient wisdom, and teased out medical advice from the more recent body of binding halakhic norms.[8] Later authors who compiled collections of traditional remedies (*segulot urefuot*) were also fairly sparing in their citation of the Gemara. Nonetheless, some members of the traditional community, especially those who practised as feldshers or barber-surgeons, saw the study of talmudic-era medicine as an important facet of their knowledge of their own profession and of available treatment methods. 'He was extremely well versed in the work of the feldsher . . . He would spend winter evenings sitting in the *beit hamidrash* [study hall] and . . . studying the Gemara. He was particularly keenly interested in the passages of the Talmud which discussed the limbs of cattle and animals',[9] runs the description of a local feldsher written by a former resident of the town of Turzec. The knowledge acquired in the course of such study was of a rather general nature. It was the legacy of the medicine of the ancients, both Jewish and Graeco-Roman, and many of the concepts this espoused had lost nothing

   [8] Barilan, *Jewish Bioethics*, 33; Efron, *Medicine and the German Jews*, 14.
   [9] Trayevitski, 'Geshtaltn', 203. See also Gordon, *Between Two Worlds: The Memoirs of a Physician*, 20.

of their currency in European popular culture, even as recently as the twentieth century. It is noteworthy that part of the medical and paramedical
vocabulary of Yiddish was derived from the language of the Talmud; this
component, if not large, was certainly perceptible. Thus, taking the pulse
was *tapn doyfek* (Heb. *dofek*); someone with sexual attributes of both sexes
was termed *androygines* (Heb. *androginos*, from the Greek *andrógunos*); and
several common complaints had their roots in Hebrew names, including
fever, or convulsions (*nikhpe*, Heb. *nikhpeh*), and diarrhoea (*shilshl*, Heb.
*shilshul*).

The health-related passages of the Talmud eventually found their way
to less educated readers, in particular via the medium of ethical literature
written in vernacular languages. Around 1900 many such volumes were
still being published. Among the most widely read was *Sefer ets ḥayim*, an
abridged edition of the work *Shenei luḥot haberit* by Isaiah Halevi Horowitz
(d.1630), which ran into many editions. Aside from striking fear into the
hearts of readers by enumerating the inevitable consequences of sin and
demonstrating a direct causal link between health-related problems and
moral weakness, the author also employed the words of the talmudic rabbis
to support his theories on matters such as proper diet:

Our sages say: to eat and not wash it down with drink is to eat one's own blood; it
leads to disease of the intestines. This was all spoken in connection with the
morning meal; while at the evening meal, if one eats and does not stand up and
walk four cubits, the viscera rot and the breath is foul. And if one needs to empty
one's bowels but does not do so and goes instead to eat more food, it is akin to
lighting a stove which one did not previously empty of ashes, causing the fire to
be smothered and not take well; so too the food will not break down, and this is
the source of major diseases.[10]

According to Regina Lilientalowa, there was widespread awareness in
Jewish folk culture of talmudic warnings regarding conception.[11] Their
popularity was due not only to intensive study of dedicated passages of
the oral Torah, but equally to the ubiquitous presence of similar guidance in
moralizing texts. The recommendations forthcoming from rabbis, some
of which dated from the days of the Second Temple, were passed on to
their audiences via channels including matrimonial manuals such as *Imrot
shelomoh*.[12] In east European ethnographic material and books of customs,

---

[10] *Ets ḥayim*, 64–5; cf. BT *Shab.* 41*a*.
[11] Lilientalowa, *Dziecko żydowskie*, 20.
[12] See Wilff, *Imrot shelomoh*, 54–6.

the fear of pairs and even numbers that is also present in the Talmud recurs
repeatedly.[13] Popular belief warned against passing between two women or
two trees, for example; infants were to be weaned only in odd-numbered
months; and patients were advised to take odd numbers of therapeutic
baths.[14] The examples cited here of the centuries of influence of rabbinic-
era medicine and mores are evidence of the constant presence of the Talmud in the sphere of Ashkenazi health-related beliefs and practices, despite
the reserve with which some treated the medical advice of the early rabbis.

The wealth of Bible-related resources grew larger the further one
departed from a literal interpretation of words and quotations. Judaism
recognizes four methods of Torah exegesis: the basic, or literal (*peshat*); the
comparative rabbinic (*derash*); the allegorical symbolic (*remez*); and the eso-
teric (*sod*). While the most direct interpretation of Scripture yielded a certain amount of early medical knowledge, each of the other three offered a
new reading of the text, equally applicable to the functioning of the human
body and to sickness. The Bible constituted a boundless reservoir of quotes
which might be used in conjurations against illnesses or on amulets. These
were seen not only as guidance for action, but also as integral elements of
sorcery. It is often impossible to understand the meaning of such quotations on the basis of a literal reading of the text, and it is necessary to seek
a rabbinic or kabbalistic interpretation. This is superbly illustrated by the
tale of a man suffering from nosebleeds, who was advised to drink a measure of good wine 'down in one'. This remedy, popular in a number of cultures, was doubtless based on the symbolic bond between the two red
liquids. In the Jewish tradition, however, the story is interpreted as having
its roots in the Torah. The tsadik Pinhas of Korets (now in north-western
Ukraine) noted that when Jacob the patriarch prophesied to Judah that
he would wash 'his robe in the blood of grapes' (Gen. 49: 11), he was also
pointing out the blood-staunching property of wine.[15] In another instance

---

[13] See BT *Pes.* 110*a*–111*a*; Bastomski, *At the Source: Jewish Proverbs* (Yid.), 104. Pairs were
avoided above all on the basis of the conviction that they were ruled by Asmodeus, the king of
the demons.

[14] Trachtenberg, *Jewish Magic and Superstition*, 118–19. The customs relating to weaning
babies and taking baths were noted by Fels, 'Zabobony lekarskie u Żydów', 2–3. Cf. Moszyński,
*Kultura ludowa Słowian*, 286.

[15] Sperling, *Ta'amei haminhagim oyf ivri taytsh*, ii. 15. Rosenberg (*Der malekh refoel*, 22), com-
menting on the same verse in Genesis, explains the meaning of *suto* (his robe) thus: 'The word
*suto* means to heal, from the medical language of the Gemara.'

the connection between the ailment and the choice of quotations seems slightly more obvious: someone suffering from a nosebleed was advised to repeat the words from the book of Isaiah (19: 6): 'Channels turn foul as they ebb, and Egypt's canals run dry. Reed and rush shall decay', and from Genesis 8: 2: 'The fountains of the deep and the floodgates of the sky were stopped up, and the rain from the sky was held back.'[16] A barren woman, in turn, was advised to be joyful and not to succumb to melancholy, for it was written in the prophetic texts: 'Shout, O barren one, you who bore no child! Shout aloud for joy, you who did not travail' (Isa. 54: 1).[17] Some recommendations are a subtle reflection of the mores common among both the Jews and their Slavic neighbours. The commandment issued to the Israelites to remove the lepers from their camp (Num. 5: 2) might be interpreted as justification for the custom of transferring misfortunes onto outsiders.[18] According to one collection of customs, even the therapeutic properties of chicken broth had biblical roots. The Yiddish name for this panacea, *yoykh* (which is cognate with the Slavic *yukha*, meaning broth or animal blood), was interpreted as an abbreviation composed of the last letters of the Hebrew words of the psalm: 'For He will order his angels to guard you wherever you go' (Ps. 91: 11).[19]

A key preventative role in the folk culture of east European Jews was played by mezuzot. These tiny scrolls of parchment prepared according to the rules of writing sacred texts, and contained in little cases, are inscribed with passages from the book of Deuteronomy (6: 4–9; 11: 13–21), including the words of the creed 'Shema yisra'el'. The exhortation to affix a mezuzah on the door frame of the house in obedience to the words 'to the end that you and your children may endure' (Deut. 11: 21) was commonly interpreted as a promise to protect the members of the household from all ills.[20] If damaged or worn out, the mezuzah was to be replaced as a matter of urgency, for aside from its ritual significance it would lose its protective

---

[16] Rosenberg, *Rafa'el hamalakh*, 104. This latter quotation, often distorted, recurs in conjurations for bleeding after circumcision (e.g. Lifshits, *Sefer sharbit hazahav*, 96a) and for overly heavy menstrual bleeding (e.g. Khotsh, *Segulot urefuot*, 6).

[17] J. Ashkenazi, *Tsene urene fun harav hekhasid*, 2.

[18] Kanarvogel, *Ta'amei mitsvot*, 18b (194). This custom, attributed to the tsadik Menahem Mendl of Rymanów, was sourced from the book *Igra depirka* by Tsevi Elimelekh of Dynów.

[19] Lipiets, *Sefer matamim*, 30.

[20] It was said that children could die of 'mezuzah sin' (BT *Shab.* 32b; Lipiets, *Sefer matamim*, 72).

functions. The literature has preserved many descriptions of the custom of checking the text of the mezuzah in situations where a house or a town had been visited by misfortune, such as an epidemic or possession by a dybbuk.[21] Indeed, regular checks were considered the responsibility of both individuals and the community organization.[22] The fact that the mezuzah was to be mounted in a visible position inside the house—on a door frame, right over the threshold—amplified these magical functions further still. Many therapeutic and prophylactic practices would be enacted in its immediate vicinity. The husband of a woman enduring a difficult birth would recite a portion of the *haftarah* (a selection from one of the prophetic books of the Bible, read out in the synagogue following the Torah reading) and the appropriate incantation while standing by the mezuzah.[23] For whooping cough, the collection *Rafa'el hamalakh* recommended standing the sick child on the threshold beneath the mezuzah and making an incision in the wood immediately above its head; the illness would pass when the child grew to be taller than the marked place.[24] It was also believed that anyone afraid of lightning and hearing voices on a stormy day should say the name of the archangel Gabriel three times, and stand by the mezuzah and recite the text it contains three times, followed by passages from Habakkuk[25] and Psalms.[26] In cases of infantile convulsions it was said that reciting the text of the mezuzah over the sick child's right ear was efficacious.[27] Tiny *mezuzelekh*, as they were known, might also serve as amulets worn in a metal or leather case, and would provide protection from a range of demonic afflictions, from fright to cholera.[28] The strips of parchment trimmed from the scrolls were known as *gilyoynes* and themselves could be used as amulets for boys.[29]

[21] See e.g. Rechtman, *Jewish Ethnography and Folklore* (Yid.), 333; Ginzburg, 'How Our Forefathers Fought Cholera' (Yid.), 231–2.

[22] BT *Shab.* 32*b*. Private mezuzot were to be checked twice in a seven-year period, and public ones twice in a fifty-year period; see Ganzfried, *Keset hasofer*, 39*b*.

[23] Rosenberg, *Rafa'el hamalakh*, 63; Wilff, *Imrot shelomoh*, 101.

[24] Rosenberg, *Rafa'el hamalakh*, 44.

[25] Hab. 3: 10: 'The mountains rock at the sight of You, a torrent of rain comes down; loud roars the deep, the sky returns the echo.'

[26] Ps. 77: 18–19: 'Clouds streamed water; the heavens rumbled. Your arrows flew about, your thunder rumbled like wheels. Lightning lit up the world; the earth quaked and trembled.' Ps. 84: 13: 'O Lord of hosts, blessed is the man who trusts in You.'

[27] Plaut, *Likutei hever ben hayim*, 6*b*; Berger, *Imrei yisra'el*, 10*a*.

[28] Rosenberg, *Rafa'el hamalakh*, 79; Lilientalowa, *Dziecko żydowskie*, 75.

[29] Lilientalowa, *Dziecko żydowskie*, 76.

Biblical stories and figures, like heroes of the talmudic age, recurred again and again in the folklore of the Jews. Every character that had an association with healing, such as King Hezekiah, the Syrian Na'aman,[30] or the prophetess Miriam, might be incorporated into the words of popular incantations.[31] Motifs such as the imperviousness of a hero to flames were used in treating ailments associated with fire, as in the case of conjurations against erysipelas, which featured the names of Hananiah, Misha'el, and Azaryah from the book of Daniel (Dan. 1–3).[32] One of the most popular biblical figures was the prophet Elijah. A widespread schema for removing the evil eye incorporated a dialogue between the suffering Job[33] (who was afflicted by toothache[34] or headaches[35]) and Elijah, who advised him to seek healing in the fiery river Dinur.[36] Another conjuration, this one against demons, took the form of stories of how the prophet succeeded in preventing Lilith (also known as the Queen of Sheba),[37] the angel Dumah,[38] or Ashtruvi[39] from causing harm to a sick person (usually a child). Elijah stood out among all other figures of the Bible, and was so prominent in the folk imagination as often to take the place of other biblical characters in narratives traditionally associated with them. Rabbi Elimelekh of Leżajsk once stated that the revelations of Elijah were possible because the soul of the prophet contained the souls of all Jews—just as the soul of Adam, the first man, was said to contain the souls of all future people.[40] According to the author of *Berit avot*, a circumcision manual, in order to ease a woman's pain

[30] Benet, *Sheloshah sefarim niftahim*, 75b.

[31] Lilientalowa, *Dziecko żydowskie*, 55–6.   [32] *Segulot urefuot*, JTS, MS 9862, 8.

[33] Sometimes Job would be replaced with a nameless sick person; see Benet, *Sheloshah sefarim niftahim*, 75b.

[34] Kanarvogel, *Be'erot hamayim*, 73a; Rubinstein, *Zikhron ya'akov yosef*, 69b.

[35] 'Items' (Heb.), 381.

[36] Sometimes the river of flames is nameless. See Avida [Złotnik], 'Incantations and Remedies in Arabic and Yiddish' (Heb.), 6. In the specialist literature there are similar Latin, Russian, and German conjurations featuring Jesus and St Peter; see Vietukhov, *Zagovory*, 276–8.

[37] Benczer, 'Jüdische Volksmedizin in Ostgalizien', 120–1. For similar German conjurations featuring Jesus and 'a certain type of ailment' ('ein kaltes Gesicht'), see Vietukhov, *Zagovory*, 280.   [38] See Lilientalowa, *Dziecko żydowskie*, 54; ead., *Obrzędy pogrzebowe*, fos. 21, 211, 217.

[39] Lilientalowa, *Dziecko żydowskie*, 53–4; *Segulot urefuot*, JTS, MS 9862, 12–13; Goldberg and Eisenberg, *Sefer lahashim usegulot*, 9a–b. The name appeared in many variants (e.g. Ashtrugi, Astrige). According to Gershom Scholem it was the female demon Lilith or a witch (*astariga*); *Gnosticism, Mysticism and Talmudic Tradition*, 72–3 and 134.

[40] Unger, *The Hasidic World* (Yid.), 17; Schwartz, *Tree of Souls*, 162–3. According to yet others, Elijah was the incarnation of Pinhas, grandson of Aaron; see Lilientalowa, *Śmiecie*, fo. 35, no. 226.

during childbirth, the thing to do was to invite poor people to an 'Elijah's feast',[41] though this was more usually associated with the figure of the prophet Be'eri or his son Hosea.[42] The dialogue with Job cited above was, in some variants, conducted not by Elijah but by God himself.[43]

These conjurations accord with the widespread tales and legends in which the prophet watches over the people of Israel. Their customary retelling on Saturday evenings, after the end of the sabbath, was considered a worthy pastime.[44] In these tales, Elijah features either awake or asleep, in the garb of a vagrant or a tramp, dressed in rags, or more rarely as a noble-man, a peasant, an Arabian merchant, an animal, or a rabbi, and rescues the protagonist from the dangers threatening his life and health. As Lilien-talowa noted, 'The common people believe that the prophet Elijah some-times appears in the person of an ordinary mortal, and that with his entrance into a house remarkable happenings occur, such as the sudden dis-appearance of a case of impotence which had been considered incurable.'[45] In other readings, he was said to take upon himself and atone for the sins of the righteous, and thus indirectly protect them from divine punish-ment.[46] Moreover, he was associated with a number of objects of ritual sig-nificance, which could also be used for curative purposes. For instance it was traditionally held that a man faced with the problem of childlessness should present the community with a new Elijah's chair, a requisite during the circumcision ritual.[47] It is also interesting to note the presence and role of Elijah in the mythology of the eastern Slavs, where he was associated with fire and lightning.[48]

Many curative practices employed by the Jews necessitated the use not merely of quotations but of extensive passages from the Hebrew Bible, such as a whole chapter of one of its books, or even a whole book. The tsadik Nahman of Bratslav (now in Ukraine) believed that every type of medication was mentioned in the Song of Songs. Furthermore, in one book of customs we find the advice: 'It would be well for someone, God forbid,

[41] Lifshits, *Berit avot*, 2b.

[42] Kanarvogel, *Ta'amei mitsvot*, 17b (192); Berger, *Imrei yisra'el*, 13b.

[43] Rosenberg, *Rafa'el hamalakh*, 109.

[44] The figure of Elijah as a wanderer prepared to come to the aid of the sick and wounded was known as early as talmudic times; see Segel [Schiffer], 'Eliah der Prophet', 11–14, 42–5; Lehman, 'The Prophet Elijah in Folk Imagination' (Yid.), 115–78.

[45] Lilientalowa, *Święta żydowskie*, i. 35.          [46] See Lilientalowa, *Śmiecie*, fo. 37, no. 235.

[47] Rechtman, 'Some Customs and Their Folk Explanations' (Yid.), 250.

[48] See Moszyński, *Kultura ludowa Słowian*, 258.

having a sick person in the house, to recite the entire Song of Songs before daybreak.'[49] Nonetheless, the book with the greatest significance in matters of health was Psalms, which Jewish tradition held to be the work of King David. *Tey un thilim shat nit* (Tea and psalms will do no harm),[50] went the saying reflecting belief in their curative properties, though sometimes this was followed, with a note of disappointment in the voice, by the remark that if they really did work, 'they'd be on sale at the pharmacy'.[51] Reciting the book of Psalms in its entirety was perceived to be a path to redemption and a tried and tested way of obtaining the grace of heaven.[52] A salvific effect was also attributed to cyclical readings of the psalms, and in some cases even to readings of individual psalms. For protracted menstrual bleeding the matrimonial handbook *Imrot shelomoh* recommended that the husband of the afflicted woman study the psalm for the day, which was recited at the end of morning prayers each day of the week.[53] He might cleanse himself from nocturnal emissions by taking a ritual bath and reciting with a heavy heart Psalms 16, 32, 41, 44, 49, 77, 90, 105, 136, and 150.[54] In the nineteenth century a commentary in the Ashkenazi prayer book of Meir Ganz (which followed the rite of the Polish Jews) mentioned the particularly beneficial role of Psalm 20 in cases of difficult childbirth.[55] The tsadik of Velidniky in Ukraine (Polish: Wieledniki), in turn, is reported to have directed a convalescent mute woman to recite Psalm 130—'Out of the depths I call you, O Lord'—every day.[56] The custom of turning to the songs of David in situations of crisis also had a communal aspect. Yehudah Yudl Rosenberg, the author of the manual of curative remedies *Rafa'el hamalakh*, suggested that a sick person could be helped by psalms recited by a *minyan* (quorum of ten men) with emotional ties to the patient (*shehem ohavim lehaholeh*), and if there were not that many, boys from the *ḥeder* should be asked.[57] In emergencies such as difficult births, the local psalm fraternity would be called in to pray.[58]

---

[49] Sperling, *Ta'amei haminhagim oyf ivri taytsh*, ii. 51.

[50] Einhorn, 'Folk Proverbs in Yiddish' (Heb.), 207; 'Useful Proverbs' (Yid.), *Yidishe shprakh*, 14, p. 61.   [51] I. Bernstein, *Jewish Proverbs and Sayings* (Yid.), 291.

[52] Sperling, *Ta'amei haminhagim oyf ivri taytsh*, ii. 101; Rosenberg, *Rafa'el hamalakh*, 82 (who associates the custom with the tsadik Pinhas of Korets).

[53] Wilff, *Imrot shelomoh*, 97. On Sundays the psalm for the day was Ps. 24, and thereafter in succession: 48, 82, 94, 81, 93, and 92.

[54] Rosenberg, *Rafa'el hamalakh*, 86.   [55] Ganz, *Maḥzor mikol hashanah*, 31b.

[56] Rotner, *Sipurei nifla'ot*, 11.   [57] Rosenberg, *Rafa'el hamalakh*, 34.

[58] Shlaferman, 'The Folklore, Customs, and Stories of Kazimierz' (Yid.), 173.

The book of Psalms was one of the central pillars of Jewish education in eastern Europe. Most children were able to read it by the time they left *ḥeder*. In common parlance the term *thilim-yid* (lit. a psalm Jew) became the standard designation of a simple man with no prospect of devoting himself to talmudic study, and whose knowledge of Hebrew was thus limited to the contents of Psalms. For Jews living in rural areas and practising few of the rituals, this was one of the limited available ways of communing with the God of Israel. The tradition of using psalms in curative practices had been systematized to a certain extent as early as the Middle Ages. It was then that the anonymous collection *Shimush tehilim*, attributed to Hai Gaon (939–1038), was compiled; this book contained numerous ways of using psalms for the benefit of the human body and soul. Aside from explaining the 'efficacy' of each chapter, it also included descriptions of the actions to be performed while reciting them.[59] The modernizing processes that extended to the Jewish populace in the second half of the nineteenth century did nothing to diminish the popularity of this book. Excerpts from the *Shimush tehilim* are to be found in other works, including Rosenberg's *Rafa'el hamalakh*,[60] and it was still being reprinted as an autonomous volume in Poland in the interwar period.[61]

The fear that surrounded rapidly progressive incurable diseases and epidemics was incentive enough to promote the practical use of sacred texts. Books and pamphlets on miasma (Yid. *ipesh*, *aver*), such as the eighteenth-century *Zevaḥ pesaḥ* by Jacob Pesah of Zhovkva (now western Ukraine),[62] or the *Shemirot usegulot nifla'ot* from a century later, were an amalgamation of resources from biblical and talmudic literature, many of which made reference to practices first performed in the Tabernacle. They recommended, for instance, reciting three times Exodus 30: 34, which reads: 'And the Lord said to Moses: "Take the herbs stacte, onycha and galbanum—these herbs together with pure frankincense; let there be an equal part of each"', and then repeating it three times backwards.[63] Other Hebrew and Yiddish sources confirm the practice of reading passages about incense at the four corners of the town in times of plague.

---

[59] See also e.g. Grunwald and Kohler, 'Bibliomancy', 202–5; Trachtenberg, *Jewish Magic and Superstition*, 109.                              [60] *Rafa'el hamalakh*, 97–8.

[61] See e.g. *Kuntres shimush tehilim*. For more on this subject see Ben-Ezra, 'The Book of Psalms—A Book of Remedies' (Heb.).

[62] The title *Zevaḥ pesaḥ* (The Paschal Offering) is a reference to the story about the deaths of the Egyptians' firstborn sons.                    [63] Pesah, *Zevaḥ pesaḥ*, 8; *Shemirot usegulot nifla'ot*, 6.

At such times the words describing the burning of incense took on a truly physical dimension. The symbolic barrier thus created would encircle the human settlement, protecting it from the danger advancing on it from the outside world.[64] The tradition of manipulating passages about incense had its roots at least as far back as the sixteenth century; it was used as a protective measure in the kabbalistic community in Safed.[65] The pamphlet *Shemirot usegulot nifla'ot* also cites popular amulets employing biblical quotations in written form. In one of these the letters of the words 'Pinhas stepped forward and intervened, and the plague ceased' (Ps. 106: 30) were arranged in five lines and columns, and the letters forming the Tetragrammaton were added to the first four columns.[66] In another pamphlet, attributed to Eliyahu Guttmacher, the tsadik of Grätz, the main text of the amulet began with the phrase: 'For he will order his angels to guard you wherever you go' (Ps. 91: 11). This was followed by the encoded content, arranged in sixteen lines and seven columns, comprising a series of quotations from the Bible (including Exod. 8: 1–2 and 49: 18) and ringed by a series of excerpts from Psalms.[67] The booklet also contained information on the ingredients of incense to be burned in the home during an epidemic (these included sage, juniper, mint, red deer horn, and the peel of a tart apple),[68] and a short list of herbs recommended by the Roman physician Jacob Tsahalon (1630–93). The author further mentioned hanging onions, garlic, and toadstools in windows and doorways as a protective measure as well as other methods described in contemporary sources.[69]

The *Shimush tehilim* and *Zevaḥ pesaḥ* are examples of the creative exploitation of biblical texts in a kabbalistic spirit. Their beneficial power was believed to lie in the sacred words representing the names of God or of angels. These might be cited overtly or by way of manipulations to the text designed to reveal hidden content. Methods such as gematria, *notarikon*,

[64] Rosenberg, *Rafa'el hamalakh*, 54; see Veynig, '*Mageyfe* Weddings' (Yid.), 29.

[65] See Bos, 'Hayim Vital's Practical Kabbalah and Alchemy', 61.

[66] *Shemirot usegulot nifla'ot*, 5. This amulet is found in many sources, either as an autonomous whole or as part of a more complex compilation of sacred names. It has sometimes been attributed to the tsadik Moses Teitelbaum. See Pesah, *Zevaḥ pesaḥ*, 9; Rosenberg, *Rafa'el hamalakh*, 54 and 55; Veynig, 'Medicaments and Remedies among the Jews' (Yid.), 29; Schmid, 'Jüdische Amulette aus Osteuropa', 290, 292.

[67] *Shemirot usegulot nifla'ot*, 26. The same amulet, with minor alterations, was reprinted in Rosenberg, *Rafa'el hamalakh*, 56.

[68] Cf. Rosenberg, *Rafa'el hamalakh*, 51; id., *Der malekh refoel*, 47.

[69] Rosenberg, *Rafa'el hamalakh*, 52.

and *temurah* became a permanent element of popular kabbalistic literature. As far back as the Middle Ages, when the Ashkenazi diaspora was migrating to eastern Europe, it already had a number of important titles of this type in its collections. Both the *Sefer yetsirah*, which describes the creation of the world on the basis of the ten *sefirot* and the twenty-two letters of the Hebrew alphabet, and the Zohar, which was the foundational work for mystical speculation in later periods, found a sizeable body of readers and adherents in the lands along the Vistula and the Bug in the early modern period. In the golden age of Jewish history in Poland this fact was bemoaned by Rabbi Moses Isserles. Though he himself held a profound interest in mystical ideas, he was nonetheless critical of their vulgarization and dissemination among the common people.[70] It was no coincidence that the author of the *Ma'aseh tuvyah*, a physician educated in western Europe, exclaimed in the early eighteenth century that 'there is no other country where so much attention is afforded to demons, amulets, conjuration, names, and dreams' as the Polish Commonwealth.[71] The *Shivhei habesht* (In Praise of the Ba'al Shem Tov), the first hagiographical work on the founder of Polish hasidism, was testimony to the fact that this statement was still true a century later. The work made no secret of the Ba'al Shem Tov's attachment to the Zohar as a magical instrument, reporting, for instance, that he used it to ward off brigands.[72] The Zohar remained one of the most important books for the leaders of the hasidic movement. It also inspired popular ethical literature, in which elements of folk healing were interwoven with visions of the world of demons. Another book with a particularly large readership was the *Kav hayashar* by Tsevi Hirsh Koydanover (d.1712). Based on the zoharic doctrine of the powers of good and evil (*sitra dikedusha* and *sitra ahra* respectively), this book devoted considerable space to descriptions of the influence of unclean forces on the human body. It included warnings against such potential dangers as bloodletting on inauspicious days, demons spreading diseases, and people capable of casting spells, and also listed certain times of the year when parents should take particular care over the safety of their children.[73] At the same time it incorporated medical concepts from the ancient world, mentioning for instance the notion that sperm (white fluid, or phlegm) was produced in the brain and

[70] Isserles, *Torat ha'olah*, 72b. See Bałaban, *Żydzi w Krakowie i na Kazimierzu*, 149.
[71] Hakohen, *Ma'aseh tuvyah*, 99b.
[72] Ben-Amos and Mintz, *In Praise of the Baal Shem Tov*, 165–6.
[73] T. H. Koydanover, *Kav hayashar*, 94–5.

drained down through the eighteen segments of the spine, which were said to correspond to the eighteen blessings in the daily liturgy.[74]

The kabbalistic ideas formulated in the school that grew up around the sixteenth-century thinker Isaac Luria of Safed (the Ari, 1534–72) likewise left an indelible impression on folk healing practices. Their echoes were still discernible in popular publications around 1900, as well as in Jewish ethnographic material. The collection *Rafa'el hamalakh* cites the Ari as the source for its recommendations to rub the eyes with the knots of the *tsitsit* as a method for preventing blindness,[75] to avert all misfortune by looking down at one's fingernails while reciting Exodus 33: 23, as well as to pronounce the sacred names Agaf Sagaf Nagaf and Peniel Uriel when performing the Havdalah ritual.[76] The extent to which Lurianic kabbalah had become an inextricable element of Ashkenazi curative practices is visible in the context of the activities of the *ba'alei shem* (sing. *ba'al shem*, lit. master of the name, i.e. one who is versed in the use of sacred names), who, in the period around 1700, were the dominant actors in traditional Jewish healthcare in eastern Europe. When Joel Halpern, the author of the work *Mifalot elokim*, examined the question of the ban on using the divine names without purification in the ashes of a red heifer (cf. Num. 19: 2), his aim was to elaborate on Luria's prohibition of such practice. Halpern's conclusion that some names, in view of their exceptional holiness, might be employed to counter the actions of demons without the need for extra ablutions, however, opened up a broad scope for the practical application of kabbalistic ideas.[77] Nonetheless, even numerous examples of mystical techniques cannot fully reflect the significance of Lurianic and zoharic thought for the commonly held beliefs of Ashkenazi Jews relating to this—and, more significantly, the next—world.

It is also worth devoting a few sentences to *Sefer razi'el hamalakh*, not so much for its content as in view of the respect accorded it in Jewish folk

[74] Ibid. 180.     [75] Rosenberg, *Rafa'el hamalakh*, 74; id., *Der malekh refoel*, 9.

[76] Rosenberg, *Rafa'el hamalakh*, 26. The names of the guardian angels Peniel (Paniel) and Uriel would also be spoken in other circumstances as a protective measure against enemies, spells, and misfortunes; see Goldberg and Eisenberg, *Sefer laḥashim usegulot*, 1b. The sacred name Agaf Sagaf Nagaf, sometimes in other, variant forms, aside from providing protection from the actions of enchanters (Simner, *Zekhirah*, 27b), was also used to prevent bleeding (Halpern, *Mifalot elokim*, 14b), children dying (Lifshits, *Berit avot*, 3b), and the plague (Rosenberg, *Rafa'el hamalakh*, 52). See Schrire, *Hebrew Amulets*, 125; M. Bernstein, 'Two Remedy Books in Yiddish from 1474 and 1508', 297.

[77] Halpern, *Mifalot elokim*, 3a–b. See Etkes, *The Besht*, 40–1.

culture. This work was probably compiled by Eleazar of Worms, and most of its sections originated in the Middle Ages. It was not released in print until a relatively late date, 1701, in Amsterdam. The content of *Sefer razi'el hamalakh* was rather hermetic in character, and demanded not only fluency in Hebrew but also a strong command of the extensive mystical terminology. It was in fact a collection of highly varied texts, including lengthy excerpts from the *Sefer harazim* (third–fourth centuries CE) and the *Sod ma'aseh bereshit* (thirteenth century, Ashkenazi Pietists).[78] In the popular consciousness it was believed to have been the gift of the angel Raziel to Adam, the first human. It offered aid in cases of difficult childbirth, when it would be placed under the head of the birthing woman, and was said to protect the house from fire.[79] Its vast influence on the richness of Jewish health-related folklore was also visible in the context of amulets. The twentieth-century collection *Rafa'el hamalakh* contained a few reproductions of prints that had originally appeared in *Sefer razi'el hamalakh*. In *Berit avot*, an anthology on circumcision, there are instructions for making an amulet from red deer hide, containing the names Kof, Okf, Ofk, and providing protection from a difficult birth.[80] Another amulet from *Sefer razi'el ha-malakh* portrayed the figures of three guardian angels protecting an infant and its mother from the female demon Lilith. Sanoi, Sansanoi, and Semangalof on this amulet resembled birds, and each had such distinctive characteristics that in time they became autonomous figures, and their portraits and names were printed individually, written out by hand, and engraved.[81]

One deeply entrenched element of Jewish cultural heritage in the Polish lands was the legacy of the medieval Ashkenazi Pietist movement. The authors of printed medical manuals, like those who compiled collections of customs, made multiple references to *Sefer ḥasidim*, a product of the

---

[78] See Dan, 'Raziel, Book of', 129.

[79] Other sacred books, such as psalters and prayer books, would also be placed under the head of a woman in childbirth. See e.g. Maimon, *An Autobiography*, 103 (noted as *Book of Raphael*). Elzet [Złotnik], 'Some Jewish Customs' (Heb.), 363; Lilientalowa, *Dziecko żydowskie*, 31; Pulner, 'Obryadi i povirya', 106; Lifshits, *Berit avot*, 6a; Unger, *The Hasidic World* (Yid.), 34. The acolytes of particular tsadikim would also use works by their own masters for the same purpose; see Zandvays, 'Sarny—Its Foundation, Existence, and Decline' (Yid.), 96.

[80] *Sefer razi'el hamalakh*, 43a. After the amulet was placed on the birthing woman, the following, slightly modified words from Exod. 11: 8 were to be whispered into her right ear: 'Depart, you and all the people who follow you'; Lifshits, *Berit avot*, 2a.

[81] See Schmid, 'Jüdische Amulette aus Osteuropa', 184; Patai, 'Lilith', 296.

thought of that movement, using the information it contained as justification for certain popular views on health. Among the snippets that filled its pages, there was a remark on the auspicious nature of being born in the caul;[82] a warning, found in several ethnographic sources, against eating bulls' hearts (which was said to cause malice, stupidity, or memory problems);[83] and a description of the custom of 'selling off' a sick child so that the sins weighing on its biological parents would no longer affect its health.[84] In many cases these convictions had parallels in the folklore of local Christians. The spectrum of remedies traditionally associated with key figures among the Ashkenazi Pietists was not confined to the sphere of mysticism. Two examples will suffice as illustration. The editor of the printed anthology *Likutei me'ir* recorded as 'tradition received from Rabbi Judah Hehasid' a 'great cure for toothache', which involved buying from a pharmacy and then boiling the herbs known as *Ochsenzunge* (ox tongue) and serving them to the patient.[85] Similarly, a recipe in one nineteenth-century manuscript for treating macular pucker using powdered camphor was described as having been revealed to Judah Hehasid by an angel.[86]

The rabbinic authorities had long battled the infiltration into Jewish therapeutic tradition of culturally alien elements. They tended to be relatively tolerant of natural methods, but remained deeply suspicious of magical practices. These were placed in the category of 'ways of the Amorites' (*darkhei ha'emori*) in the Talmud, and were condemned as 'foreign' and deprecated as a 'foolish custom' (*minhag shetut*) by the rabbis, but this stigmatization did not prevent such practices from surviving in folk culture. On the one hand the rabbis produced detailed descriptions of acts which they perceived to be magic of alien provenance and thus forbidden, but on the other, as these were intended to save lives, if they did not involve the sin of desecrating the divine Name or murder, either of which precluded any form of acceptance in the context of halakhah, their status remained ambiguous.[87] Successive generations of Jews living in various centres of

[82] Judah Hehasid, *Sefer ḥasidim*, 255; Lifshits, *Berit avot*, 5b.
[83] BT *Hor.* 13b; Judah Hehasid, *Sefer ḥasidim*, 436. Cf. *Ets ḥayim*, 29; Bastomski, *At the Source: Jewish Proverbs* (Yid.), 107; Benczer, 'Volksglaube galizischer Juden', 274; Rechtman, 'Some Customs and Their Folk Explanations' (Yid.), 263.
[84] Judah Hehasid, *Sefer ḥasidim*, 160.
[85] This may have been a reference to Anchusa officinalis or the rhizomes of Bistorta officinalis. See Arends, *Volkstümliche Namen der Drogen*, 218.
[86] *Segulot urefuot*, Bibliotheca Rosenthaliana, HS. ROS. 444, 14b.
[87] BT *Shab.* 37a, *Ḥul.* 77b; also JT *Shab.* 6: 10.

the European diaspora departed further and further from the strict prohibitions imposed by the early sages. Among the medieval Ashkenazi Pietists the prevailing opinion was that the ban on employing 'the ways of the
Amorites' had had real justification in antiquity because it was founded on a
fear of idolatry. Since the pagan cults had died out, however, these methods
had lost the odium of heresy and had become permissible.[88] Many practices
that fell in both categories are mentioned in ethnographic material or folk
medicine collections of the period around 1900. One interesting example is
the custom of seeking protection from spells by tying a red thread around
one's little finger. This was mentioned explicitly as one of the 'ways of the
Amorites' and was unequivocally condemned. For precisely this reason the
author of *Rafa'el hamalakh* devoted a paragraph to criticizing it, adding that
it was a widespread custom among the people.[89] Yet the book *Sefer hahayim
hanikra segulot yisra'el*, published in Munkács (now Mukachevo, Ukraine)
at a slightly earlier date, recommended tying red silk thread around two
fingers of one hand to guard against choking,[90] and around one finger as
protection from nosebleeds.[91] This meant that not only did this work confirm the existence of the custom, but it even approved of it as an effective
remedy. There are several other similar examples of customs which by this
period had become firmly entrenched in Ashkenazi culture, such as killing
a hen which crowed like a cockerel,[92] or warning the demons before pouring waste water out onto the street.[93] One popular tradition cited as *minhag
shetut* by Joseph Karo, the author of the *Shulhan arukh*, was *kaparot*, the
ritual slaughter of a white cockerel (or hen) before Yom Kippur as a sacrifice to atone for sins. Among the Ashkenazim the custom proved to be so
entrenched, however, that this comment disappeared from subsequent
editions of the work.[94]

[88]  See Jakobovits, *Jewish Medical Ethics*, 34.
[89]  Tosefta *Shab.* 7: 1; Rosenberg, *Rafa'el hamalakh*, 46.
[90]  Lifshits, *Sefer hahayim hanikra segulot yisra'el*, 128b.                    [91]  Ibid. 20b.
[92]  Tosefta *Shab.* 7: 3; Bastomski, *At the Source: Jewish Proverbs* (Yid.), 105. An analysis of this
Ashkenazi practice from the angle of rabbinic judicature is to be found in Benin, 'A Hen Crowing like a Cock', 261–81.
[93]  Tosefta *Shab.* 7: 6. In the Polish lands the warning used was not the talmudic *Hada!*, but
the Yiddish *Hit zikh!*; see Sperling, *Ta'amei haminhagim oyf ivri taytsh*, ii. 70; Bastomski, *At the
Source: Jewish Proverbs* (Yid.), 102; Buchbinder, 'Jewish Omens' (Yid.), 257. There were also
local variations of this cry; see Fayvushinski, 'Pruzhener folklor', 199; Shlaferman, 'The Folklore, Customs, and Stories of Kazimierz' (Yid.), 174.
[94]  See Benin, 'A Hen Crowing like a Cock', 263–4; Gordis, *The Dynamics of Judaism*, 108.

# CHAPTER THREE

# IN THE FAMILY CIRCLE

A T THE END of the nineteenth century, large, multi-generational families were a common phenomenon in Europe, especially in its eastern areas; this meant that people were rarely left alone to struggle with physical afflictions. They were surrounded by both immediate and more distant relations as well as neighbours, among whom there was usually no shortage of home-grown specialists or concerned advisers. People lived within the orbit of not a single system of medicine but several at once: they could seek relief from practices based on folk beliefs or those founded upon conventional medicine. Similarly, they could choose cheap or more expensive options, close to home or further afield, offered by acquaintances or strangers. In examining the decisions taken in this sphere by east European Jews on the threshold of modernity it is easy to fall into the trap of looking at them from our contemporary perspective. In order to avoid this, we need to remember that we are talking about a society without access to universal, free healthcare or many of the social benefits available nowadays. In the western guberniyas of Russia, rudimentary elements of an opt-in health insurance system were introduced in the late nineteenth century for industrial workers. The changes in this area, which passed into law in 1912, never came into force, however, owing to the outbreak of the First World War. In Galicia a mandatory sickness insurance scheme and system of patient funds was introduced in 1888 for certain categories of employees, but by the end of the disintegration of the Habsburg empire the goal of universal insurance had still not been achieved.[1] Moreover, this was a populace for which contact with an educated physician was often not only a logistical and economic challenge, but also a psychological one, the more formidable as it frequently entailed a confrontation between traditional culture and the biomedical approach. Anyone undertaking such treatment had to relinquish control over the treatment process to a degree unprecedented

---

[1] Grzybowski, *Galicja 1848–1914*, 141; Szubert, *Ubezpieczenie społeczne*, 25.

in previous generations, and to people whom they did not particularly trust.

Early modern medicine, while recognizing a number of different treatment alternatives, nonetheless prioritized the decisions taken by the patients themselves. Doctors subordinated their judgement to their patients' narratives, and were expected to pay more attention to the sick person's interpretation of their own illness than is the case today.[2] Folk culture perpetuated this model for a long time, even in an age when it was coming up against increasing pressure from proponents of new developments in medicine. This need to retain control of the treatment process found expression in colloquial parlance. Even as late as the beginning of the twentieth century, Jews would say, *Freg nit bam royfe, freg bam khoyle* ('Don't ask the doctor, ask the patient'),[3] revealing the considerable weight carried by the patient's opinion on any subject connected to their condition. For this reason, any attempt to explain the system of Jewish folk medicine in this period must cover the full range of alternatives, none of which was entirely dismissed or rejected by the Jews.

Don Yoder, who researched the ethno-medical aspects of the culture of Pennsylvania, listed four basic 'grades' of action in case of ailments: ignoring them, taking a home-made remedy or tried and trusted medication, treatment by a healer, and, if all else failed, consultation with a medical professional.[4] A similar scale of behaviour in seeking treatment can be found in many other societies and ethnic groups. It is no less applicable in the study of Jewish folk medicine in eastern Europe, with the reservation that it should be treated only as a general pattern rather than as an incontrovertible algorithm. The choice of treatment procedure depended on a range of factors, among which the following should be mentioned in particular: the severity of the illness, the patient's personality, their familiarity with treatment methods and the range of remedies stocked in the medicine cupboard at home, the availability of official and unofficial medical or paramedical services, and the financial standing of the patient and those in his or her immediate circle. Decisions regarding healthcare were always a personal matter to some extent, and, while they were largely conditioned by one's community and its traditions, this dependence was by no means absolute. People were eager to seek out new cures and treatment methods outside

---

[2] See Lindemann, *Medicine and Society in Early Modern Europe*, 275.
[3] I. Bernstein, *Jewish Proverbs and Sayings* (Yid.), 256.          [4] Yoder, 'Folk medicine', 208.

their own milieu in hope of the best possible results, even if the novel methods contradicted the traditional world-view.[5]

If we analyse the variety of remedies used on the level of popular treatment we will notice a clear gradation in their degree of availability and magical potential. For the most part they were perceived to be natural, though this statement must be accompanied by the caveat that there was a ubiquitous supernatural element, in the form of daily prayer, almsgiving, and other actions (such as those performed when gathering or applying herbs). Deliberate use of magic was limited in scope and was most common in preventative practices used on children (blowing on them, licking their face, spitting, etc.). It was not until life-threatening diseases, such as cholera, or incurable conditions such as epilepsy or infertility arose that the methods adopted to fight them were significantly reinforced by magic. In the first place, methods that were readily available in the immediate environment were used. Only afterwards was outside knowledge called upon, in a gradual progression away from the centre (the home, the street, the town), and engaging an increasing number of people in the treatment process. At later stages help was often sought beyond the boundaries of the community, and the quest was accompanied by a growing readiness to try methods which were taboo, from sacred names of angels and God to others that were alien, ritually forbidden, and even abhorrent. At this point the sufferer also became increasingly willing to expend extreme effort, both financial and physical, such as travelling to a professor of medicine in a distant city.

Most people tended to have firmly entrenched views on the competence of the various categories of health practitioners. Common parlance attested the opinions that *Doktoyrim veysn khoylas ineveynik un royfim a make oysnveynik* (Doctors understand sickness within, and *royfim* [healers] a carbuncle on the outside), *Tsu a vund un tsu a bloter—az es helft nit keyn dokter, helft a toter* (For wounds and ulcers, if a doctor cannot help, a Tatar will), or *A royz kurirn doktoyrim nit* (Doctors cannot heal erysipelas).[6] Motivating factors in the decision to find a different path or embark on a new stage of treatment included severe chronic symptoms or a deterioration in one's condition to the degree that normal day-to-day functioning became difficult. Sayings such as *Se geyt mir op vi a tsonveytik* (It concerns me as much as

[5] Pelto and Pelto, 'Studying Knowledge, Culture, Behavior in Applied Medical Anthropology', 153.      [6] Shabad, 'On Erysipelas' (Yid.), 53–4.

a toothache)[7] or *Purim nie sviata, trastsa nie khvaroba* (Purim is not a feast day, a fever is not an illness)[8] reflect the view that minor ailments should be suffered in silence and ignored. The only medication that would be taken in such circumstances was familiar home-made remedies. 'When you had a cold you didn't go to the doctor. For the most part you pretended that there was nothing wrong', one resident of the town of Wojsławice remembers. 'If it was really causing discomfort, you would procure a slab of marble from somewhere, heat it up over the fire, pour vinegar on it, and inhale the vapour through your nose. You had to move your head in all directions as you did so.'[9] Aside from obvious cases (such as removing a splinter or setting bones), the methods used were designed to eliminate symptoms, above all to relieve pain. Once this was achieved, the patient was happy to take no further action.[10] As long as the illness was bearable, no help was usually sought beyond one's immediate circle. It would be ignored due to ignorance of the severity of the condition, or accepted as other needs were prioritized, such as supporting the family. If the decision was made to take the search for treatment further, then a practitioner would be approached—a proponent of either folk or official medicine. Many testimonies suggest that, unlike in contemporary societies, the former was preferred.[11]

The first reaction to an illness that could not be ignored was to seek help within one's immediate environment. Home remedies played a primary role in the case of ailments which were not perceived to present an immediate mortal threat, or those which brought cyclical relapses such that it was possible to predict the need to have specific medications to hand. The predominance of self-medication is a characteristic feature of traditional cultures, though this does not mean that home medicine cabinets contained only items popularly perceived as folk remedies. Naturally, this

---

[7] G. Bernstein, 'Expressions and Proverbs' (Yid.), 54.

[8] Hurvits, 'My Mother's Sayings' (Yid.), 121.

[9] From, 'The Doctor and Domestic Remedies' (Yid.), 345; Sperling, *Ta'amei haminhagim oyf ivri taytsh*, ii. 120. One common treatment for a head cold was smudging (burning a variety of objects to create a curative smoke) using a goose or turkey feather, Roman coriander (blackseed), a piece of hide, asafoetida, or even a cat's tail. See Lew, 'O lecznictwie i przesądach', *Izraelita*, 49, pp. 475–6.

[10] For an interesting description of a case of tooth decay which the sufferer stopped treating with home remedies after the pain subsided, see Groer, 'Szpital Starozakonnych w Warszawie', 89.

[11] See Miller, 'Once Upon a Time in Our Town' (Yid.), 210; Moysheles, 'Singer the Feldsher' (Yid.), 246.

form of treatment was non-specialist and far more general than treatment by a healer or physician; its aim was to offer rapid solutions to the challenges presented by life. Home therapies nonetheless covered an extremely broad catalogue of actions and remedies, including many which had filtered through from practitioners of biomedicine.[12]

The vast majority of domestic cures were seen as standard, even if their selection was to some extent influenced by magical thinking. Those that fell into this category were above all the herbs, vegetables, and fruit growing in one's own garden, stocked in one's pantry, or readily available at the local market, as well as infusions or preserves made from the above. Besides fruit preserves and cordials, there was also no shortage of vodkas, liqueurs, vinegars, and ingredients for tea- or coffee-type infusions. Other products in the home medicine cabinet included mineral-based preparations (clay and soap) and animal products (eggs, fresh milk, butter, and eggnog); the common denominator was ease of procurement, preparation, and storage. This list should be extended to include everyday items, such as the cold knife placed on a swelling,[13] the scrap of fabric used as a bandage,[14] and other remedies used as necessary—chicken broth,[15] for instance, or a hot bath.[16]

All the above-mentioned cures came under the somewhat derogatory Yiddish term *babske refues* (women's cures), because their preparation and application were primarily the woman's task. It was the woman who was in charge of the kitchen, garden, and forays to the market. From their childhood years girls were trained for motherhood by being expected to care for their younger siblings, and this included performing hygiene-related and simple curative tasks. A good wife—as Isaac Bashevis Singer wrote of Esther, the wife of the magician of Lublin—'knew how to knit, sew a

[12] Saillant, 'Home Care and Prevention', 188–90.

[13] This was known as *odciskanie*, or 'impressing' (Yid. *opkvetshn*).

[14] Including also cotton wool and gauze, available from pharmacies.

[15] Consumption of chicken broth was recommended for ailments including chicken pox, measles (the broth was to be hot, *Segulot urefuot*, Bibliotheca Rosenthaliana, HS. ROS. 444, 3*b*; but not fatty, Schneersohn, *Sefer refuot*, 27), consumption (using mutton shank, Rosenberg, *Der malekh refoel*, 42), and typhoid fever (Sperling, *Ta'amei haminhagim oyf ivri taytsh*, ii. 108), as well as diarrhoea (using fresh beef as the stock base; Lew, 'Lecznictwo i przesądy', *Izraelita*, 47, p. 494).

[16] Used for ailments including lower back pain (with salt, Rosenberg, *Rafa'el hamalakh*, 19; id., *Der malekh refoel*, 57), rheumatism (with washing soda, *Rafa'el hamalakh*, 89; *Der malekh refoel*, 58), scabies (Lilientalowa, *Dziecko żydowskie*, 68), haemorrhoids (*Rafa'el hamalakh*, 38; *Segulot urefuot*, JTS, MS 9862, 89), and kidney stones (*Rafa'el hamalakh*, 8; *Der malekh refoel*, 60).

wedding gown, bake gingerbread and tarts, tear out the pip of a chicken, apply a cupping-glass or leeches, even bleed a patient'.[17] Treatment of minor ailments at home was a tradition passed down from mother to daughter.[18] The Yiddish saying *A mame iz vi a mezuze* (A mama is like a mezuzah) expressed the conviction of the vital role of maternal care.[19] The echoes of this time-honoured role continued to reverberate long after the medical sphere had been taken over by the biomedical paradigm. The stereotype of the over-protective Jewish mother, which remains vibrant in contemporary Jewish culture, is said to have had its roots in the positive image of the *yidishe mame* familiar from many testimonies of life in the east European shtetl.[20] The following is a description of the wife's room in a relatively well-to-do Jewish household in this period:

When there was no more space on the wall, pictures were stood on the chest of drawers, which held smaller household utensils, with a compartment for medications, home-made tinctures, and all manner of women's oddments for *segulot*, conjurations, and popular treatments, such as cupping cups, enema equipment, and so on. A bottle of spirit was also kept there, for serving to a goy—or, for that matter, a Jew: a tried and tested aid to a successful transaction. At the top . . . in a glass or under a plate, for some considerable period of time a *shir-hamaylesn* would be stored, such as it is customary to hang up by the bedside of a woman in childbirth.[21]

In the reminiscences of one resident of Szydłowiec we read: 'In better homes women's time was taken up with making all manner of preserves: bilberry cordial for stomach ache, raspberry cordial for perspiration, plum jam for spreading on the children's bread, and the like.'[22] Other Jewish sources confirm the immense popularity of home-made products. Infusions of elderberry and linden fruits with the addition of dried raspberries, or raspberry cordial, were all considered reliable methods of provoking perspiration, which was linked to the conviction that it was vital to draw the disease out of the body.[23] One author of a Yiddish memoir wrote: 'When

---

[17] Bashevis Singer, *The Magician of Lublin*, 4.

[18] Lew, 'O lecznictwie i przesądach', *Izraelita*, 37, p. 316.

[19] I. Bernstein, *Jewish Proverbs and Sayings* (Yid.), 149.

[20] See e.g. Dundes, 'The J.A.P. and the J.A.M. in American Jokelore', 456–75.

[21] Taub, 'The Appearance of a Jewish Home' (Yid.), 279. *Shir-hamaylesn* (Yid.) were Hebrew amulets containing the text of Psalm 121, which starts with the superscription *Shir hama'alot*.                    [22] Schwarzputter, 'From Years Gone By' (Yid.), 107.

[23] Rosenberg, *Rafa'el hamalakh*, 31; id., *Der malekh refoel*, 59; Lew, 'O lecznictwie i przesądach', *Izraelita*, 49, p. 476; Cf. Simon, *Medycyna ludowa*, 342.

[the fever was such that] your bones ached, you would be rubbed all over with turpentine, given raspberry cordial with two or three glasses of hot tea to drink, and covered with several quilts and an eiderdown'.[24] Products of this type were used above all as treatments, almost never for prevention. One testimony from Horodenka not only cites their gradation (the mildest being bilberry cordial and the strongest raspberry), but also states that they were primarily produced for the medicine cabinet.[25] The possible exception to this rule was jam, which was treated as a sweet delicacy. 'There are days in summer when all the children in town go about with smeared mouths, sticky cheeks, and black teeth and fingers', Itsik Kipnis wrote in his reminiscences of Ukraine, and recalled several other uses of fruits by his mother: 'The rest would be sprinkled with sugar in bottles or small jars . . . Liqueur is sometimes good in tea, sometimes for making Kiddush, but above all as medication. If anyone in the house has an upset stomach, this is the best remedy for strengthening them.'[26]

As mentioned above, the contents of the kitchen store cupboard were not the only domestic remedies employed:

For instance, if a child felt a churning in their belly [*gegrimt un gedreyt in boykh*], this was a sign of worms. A batch of *veremkroyt*[27] would be boiled up at once and the infusion given to the child to drink. If anyone had to dash too often with their stomach, paradise leaves [*gan-eydn-bletlekh*] would be steeped [in water] for them.[28] And that cured their stomach to such an extent that it stopped them up entirely. If anyone got a boil [*make*], a gobbet of putty—the mixture of oil and chalk used by glaziers to seal panes of glass—would be laid upon it and the boil would open up. If anyone had an earache a camomile infusion would be made . . . and injected directly into the patient's ear, which would then be stopped with a bit of cotton wool, and additionally bound up with a broad kerchief to stop the air getting in. He would go about like that with his chin bound up for several

[24] Zandvays, 'Sarny—Its Foundation, Existence, and Decline' (Yid.), 95.

[25] Farber, 'Folk Healing' (Yid.), 180.    [26] Kipnis, *My Town Sloveshne* (Yid.), 79.

[27] Various herbs were known as *veremkroyt* (Ger. *Wurmkraut*), among them tansy. Cf. Arends, *Volkstümliche Namen der Drogen*, 323.

[28] The name *gan-eydn-bletlekh* is difficult to identify with any certainty, though it invites associations with the leaf of the fig plant, which was used in folk medicine for stomach upsets and wounds among other things. In the Jewish tradition paradise leaves feature in a number of parables about the prophet Elijah, who was said to have presented them as a fragrant and extremely precious gift to Rabah son of Avuha, a talmudic rabbi. See Zevin, *All the Stories of the Talmud* (Yid.), 40.

days, looking like a war invalid. For none of those remedies was it necessary to go to the pharmacy. They could all be had at Peysakh Gelmer's little shop.[29]

A domestic medicine cabinet in the hands of a capable housewife would be famed beyond the immediate family. For procedures such as setting broken bones, cupping, and bloodletting, an external practitioner was usually called in; likewise for the 'removal' of the evil eye or fright. On occasion, however, someone from the immediate circle who was able to perform such acts was called upon. Neighbourly assistance was requested in emergencies, but also in minor matters, which strengthened good relations with those living nearby: 'In those days virtually every Jew, man or woman, could diagnose an illness and directly apply a *woman's* cure. And if one wasn't sure oneself, one sought the advice of a neighbour or an elderly aunt, and acted on their *diagnosis*.[30] Another memoirist wrote:

It was difficult to get to the feldsher. So my mother set about seeking out her own methods and using domestic cures. This involved her telling me to stick my tongue out and getting our neighbour, who was well known for doing such things, to remove the *ayn-hore*. [The woman] licked my temples, spitting each time, and comforted me by saying that if nothing else helped she would give me castor oil.[31]

Not only did such neighbourly connections increase the scope of available natural remedies, but they also made access to various types of medical books, from *segulot urefuot* to medical encyclopedias, easier.[32]

The work of the Jewish fraternities embraced a somewhat broader circle, though it was still classifiable as neighbourly assistance. In most communities in eastern Europe there was at least one such organization, whose members regularly performed a range of *mitsvot* without remuneration. Over the years they grew in number, and their competences began to overlap.[33] They brought together people of a religious bent, often under the spiritual care of the local rabbi. In the period around 1900 the fraternities that played the greatest role in health-related matters were *bikur holim* ('visiting the sick') and *linat hatsedek* ('night watch of the righteous'), though

[29] Shuster, 'The Grandfather Healer' (Yid.), 177.
[30] Ibid. 176–7. Emphases in the original.     [31] Milkh, *Autobiographical Sketches* (Yid.), 33.
[32] See e.g. Bergner, *In the Long Winter Nights* (Yid.), 99.
[33] In the town of Mława, for example, in the early twentieth century there were two rival fraternities aiding the sick, Bikur Holim and Ezrat Holim, run by social activists who were often in conflict with members of the other fraternity; Yunis, 'The Old Homeland' (Yid.), 59–60.

these were usually the same people, who were also active in the funeral fraternity, the *ḥevrah kadisha* ('sacred society'). In view of the strong aversion to mixing the sexes that was present in Jewish culture, there were usually separate groups for the care of sick men and women within such fraternities. Among their duties were tending the bedbound sick and invalids in the most general sense: supplying them with food, fuel, care of minors, and also basic medications already familiar to us from the domestic medicine cupboard: soups, herbs, cordials, and preserves. Some of them would also carry out procedures in which they had experience due to their professional background: feldshers and midwives were often members of these associations, as were people who ran pharmacies or were simply known for removing charms.[34] Among the services they performed were hygiene-related tasks such as washing, applying compresses, and massages, as well as procedures usually performed by *royfim*, such as cupping or enemas. Furthermore, the fraternities helped those who had no other source of assistance, who were poor and alone, by paying for medical consultations, travel to the hospital or sanatorium, and the stay itself. But the work of these associations was not restricted to provision of 'natural' treatments or mediation in contact with biomedical practitioners. Their members also took it upon themselves to protect the patients in their care from the actions of unclean forces. The most important tasks in this respect were keeping constant watch over the patient after dark, checking their mezuzot, and reciting psalms.[35]

In some towns in the Polish lands there were also other fraternities established by the traditional Jewish community to perform various types of healthcare. In Sokal (now western Ukraine), for instance, the Ezrat Nashim (Women's Aid) society undertook to supply kosher meals to the local hospital.[36] In Zelów and in other communities, the members of the *ḥevrat tehilim* ('psalm fraternity'), who were called out to all kinds of crisis situations—such as difficult births, the seriously ill, and the dying —enjoyed considerable prestige.[37] In Łódź and other large cities, the work of such fraternities, of which there were a great many, often took a more

---

[34] Kossoy and Ohry, *The Feldshers*, 169.

[35] See e.g. Klagsbrun, *The Jews of Mielec* (Yid.), 130–2. An example of neighbourly assistance in time of cholera, in the form of impromptu 'massage fraternities' (*khevre raybers*), is to be found in the authobiographical novel by Sholem Aleichem, *From The Fair*, 100.

[36] Kindler, 'Jewish Philanthropic Organizations and Institutions in Sokal' (Yid.), 206.

[37] Dinari, 'When Jewish Zelów was alive' (Yid.), 121–2; Shlaferman, 'The Folklore, Customs, and Stories of Kazimierz' (Yid.), 173.

modern form, even to the point of running well-equipped care institutions.[38] The Jewish communities also operated establishments such as shelters for the homeless (*hekdesh aniyim*) and homes for the elderly (*moshav zekenim*), which took in the infirm, the homeless, and those with no family to care for them. They were usually housed in old, poorly heated, and poorly situated community-owned buildings (for example close to the slaughterhouse). Many testimonies contain extremely negative descriptions of these places, and the very word *hekdesh* in Yiddish came to be synonymous with disorder. The members of the fraternities described above, in the first place the local feldsher and physician, would visit these institutions to provide basic care to their residents. It was no coincidence, though, that those of the homeless who enjoyed some respect among residents would often be tolerated in the synagogues, where the conditions offered better hope of surviving difficult times. The work performed by organizations of this type was sometimes subjected to criticism, either out of personal animosity or due to their failure to properly discharge their duties. As the saying went, where there are too many officers of charity jostling for space in the pew, you may be sure that the local paupers will go hungry.[39]

[38] Puś, *Żydzi w Łodzi*, 180–3.　　　　[39] Golenpol, *Lexicon of Hebrew Folklore* (Heb.), 30.

# CHAPTER FOUR

# FELDSHERS AND HEALERS

FELDSHERS (Yid. *feldshers*, *feltshers*) are the most undervalued group of practitioners whose services were used by the Jewish populace, at least from the perspective of historical studies.[1] Their negative image was, to a certain extent, a product of the strong standing of biomedicine and of the criticism with which they met from educated doctors. In part it is also due to a relative confusion of terms, since the same name was often applied to individuals who performed procedures typically carried out by feldshers, but without official authorization. This creates additional obstacles for the few researchers who are studying this Jewish activity in nineteenth-century medical systems. However, on the basis of testimonies sourced from memoiristic literature one gains the impression that feldshers were the group most devoted to offering medical aid, and occupied a position somewhere on the borderline between official and folk medicine.

The Talmud lists physicians among the institutions vital to the functioning of the Jewish town.[2] The Hebrew noun *rofé* (one who heals), however, was often used in the nineteenth and early twentieth centuries in respect of people employed in treating sickness in any way, and might equally well designate an educated medic or a barber-surgeon performing simple procedures and treating primarily external problems. The rabbis of the Talmud did not specify what type of qualifications a physician should have; in fact, they go no further than stipulating that he should conduct his practice *bederekh hateva*, i.e. in accordance with the natural order, without recourse to sorcery. In the period around 1900 the term *royfe* was used in Yiddish to refer primarily to men holding the function of feldsher. Practically speaking, every Jewish feldsher in eastern Europe was referred to as a *royfe*, which makes it somewhat difficult for scholars to distinguish them from physicians on the one hand and from unofficial practitioners and

---

[1] The most comprehensive—though not exhaustive—monograph on Jewish feldshers is Kossoy and Ohri, *The Feldshers*.  [2] BT *San.* 17*b*.

quack healers on the other. To make matters yet more unclear, this term was sometimes 'contemporized' and translated as *doktor*.[3]

Contemporary sources tend to echo the nostalgic, stereotypical image of feldshers as autodidacts with little or no knowledge of official medicine. To some extent their work was a continuation of the practice of the earlier barber-surgeons. It was they to whom one went with broken bones, sprains, dislocations, and other mechanical injuries. They were also considered the experts in taking the pulse, bloodletting, applying leeches, performing dry and wet cupping, applying iodine to the throat, pulling teeth, and giving enemas. In the late nineteenth century a large proportion of this group of practitioners were Jews. In 1887 there were 181 Jews officially registered as feldshers in Galicia (75.1 per cent of the total number), though by the outbreak of the Great War this number had fallen sharply.[4] For the whole of the Russian Empire, by contrast, there were 1,971 Jewish feldshers (28 per cent of the total), of whom only 6 per cent lived outside the Pale of Settlement.[5] These data do not take into account private feldshers. Without underestimating the importance of the figures cited in the statistics, a reading of the memoiristic literature is sufficient to be able to establish that the vast majority of communities in the former Polish lands had access to the services of a Jewish feldsher. Many of them combined their medical activities with those of a barber and shaver in their own shop. This is described colourfully by Abel Yarmush in his sketch of Reb Shoel, an elderly feldsher from the Kalisz guberniya, who shaved the peasants who drove into town for the market, and issued them with prescriptions for various ailments at the same time.[6] The Dębica barber Judah Leib, who even went by the title of 'doctor', was said to hold consultations with the local physician, Dr Reis, in his own shop.[7] In Jewish reminiscences these figures feature mainly in treatment-related contexts. Their primary role was assistance in emergencies. As Edward Kossoy has noted, their reception rooms had to be situated in easily accessible places, on the ground floor, and equipped for night-time visits.[8] Feldshers were also the first point of contact within the official medical system, and directed patients requiring more

[3] One feldsher was Berish (Bejrysz) Doktor of Nowy Sącz; see Kac, *Nowy Sącz*, 131–5.
[4] Friedman, 'Dzieje Żydów w Galicji', 406.        [5] Kossoy and Ohry, *The Feldshers*, 154.
[6] Yarmush, *Of Two Homes* (Yid.), 25. A similar image of the Jewish barber is found in reminiscences from the Podlasie and Red Ruthenia regions. See Garbuz and Tumiel (eds.), *Obraz wsi sokólskiej połowy*, 54–5; Zawadski, *Obrazy Rusi Czerwonej*, 52.
[7] Shneyer, 'Fools' (Yid.), 54.        [8] Kossoy and Ohry, *The Feldshers*, 98.

advanced care to specific doctors or to the hospital. On occasion they also worked in hospitals, or had at least done some training or internships in such establishments in order to gain their professional qualifications.[9]

In the period that interests us here, feldshers were not simply random manually skilled individuals offering basic surgical procedures. Some of them had completed nursing training in community institutions such as homeless shelters or public baths. Yankev Milkh remembered: 'Shaye-Itshe was a famous feldsher. Before that, he had spent twenty years working as a guard in the *hekdesh* [the local poorhouse]. It was thus obvious that he was a great specialist, and that there was no point in going to see him with less than a zloty.'[10] Many of them were said to have gained their experience during epidemics, while serving in the army, or as auxiliaries in military hospitals. This latter form of service, unlike serving at the front, offered the chance to remain connected to the local Jewish community, and thus to maintain a traditional lifestyle.[11] Lastly, they might also have taken state-run feldsher's courses, though this route was clearly a minority option in our period. Those in the majority were practitioners who had obtained official status by sitting the necessary examinations.[12]

Most feldshers based their treatment on traditional views of anatomy, attributing illness to 'bad blood'.[13] Over the years, however, this gradually changed, so that by around 1900 they had begun to bring elements of bio-medicine into Jewish folk medicine. One testimony from Turzysk (now Turisk, western Ukraine) is proof of the popularity in this period of en-lightened publications such as *Marpe le'am*, the Hebrew translation of the Polish edition of *Anleitungen für Landleute zu einer vernünftigen Gesundheits-pflege* by Heinrich Felix Paulizky.[14] Then there was Leyzer Fried, the oldest feldsher in Mława, who was said to 'treat from a book' which contained descriptions of all kinds of medications and *segulot* (charms).[15] For the next

[9] Alter, the feldsher in the town of Olkusz, often performed post-mortems in the municipal hospital at doctors' request. This in no way interfered with his barber shop business. See Blumenfeld, 'Characters from Bygone Days' (Yid.), 245.

[10] Milkh, *Autobiographical Sketches* (Yid.), 33.

[11] F. Tsherniak, 'Medical Assistance and Medical Institutions' (Yid.), 528; Gingold, 'The Ostrołęka that Is No More' (Yid.), 215; Kac, *Nowy Sącz*, 131–5.

[12] Kossoy estimates that at the end of the nineteenth century just 14 per cent of feldshers in the Congress Kingdom of Poland had had a formal education and were eligible for a state position. Nonetheless, many had private practices; see Kossoy and Ohry, *The Feldshers*, 101–3.

[13] Harkavy and Gesik, 'Medical Care in Our Town' (Heb.), 43.

[14] Rozovski, *Collected Writings* (Yid.), 18.          [15] Yunis, 'The Old Homeland' (Yid.), 74.

generation, combining traditional treatments with modern ones was nothing out of the ordinary. One Shimshen, a *royfe* from Horodenka (now in
western Ukraine), in addition to the familiar range of feldsher's remedies
would also give his patients aspirin.[16] There are many testimonies attesting
to the fact that such practitioners attended regular physicians' case con-
ferences. Jewish feldshers sometimes wrote out their prescriptions in
Yiddish, signing them with their local byname, such as 'Tevye the doctor',[17]
or even—in spite of their lack of a university education—in Latin. Knowledge of Latin was significant in light of the requirements for the state
examinations, and so some feldshers learned to read and write out prescriptions in this convention in the course of their regular visits to hospitals,
often in quite distant localities.[18] In fact, the Latin on prescriptions seemed
more important to patients than to pharmacists. In the late eighteenth-
century, Moses Markuze bemoaned the naivety of a populace who took the
feldshers' 'hocus pocus' for learned Latin.[19] Later proponents of biomedicine poked fun at feldshers' prescriptions, written in a peculiar Yiddish-
Latinesque jargon and reading something like this: *Khininum sulfus, untses
dues, royte proshkes, di vayst shoyn vues* ('Khininum sulfus, ounces two, and
those red powders, the ones you do').[20]

   In the eyes of the common people, feldshers had a number of advan-
tages over other practitioners. First of all, they were closely connected with
their local communities and, unlike most physicians, had not moved away
from Jewish Orthodoxy. The image that emerges from the literature is that
of a man mature in years, with a clipped beard, dressed like his neighbours,
and carrying a leather bag filled with implements and medications. 'When
nothing else helped, the feldsher would be called; he was popular in the
town. You could talk to him in simple Yiddish, so you could tell him in
detail what hurt, and where', one resident of Mława recalled. The same
author noted that the feldsher behaved in such a way that the patient felt in
control of the treatment process: 'The neighbours, the family, and the
patient himself would try to explain and advise him what to do. The feldsher, a familiar figure, listened patiently to all the advice; it was no stain on

[16] Lindenberg, 'Our Town as I Remember It' (Heb.), 45.
[17] Veynig, 'Hygiene and Sanitation Services' (Yid.), 25.
[18] Emiot-Goldwasser, 'Reb Mordecai Leyb Goldwasser' (Yid.), 209.
[19] Markuze, *Sefer refuot*, 71*b*–72*a*.
[20] Blumental, *Reminiscences* (Yid.), 168; For other instances of Jewish feldshers who made
out prescriptions in Latin, see e.g. Shneyer, 'Fools' (Yid.), 54.

his honour.'[21] Most of the remedies used by feldshers in their daily work corresponded to popular ideas of how treatment should be conducted. Another factor that contributed to the popularity of feldshers may have been the economic argument: their services cost less than a physician's visit, and poor patients could even expect to be treated free of charge.[22]

A further fact that was almost certainly of significance was that these practitioners usually continued family traditions, or had in some other way taken over the practice of someone who had worked as a feldsher or barber-surgeon before them. Thus they were recommended not only by the fact that they shared the same values as their patients and were accepted as one of their own, but also by ties of family and familiarity. There are numerous testimonies of a son or a daughter inheriting their vocation from their feldsher father or midwife mother. Even as the younger generation acquired their parents' knowledge, however, they also looked to modernize it, and aspired to climb the social ladder. The son of Fayge of Bursztyn in Galicia, a woman who assisted at births, was the feldsher Petahyah there.[23] The feldsher Moyshe, *royfe* of Zamość, himself a son of the town's leading midwife, passed on his knowledge to one of his own sons, who studied at the feldsher school in St Petersburg, while his second son owned a pharmaceutical warehouse.[24] Eliezer Pas of Brzozów, who was said to make out prescriptions that were regarded by pharmacists as being on a par with those issued by doctors, had his son educated as a physician.[25]

If distinguishing between feldshers and quack healers—who were also on occasion known as *royfim*—is problematic, making distinctions between the activities of quacks, wise women, and midwives is often virtually impossible. In the nineteenth-century shtetls in the Pale of Settlement and Galicia there were instances of one woman doing the work of feldsher, midwife, and diviner, as well as removing charms, treating illnesses, making candles, measuring graves,[26] mourning the dead, working in the *mikveh*, and the

---

[21] Yunis, 'The Old Homeland' (Yid.), 74. Cf. the character of Yenkel the Medic in Sholem Aleichem, *From The Fair*, 101.

[22] See e.g. Sholem Aleichem, *From The Fair*, 101; Blumenfeld, 'Characters from Bygone Days' (Yid.), 245; Kac, *Nowy Sącz*, 131–5.

[23] Schwarz, 'Characters and Personalities' (Yid.), 264.

[24] Gevat, 'Thousands of Memorial Candles' (Heb.), 279.

[25] Vilner, 'People from the Shtetl' (Yid.), 156.

[26] There was a widespread custom among women of measuring graves with wicks that they then used to make candles for the synagogue for Yom Kippur.

like.[27] The above-mentioned Fayge, 'the *bobe* of Bursztyn', was much sought after in her town as a midwife (*bobe, heybam*). She was also said to have something in the nature of a first-aid box, the contents of which she application to treat swellings and 'the English sickness' (rickets); what is more, she did not take money from the poorest.[28] Jewish wise women tended to be older women who had acquired their skills through a lifetime of experience.[29] They knew about perinatal and post-partum-related illnesses; they knew what might be wrong with a child, and how to care for infants. They could also offer advice on gynaecological problems. Hantshe of Gliniany (now western Ukraine) was known as a 'paediatrician' (*kinderdoktorin*) despite never having studied medicine of any sort or having had any vocational experience in a hospital. Her knowledge was gleaned from her personal tragedies: she had lost ten children, none of whom lived to the age of 3. This misfortune did nothing to damage her reputation, and the local women saw Hantshe as an excellent wise woman. She would be called out at all hours of the day and night, in all weathers. In addition to assisting at births, she offered treatment based on *babske refues* (women's cures): she made a beverage from dried dog faeces with hot milk; used coals to remove the evil eye; and when she could tell that a child had a temperature she would borrow a sharp knife from the cobbler, make small incisions in the child's ears, and let a little blood. For greater effect she would then smear its face with the blood.[30]

In the second half of the nineteenth century, women educated in midwifery schools gained the recognition of the rabbinic authorities. They were cited in the responsa as specialists, the more so since the scope of their competencies went far beyond assisting at births and they were practically comparable in their functions to feldshers.[31] At this point it is worth quoting Nakhmen Blumental's description of the kit carried by a midwife called Sore, whom he remembered from Borszczów (now Borshchiv, western Ukraine). The collection of implements that she used differed vastly from the basic items with which the stereotypical wise woman was equipped:

And then her [Sore's] medications of choice: lysol, which is added to water when washing an injured leg; carbolic acid for disinfecting her hands; spirit for the

---

[27] Reyman, 'Notes on Women's Professions' (Yid.), 29.
[28] Schwarz, 'Characters and Personalities' (Yid.), 263.
[29] Libera, *Znachor*, 130.          [30] 'Characters Among the Jews of Gliniany' (Yid.), 173–4.
[31] Zimmels, *Magicians, Theologians and Doctors*, 32–3.

primus stove for heating up a little water; valerian proof spirit for when a woman in childbirth needs calming; cotton wool, gauze, chloroform, zinc ointment, and all manner of plasters—above all, of course, those needed by mothers and babies. But also the type that is applied to abscesses, pustules, carbuncles, to bring them out faster and cause them faster to . . . burst. Castor oil, which may be given not only to a woman in labour, but even to a man.[32]

The Jewish populace preferred the assistance offered by feldshers, wise women, and midwives from within their own community. Memories of such individuals are dominant in the literature, while non-Jewish practitioners play merely an episodic and usually anonymous role. Naturally, there were exceptions to this rule, for various reasons. Sometimes relations with Christian neighbours were cultivated precisely in order to facilitate contact in emergencies; in some circumstances a non-Jewish woman might be employed as a domestic servant or wet nurse. Officially recognized feldshers and trained midwives would be called out to Jewish homes irrespective of their faith; after all, they represented the authority of official medicine. The presence of Christian women side by side with Jewish ones at the bedside of a patient or woman in childbirth is not unusual in Jewish memoiristic literature.[33] In many cases, indeed, where there were no doctors in the area, there was little other choice. Lastly, the decisive factors might be economic considerations or personal preference, as reflected in this example from Pińczów:

Every woman in Pińczów had her babies at home—with the assistance of a midwife, of course. There were two midwives in the town: the Jewish Hanele and a Christian woman, Kubicka. The Jews preferred Hanele, but she was very high and mighty, demanded special treatment, forced her opinions at every turn, and was permanently dissatisfied with something or other. Not everyone was willing to put up with such caprice, and some would call Kubicka out.[34]

Within any traditional community there was a fairly large group of practitioners who worked outside the parameters of the law and the regulations of state bodies. The scope of their activities may be defined as healing, even quackery, though not all of them drew on magic and they were not all known as quacks. It is hard to establish with any certainty whether their involvement in healing was solely due to a lack of feldshers or physicians

---

[32] Blumental, *Reminiscences* (Yid.), 164.
[33] Kvartin, *My Life* (Yid.), 13–14; Nigal, *The Hasidic Tale*, 124.
[34] Himmelblau, 'Medical Aid in Pińczów' (Yid.), 214–15.

in the immediate area, or whether they plied their trade in spite of the existence of professional competition. The skills of such practitioners lay chiefly in their ability to use manual tools, which, aside from their normal use in crafts, were also employed to bring relief to the sick. This is illustrated clearly in a reference to a certain medic who borrowed pliers designed for pulling nails out of planks of wood from the local blacksmith to perform dentistry procedures.[35] In Mielec a cobbler by the name of Meylekh removed corns from the feet of men and women alike; he would pull out his cobbler's last, sharpen his knife, and cut out the callus without drawing a drop of blood.[36] In Baranów Sandomierski, Reb Yoyzip the tailor, who was nimble with his needle and thread, also dabbled in surgery. He would be called out to emergencies even at night, and accepted no payment for his services. During these 'operations' he would put the patient at ease by joking with them, and at the end he gave them a dab of snuff.[37] In Mława there were 'specialists' of all trades available to treat wounds: locksmiths with iron filings; carpenters, who used birch tar; and blacksmiths, who preferred red-hot metal and wheel grease.[38]

One group of practitioners unique to Jewish communities was that comprising specialists in circumcision (*mohalim*) and ritual slaughterers (*shohatim*). They played an important role in the functioning of the community, and were thus known in Yiddish, like the rabbi, as *kley-koydesh* (instruments of holiness). The *mohel* had to be capable of diagnosing sickness in an infant and know various ways of opening wounds, staunching blood, and applying dressings. The literature devoted to circumcision usually included a modicum of medical information and a catalogue of treatment methods. It is thus unsurprising that there were *mohalim*, such as Hershele from the Polesia village of Werebiowo, whose reputation as healers assured them clients among Jews and non-Jews alike.[39] In the eyes of the traditional community the *mohel*'s role was not restricted to performing a physical procedure, but also had a sacred dimension, and constituted an important *mitsvah*. According to testimonies, some *mohalim* were able to foresee during the circumcision ritual whether or not the child would survive.[40] *Shohatim* worked with animal anatomy on a daily basis and wielded

[35] Tenenbaum, *Ayzik Ashmeday* (Yid.), 247.
[36] Klagsbrun, *The Jews of Mielec* (Yid.), 134–5.
[37] Fenster, 'Characters from the Shtetl' (Yid.), 155.
[38] Yunis, 'The Old Homeland' (Yid.), 73.
[39] M. L. G., 'Hresk' (Yid.), 436.       [40] Wilff, *Imrot shelomoh*, 105.

knives masterfully, as the laws of the ritual demanded of them. To a certain extent they also adjudicated on legal issues surrounding *kashrut*. In many communities they were men with a religious education who also held the position of cantor or led prayers in the synagogue.[41] Contrary to received opinion, the medical work of these ritual slaughterers was not confined to setting broken bones. In Radom, Simhah Bunem Zuker, in addition to his duties as a butcher, 'was also fully a doctor and treated people, wrote out prescriptions accepted by pharmacists'.[42] In the pages of another memoir we read: 'In Białystok there lived a certain local dignitary, Reb Meyer Brumer. He was known as Reb Meyer *shoykhet* . . . but in addition to *sheḥitah* he had one more important trade. He was a great specialist in diseases of the eyes . . . He treated the poor for free.'[43] It was sometimes the case that the wives of *shoḥatim* were well versed in folk cures (as in Brzozów, for instance).[44]

Among the Jews there were also healers who drove out sickness and lifted the evil eye using magic formulas and practices. Their assistance was sought in connection with ailments caused by presumed charms or curses, primarily because they seemed to be the most competent in this area, but also when other methods (such as those available to the feldsher) failed to bring results.[45] The most widespread category was specialists in the evil eye and in the treatment of erysipelas and swellings; these were not hard to find in the immediate environment. According to some sources, 'wise women' sought out those whom they might be able to help, and even imposed themselves on their potential patients, motivated by sympathy and faith in the efficacy of their actions.[46] The local specialists who used magic to drive out sickness would usually be referred to by their given name, or as *opshpre-kher/ke* (remover) or *mumkhe/nte* (expert). Every Jewish community had its own specialists of this nature. They performed their work free of charge, as a *mitsvah* or a form of neighbourly assistance, or for a small fee, which was usually paid in kind. If there was no improvement as a result of the cure they proposed, however, patients had no hesitation in asking non-Jewish acquaintances for help.

[41] Pomerants, 'Reb Yankl the Ritual Slaughterer' (Yid.), 216–17. Schweizer, 'The Over-grown Path' (Yid.), 25.    [42] Zuker, 'Ritual Slaughterers' (Yid.), 59.

[43] Klementinovski, *Dr Yosef Khazanovitsh*, 84.

[44] Bank, 'Reb Yoysef Glikman', (Yid.), 221.    [45] Libera, *Znachor*, 171.

[46] Lew, 'O lecznictwie i przesądach', *Izraelita*, 37, p. 316. See Levine, *Memories Tell Stories* (Yid.), 24–5.

Quack healing was the speciality of older women, who had a 'light touch'. Women who were pregnant or menstruating, on the other hand, did not undertake conjuration or the driving out of disease owing to the possibility of causing 'complications' in their patients.[47] Men might also turn their hand to healing; the actions performed by young boys and by pious men who could write Hebrew and could recite their conjurations in the holy tongue were regarded as particularly effective. Firstborns were considered predestined for such roles. Those who were born with the gift of healing were generally thought to have stronger powers than those who had learned it as a skill,[48] though it was possible to become a healer by learning from someone more experienced. Healers took great care not to share their secrets. It was widely believed that teaching conjurations to others or passing on their words to someone who did not believe in their efficacy would not only cause them to lose their magical power, but could also be potentially dangerous to the health of the person who had previously been using it. An-sky, in the course of his expedition to Volhynia, bought charms of this type from old women, but on each occasion this necessitated lengthy negotiations and a handsome payment.[49] At the same time, however, healers believed that they had a duty to pass on their knowledge to those who came after them, but the new adept would be selected very carefully and responsibly. Often the lore would remain within the family, and in addition to oral teaching, the older generation would pass on their jottings and books to the younger. Often the search for the right candidate proved time-consuming. One healer from Zambrów only relinquished her role in extreme old age, when she had at last found her successor: a firstborn woman whose mother and grandmother had also been firstborns.[50]

There were specialists among the Jews whose reputation spread far beyond their own community. Key to the popularity of such individuals was their close contact with the non-Jewish population and utilization of items well recognized by both the healer and the sick. Franciszek Wereńko recalled a Jew who borrowed a 'rabies stone' (a 'frog stone' brought from Rome, said to draw out poison) from a peasant, and used the miraculous

---

[47] Lew, 'O lecznictwie i przesądach', *Izraelita*, 37, p. 316; Segel, 'Wierzenia i lecznictwo', 60.

[48] Cf. Libera, *Znachor*, 142.

[49] Rechtman, *Jewish Ethnography and Folklore* (Yid.), 291–2; see e.g. Presman, *The Road We Have Travelled* (Yid.), 7.                    [50] Levinski, 'Learned Women' (Yid.), 297.

object to make a living from 'healing'.[51] In the Podlasie region in the second half of the nineteenth century, there was an old Jew who neutralized viper venom by binding up the bite area with tape and chanting magic formulas. He, too, made this a source of income, predestined as he was for this role by his gift of snake charming (he kept a number of snakes in his house, which emerged from their nests at his whistle).[52] In both these cases what is immediately telling is the possession by Jewish healers of special gifts or objects believed to guarantee the efficacy of their actions—or at least perceived to do so by Jews and peasants alike.

Nonetheless, on the whole the Jewish populace seems to have preferred to use healers of this nature from outside rather than from among their own. There is information in the sources testifying to the use of ritually unclean methods as these were said to be imbued with greater magical powers. If a throat infection was to be treated by the application of a stocking, the recommendation was that it first be rubbed with *treyf* soap (the explanation for this was that 'kosher soap is not so warming').[53] In certain cases fresh animal blood would be consumed, something expressly and absolutely forbidden by the Torah.[54] 'There was a belief in and respect for both the unclean and the sacred. On the one hand the Lord God, then the *tsadik* of the given generation, the intercession of ancestors, the Torah, and the *aron hakodesh* [synagogue ark]; and on the other the *sitra ahra* of Satan, witches, healers, Tatars . . . The switch from one to the other might be made at the drop of a hat', one resident of Felsztyn (now Skelivka, Ukraine) reminisced.[55] Among the culturally alien magical items in circulation there were apparently some Christian ones, such as crosses, and medallions featuring the Virgin Mary, to which Jewish culture attributed meanings entirely different from their original ones.

Ashkenazi Jews adopted a plethora of terms used in the Slavic environment to denote unofficial therapeutic practices. In Yiddish, the word *znakher* came to mean in the first place a non-Jewish quack healer (who might also be known as a *mekhashef*, from the Hebrew for magician), and in the second a practitioner of folk medicine irrespective of origin. More

---

[51] Wereńko, 'Przyczynek do lecznictwa ludowego', 189.

[52] Gloger, 'Zabobony i mniemania', 105. See also Rulikowski, 'Zapiski etnograficzne z Ukrainy', 113.        [53] 'A Handful of Beliefs from Zhitomir' (Yid.), 63.

[54] Lew, 'O lecznictwie i przesądach', *Izraelita*, 49, p. 476.

[55] Kling, 'The Unwritten Book of My Mama's Remedies' (Yid.), 562.

popular still was the term 'Tatar' (Yid. *toter, keyder*), which retained echoes of the major role played by Tatar healers in the Polish Commonwealth. By 1900 this word no longer necessarily denoted any specific ethnic group; it was used, inter alia, to refer to Polish peasants who were quack practitioners. The Jewish populace also relied on the help of shepherds, who were known in this context by the Polish word *owczarze*, even though Yiddish had its own, more common synonyms for the word 'shepherd'. When an *owczarz* famed for his miracles arrived in the Mława area, the Jews from the town made pilgrimages to him.[56] To some extent this name also evolved into a synonym for folk practitioner and healer, though it never became as popular as Tatar. Witches and sorceresses were also often called by the same names that the Slavs used for them, such as *viedme* or *koldunie*.

Belief in the magical powers of Gypsies, Tatars, and *owczarze* was reflected in the ethnographic material, even if those reporting it did so with the caveat that 'they used to know more'.[57] These groups enjoyed immense authority; although it was undermined to some extent by practitioners of biomedicine, it remained essentially unshaken among the common people. When Mendele Moykher Sforim sketched his portraits of the residents of the stereotypical Ukrainian shtetl Tuniyadevka, he did not hesitate to outline the competencies of the local *royfe* in the following words: 'It was said that he had acquired his knowledge of the physician's art from a Gypsy, apparently a direct descendant of the Egyptian priests [*ḥartumei mitsrayim*].'[58] Healers were usually visited rather than called out. They were to be found at a certain distance from the town, like the Tatar living around ten miles from Nowy Pohost (now Novyy Pogost, Belarus), who cured madness using conjurations and the offal that was brought for him in lieu of payment.[59] Patients from Włocławek travelled to a Tatar who transpired to be a peasant from the village of Topola, near Łęczyca.[60] Healers used the whole spectrum of methods familiar to us from ethnographic sources and popular therapeutic manuals. Their operations were heterogeneous in character, combining simple and more complex natural elements with the ubiquitous magical factor. Henryk Lew saw in the Tatars

[56]  Yunis, 'The Old Homeland' (Yid.), 72.
[57]  Lilientalowa, 'Wierzenia, przesądy i praktyki', 151.
[58]  *The Travels of Benjamin the Third* (Yid.), 169.
[59]  Sosnowik, 'Material on Jewish Folk Medicine in Belarus' (Yid.), 163.
[60]  Winter, 'Tatars and Witches' (Yid.), 394.

itinerant vagabonds who healed using herbs, powders, ointments, and rectified spirit.[61] Nonetheless, all descriptions of their practices which go into any detail stress the importance of the incantations and blessings they pronounced, their gestures, and even the magical formulas they wrote on paper or parchment and then dissolved in water.

Travelling to sorcerers outside the community was frowned upon by the rabbinic authorities and most tsadikim. When the wife of one hasid, disappointed by the lack of effects of the actions of the rebbe of Boiany in Bukovina, tried to persuade him of the necessity of taking her child for treatment to an elderly peasant woman known for her healing practices, her attempts were in vain. Her devout husband, trusting only the will of the Creator and the intercession of his rebbe, would not hear of involving a witch.[62] Christian healers who consented to see Jews treated them using the same formulas and gestures as they used for their other patients. In addition to pagan elements, this included the sign of the cross, or references to Jesus, Mary, and the saints.[63] In view of the principle of *pikuaḥ nefesh*, which permitted the breaking of the Law in order to save human life, some rabbis tolerated such practices despite the evident signs of idolatry.[64] This was what happened in the case of a certain devout Jew whom the tsadik of Sampol permitted to travel to see a healer, despite the controversy caused by the condition imposed by the peasant, who demanded that his patients supply him by way of payment with wax for his local church. Jews also consulted another group of health practitioners whom they sometimes held to be sorcerers: Catholic and Orthodox priests. In one collection of responsa we read about a priest who healed people bitten by a rabid wolf. Alas, in this case the 'remedy', concocted from water and 'god

---

[61] Lew, 'O lecznictwie i przesądach', *Izraelita*, 36, p. 306.

[62] Akerman, *Oysgeloshene shtern*, 164–5.

[63] One Christian woman treated erysipelas by blowing on the sufferer's face and repeating in a whisper a formula, the only words of which the informer could remember were 'Jesus my son'; Winter, 'Tatars and Witches' (Yid.), 395–6. The *Shulḥan arukh* permitted the use of non-Jewish conjurations as long as they did not feature the 'names of gods'; see 'Yoreh de'ah', 155: 7. Jewish manuscript sources testify to the omission of the names of saints from magic texts obtained from the Slavic milieu, but this practice was not consistent.

[64] Winter, 'Tatars and Witches' (Yid.), 396. This same principle permitted the breaking of the holy sabbath, for instance by writing or travelling, if it was vital in order to save the life of a sick person. In such cases some authorities stipulated that if the journey taken in contravention of the sabbath restrictions was on horseback, the rider should dress 'not after the Jewish fashion', in order not to spread outrage. Sperling, *Ta'amei haminhagim umekorei hadinim*, 131.

powder' (perhaps made from a cross), proved ineffective.[65] It may be to these contacts that we owe a number of magic formulas that surface repeatedly in Jewish manuscripts, and which leave us in no doubt as to their connections with Latin prayers.[66]

[65] Zimmels, *Magicians, Theologians and Doctors*, 34;

[66] See Mesler, 'The Three Magi and Other Christian Motifs', 161–218.

CHAPTER FIVE

🙢

# TSADIKIM AND
# PHYSICIANS

FOR MUCH of the nineteenth century the Jewish population of eastern Europe was caught in the middle of a conflict between traditional
treatments, represented by Orthodox circles, and the modern alternatives
propagated by educated physicians. This conflict is relatively well documented in the writings left by proponents of the Haskalah. Enlightenment
and biomedical publications effectively never stopped accusing the Orthodox, especially hasidim, of peddling superstition, and the isolated cases of
doctors becoming fascinated by hasidism could do little to change this. The
hasidic perspective probably remains less explored, but it, too, has been the
subject of frequent studies for many years now. Indeed, even in the *Shivḥei*
*habesht* we find stories of the 'duels' that the Ba'al Shem Tov was said to
have fought with 'doctors'. The Besht's actions should not be interpreted as
an endeavour to monopolize the sphere of Jewish therapeutic practices:
firstly because not all the 'doctors' whom he confronted were proponents
of conventional medicine, and secondly in view of the character of these
tales themselves, which, as Immanuel Etkes has noted, were intended not
as portrayals of a conflict between natural and magical therapies, but more
as testimonies to the coexistence of different medical systems, and even to
the hasidic acceptance of this state of affairs.[1] Tradition has it that similar
situations arose in the lives of some of the later masters. Nahman of Bratslav, the great-grandson of the Ba'al Shem Tov, spent the final months of
his life in Uman (now in Ukraine). Having contracted tuberculosis, he saw
local physicians, who probably forbade him his ritual immersions in the
cold water of the *mikveh*. The tsadik's works from this period contain an
apologia for the health benefits of such baths which seems to have been
intended as a polemic against these learned professionals.[2] The attitudes of

[1] Etkes, *The Besht*, 64–9.
[2] Liebes, *Studies in Jewish Myth and Jewish Messianism*, 136. The conflict between tsadik and

hasidic leaders to biomedicine evolved with the march of the generations, and to some extent may be seen as a barometer of the popularity of new currents within the traditional Jewish community. The conflict waxed and waned depending on the circumstances, but it gradually mellowed into a kind of consensus, which permitted a considerable degree of co-operation between doctors and tsadikim.

Tsadikim were often perceived as allies in the struggle for health and life. The Hebrew word *tsadik* (righteous) has functioned in Jewish tradition since biblical times. In the Talmud this was the term used to denote individuals of exceptional piety and probity, suffused with the grace of heaven in recognition of their virtues. The belief in their especial gift of winning the will of the Creator was expressed in the proverb: 'The just man ordains and God fulfils.'[3] Legends about the thirty-six hidden righteous people, whose virtue was said to be the basis on which the Creator granted the world continued existence, sometimes portrayed these figures in contexts related to health.[4] The ethical literature expected a *mohel* to be god-fearing and a *tsadik*, otherwise his actions would be detrimental to the child's health.[5] Rabbis were also considered *tsadikim*; throughout Jewish history they would be approached for advice and prayers for the sick. The precedent for this practice is found in the Talmud,[6] and there were similar heroes, holy rabbis with the power to perform miracles, in many communities all over eastern Europe. As scholars of the Law, they could advise those who came to them on the acceptability of particular treatment methods, had access to the literature, and sometimes used practical kabbalah or even had an interest in medicine. According to legend, they continued to honour their responsibility for the health of their communities even after their death, as did rabbi Moses Isserles, for instance, when he successfully intervened to curb an epidemic in Kraków.[7] His grave in the old Jewish cemetery

physician is a multifaceted theme in hasidic writings. It could offer opportunities for the defence of traditional religiosity and lifestyle, for demonstration of the eminence of the community leader, or for a strike at heretics. See Nigal, *The Hasidic Tale*, 172–8.

[3] BT *MK* 16b; *Shab.* 59b. Cf. Job 22: 28: 'You will decree and it will be fulfilled.'

[4] BT *San.* 97b, *Suk.* 45b. The thirty-six *tsadikim* are called *lamedvovnikes* in Yiddish, from the Hebrew letters *lamed* and *vav*, which form the number 36. See S. H. Bergman, 'The Tsadik of Wolnica' (Yid.), 490–1; Ganuz, 'Thirty-Six Righteous Men' (Heb.), 28–31.

[5] Wilff, *Imrot shelomoh*, 103.

[6] BT *Ber.* 34b. See Zimmels, *Magicians, Theologians and Doctors*, 35–6.

[7] Halkowski, *Żydowski Kraków. Legendy i ludzie*, 42–3.

of the city's Kazimierz district immediately became a place of pilgrimage, and many of those who visited it were seeking cures. Making pilgrimage to and measuring the graves of great rabbis in the hope of finding a powerful intermediary before the heavenly throne were some of the most important steps one could take when faced with serious or chronic illness.[8]

In the late eighteenth century, one of the paths to healing led through contact with *ba'alei shem*. In many cases these were people who held important positions within the Jewish community; sometimes they were even rabbis. The literary descriptions of their practices, which were based on a combination of methods rooted in practical kabbalah, folk medicine, and early official medicine, are worthy of examination in a separate work. As the hasidic movement gained in significance, the star of these figures faded and they lost their prominence. The tsadikim, the spiritual heirs of the Ba'al Shem Tov, who superseded them in their role as shamanic intermediaries, started treating the sick using similar methods and often relied on the same traditions. The term *ba'alei shem* remained in the vernacular, now denoting itinerant healers, miracle-workers, and quacks employing elements of kabbalah. It was also used in descriptions of treatment methods to define a distinct category of magic: *segulot* issued by a *ba'al shem*, or *baal-shemske zgules*. Over time, the term *ba'al shem* acquired a negative connotation, mainly due to promoters of the Enlightenment. It was with a stigma of backwardness and harmfulness that it penetrated into popular literature, including modern Yiddish and Hebrew memoirs. In his memoir, Kalmen Marmor described his mother's attempts to have her paralysed daughter healed. Among the methods used were amulets inscribed by an itinerant *ba'al shem* and rubbing the girl's body with fresh pigeon blood, also recommended by him.[9] Marmor's enigmatic description of the person of the healer ('a tall, pale youth with huge, bright eyes and a short, dark brown, pointed beard') and the things he did, and of his mother's excessive naivety in the face of her daughter's illness, produced an unequivocally negative image of *ba'alei shem*, though this was not an absolute rule.

In the communities of the former Grand Duchy of Lithuania, hasidism never became a dominant current. Aside from a very few centres, Jews remained faithful to the conventional rabbinic interpretation of Judaism, which was considered by the hasidim a rival form (they referred to rabbis

---

[8]  See Ch. 10 below.

[9]  Marmor, *My Life Story* (Yid.), 105–6. See Biegeleisen, *Lecznictwo ludu polskiego*, 224.

who did not share their views as *misnagdim*, opponents). In Lithuania
devout holy men with strong links to traditional religiosity, who were not
hasidic tsadikim but practised some form of healing, were common. In
many respects they were reminiscent of the *ba'alei shem* familiar to us from
eighteenth-century sources. These practitioners of folk healing and kabbalah, like the tsadikim, were known by the generic name *gute yidn* ('good
Jews'), the equivalent term to the Slavic 'divine people'. Bernard Abrahams, who was born in Kroże (Kražiai) in Samogitia, remembers one such
figure thus:

> He was known as Reb Itsele, but my uncle and aunt never spoke his name without
> the epithet 'holy', 'righteous', 'divine man', full of pride to be hosting him under
> their roof . . . Reb Itsele was one of those Litvak-*mitnaged* holy men that almost
> every town in that region possessed. Their influence, particularly on women,
> was boundless. If the local rabbi, or any rabbi, for that matter, any scholar, was
> respected according to his greatness in the Torah, they were respected for
> being upright, humble, modest . . . The Lithuanian divine people did not accept
> *kvitlekh*; they were given *pidyon* [*pidyon hanefesh*, 'ransom of the soul', a pecuniary
> offering]. People came to them to have spells or charms removed, erysipelas or
> swellings cured, and often simply to be listened to.[10]

Descriptions of the hasidic leaders as practitioners of healing recur in
Jewish sources from the very emergence of the movement. As a treatment
alternative, meetings with tsadikim became so important that the halakhic
literature had to address the issue of journeys made to them on the sabbath
for health reasons. The rabbis believed that it was permissible to violate the
peace of the holy day in the face of a threat to life, but only for a natural—
that is, not magical—remedy. The author of the *Ta'amei haminhagim*, however, averred, in agreement with the opinion of most hasidic authorities,
that such a journey might be made if the patient placed his hope in the
tsadik.[11] Hope (*bitokhn*) and faith (*gloybn*, *emune*) constituted the core
around which one's relationship with the community leader was built. *Az a
yid gloybt in rebn, helft got* (If a Jew believes in his rebbe, God helps),[12] it was
said in conviction of the efficacy of the ties that bound the hasid with his
spiritual intermediary. Anyone who lacked these two virtues had to face the

[10] Abrahams, *My Seventy Years: An Autobiography* (Yid.), 93–4.
[11] Sperling, *Ta'amei haminhagim umekorei hadinim*, 131; see Zimmels, *Magicians, Theologians
and Doctors*, 37.       [12] Einhorn, 'Folk Proverbs in Yiddish' (Heb.), 202.

consequences; as the saying went, *Az men fort nit tsum rebn, firt men tsum toter* (If one does not visit the rebbe, one is taken to the Tatar).[13]

However, not all those who made the journey to the tsadik's court were granted the opportunity to talk to him personally. Often they would have to be content with a handshake and a greeting, and their *kvitlekh* (or *tsetlekh*, the slips of paper on which they wrote the causes for which they asked the holy man to pray), together with the *pidyon hanefesh*, would be given to the *gabai*, the administrator of his court. The figure of the 'soul ransom' might depend on the financial means of the supplicant, symbolize his wish (for example fifty-two coins to represent the numerical value of the word *ben*—son), or allude to the name of a sick person. Most usually, however, it would be a multiple of the number eighteen (the numerical value of the letters forming the word *ḥai*, or 'alive', 'living', as mentioned above). The biblical source for the symbolism of this fee was the following passage: 'If ransom is laid upon him, he must pay whatever is laid upon him to redeem his life' (Exod. 21: 30). There were tsadikim who did not take money; nonetheless, tradition linked the efficacy of further actions to the fulfilment of the *pidyon*, though the meaning of the custom of 'ransom' might be interpreted in a number of different ways. It might be a charitable act, or even a substitute for the propitiatory sacrifice in the Jerusalem Temple.[14] The explanation for this was that ordinary people did not have sufficient merit for their pleas to be heard, and only payment of this ransom could alter that.[15] Through the medium of the donation, a person's soul could forge a bond with the soul and will of the tsadik. Thus, when a righteous man performed any kind of *mitsvah* with the donated sum, such as passing it on as alms to the poor, the merit generated by the good deed accrued to the original donor.[16] As many of those who came to the hasidic courts could not write Hebrew, the *gaba'im* were often also responsible for writing out the *kvitlekh*. These usually bore the names of relatives along with brief formulas such as *lebanim* (for children), *lirfuah shelemah min hashamayim* (for full healing from heaven), *liyshuah* (for salvation), and so on. In many cases these slips of paper also bore the names of the sufferers' illnesses, which were known to the supplicants from other sources.

The treatment process took a variety of forms, which depended not

[13]  D. Kohen, *Shpola* (Heb.), 175.
[14]  Mekler, *Fun rebns hoyf*, 246.          [15]  Ibid. 251; Nigal, *The Hasidic Tale*, 174.
[16]  Sperling, *Ta'amei haminhagim oyf ivri taytsh*, ii. 9.

only on the type of ailment but also on the healer's own preferences. Apart from the central role of the tsadik, hasidic curative practices rarely differed from the methods of others. Most prevalent were elements of kabbalah; there were also traditional *segulot*, natural remedies, and even remedies prescribed by modern physicians. The first rebbe of Belz was said to restore people to health by the laying-on of hands.[17] Shalom Shakhna, the father of Israel of Ruzhyn, helped a woman suffering a difficult childbirth with the use of a specially composed story that included mysterious explications of the Torah, sacred names, and kabbalistic arrangements of words and letters (*tsirufim*).[18] The tsadik Mordkhe David of Dąbrowa Tarnowska was said to have relieved the pain of a woman in childbirth once by ordering the door to be removed from its frame and reinstalled the opposite way round. The reasoning: read in reverse, the Hebrew word *delet* (door) gives *teled* (she will give birth).[19] Of course there were also readings of psalms,[20] prescriptions for natural remedies enhanced by mystical intentions (*kavanot*),[21] recitations of blessings reinforced by herbs and ointments,[22] and so on.

A festive communal meal headed by the rebbe was treated as a special type of ritual, during which particular significance was attributed to the sharing of *shirayim*. These morsels of food left by the tsadik were passed out to his faithful along established lines of kinship and privilege. Therapeutic properties were also associated with them, something which re-emerged in many areas of folk medicine. According to one hasidic tale, Rebbe Mordkhe of Niesuchojeże (now Vola, in north-western Ukraine) healed a man with a swollen throat by telling him to drink water containing *shirayim*.[23] Every dish or type of food consumed by the community leader would be shared, but most sought after was fish, which was considered a tried and tested remedy for infertility. According to a kabbalistic interpretation, all creatures had their spiritual 'roots' in another world. Fish were said to come from a 'very holy, exalted world', and were the carriers of the souls of the righteous after their death.[24] A hasid consuming *shirayim* would, on the one hand, be hoping for the purification and liberation of his soul from impure desires, while on the other he would be benefiting from

[17] Bakon, *The Rabbi of Sieniawa* (Yid.), 168.
[18] Rothstein, *Tsadikim and Hasidim* (Yid.), 74–7.
[19] Bakon, 'Life of the Holy Rabbi Mordkhe David of Dąbrowa' (Heb.), 81.
[20] Roker, *Toledot anshei shem*, 116.
[21] Bakon, *The Rabbi of Sieniawa* (Yid.), 196–7.       [22] Mekler, *Fun rebns hoyf*, 135.
[23] Nigal, *The Hasidic Tale*, 173.                      [24] Lipiets, *Sefer matamim*, 20.

the influence of the traditional association of fish with fertility, echoes of which are discernible in the biblical quotation 'may they be teeming multitudes upon the earth' (Gen. 48: 16).[25] Scholars of hasidic thought also draw attention to tendencies to link the figure of the tsadik with memory of the Temple cult, and to kabbalistic parallels between him and the high priest.[26] According to hasidic belief, the tsadik's table was an altar, the feast a sacrifice, and the rebbe himself the high priest making the sacrifice to the Creator. This is why the *shirayim* were considered to be sacred: these were not only ceremonial food, but also played the role of gifts intended for God.[27]

The ultimate effort that a tsadik could expend for the good of his community was the sacrifice of his life. The death of a tsadik was usually referred to as *histalkes*, departure. It did not mean the end of life, but marked the beginning of the holy man's constant, uninhibited access to the divine throne. According to hasidic tradition, in the face of danger the rebbe could choose to die a redemptory death or to liberate himself from his earthly body in order to tackle evil—the root cause of misery and misfortune—in the court of heaven.[28] Descriptions of the atonement made by the tsadik 'for all of Israel' (*kapore far kol yisroel*) are an important aspect of hasidic narratives of epidemics, which were understood as divine punishment for sins. It was in this way that Rebbe Hershele of Żydaczów (now Zhidachiv, Ukraine) was said to have protected his community.[29] According to one tale, during an outbreak of plague in the little town of Gliniany, the hasidim of the neighbouring village took in the tsadik. After a few days, however, he resolved to hide from the angel of death no longer, and returned to Gliniany, forbidding the people to call a doctor. He died, and after his death the plague passed.[30]

The legacy of a tsadik was perceived to be enveloped in a special aura of holiness. There are many accounts of items belonging to the founders of dynasties, which in the right hands could work miracles. Essentially any object with which a tsadik had had protracted contact could have this

---

[25] Mekler, *Fun rebns hoyf*, 91. The word *veyidgu* (and they shall increase) has the same Hebrew root as *dag* (fish).

[26] Green, 'The Zaddiq as Axis Mundi in Later Judaism', 327–47; Rapoport-Albert, 'God and the Zaddik', 321; Petrovsky-Shtern, *The Golden Age Shtetl*, 285–90.

[27] Roker, *The Sanzer Tsadik* (Yid.), 120–1. See Lewis, *Imagining Holiness*, 159–70.

[28] Zelkovitsh, 'Death and Its Accompanying Moments' (Yid.), 155.

[29] Unger, *The Hasidic World* (Yid.), 317.

[30] 'Rabbis and Tsadikim from Gliniany' (Yid.), 69.

status, especially if it had served the performance of a *mitsvah* (phylacteries, Hanukah candles, and so on) or the furthering of the hasidic path (such as his throne). Many tsadikim distributed amulets to their hasidim, whether in the form of pieces of kosher parchment inscribed by *soferim* (scribes) or as ordinary coins. Items of clothing were also invested with great significance. The shirt of the Seer of Lublin was the subject of a veritable war among his heirs, because it had been drenched in his sweat, said to have been induced by his bathing in the fiery mythical river Dinur.[31] In Słonim (now Belarus) men came to blows over a pair of the tsadik's padded trousers.[32] In Horodenka it was immensely popular to bathe in the *mikveh* immediately after the leader of the local hasidim had immersed himself there.[33] The tsadik's holiness could enhance the magic of any remedy, not only of amulets and coins. Various sources attest to Jewish women suffering a difficult birth or not being able to induce labour drinking a glass of their husband's urine. On occasion, if this did not help, someone might be sent for the tsadik's urine.[34]

At this point it seems appropriate to note that it was women who most frequently sought the tsadik's help, though, contrary to the opinion of the first scholars of hasidism, it was by no means easy for them to gain access to him.[35] It was received wisdom that *A rebe un a dokter vern raykh nor fun vayber* (The rebbe and the physician only get rich because of women). A dedicated term, *vaybersher rebe* (a women's rebbe), was also coined to refer to hasidic men whose only field of expertise was promising miracles. There were quite a lot of such figures, especially in large towns. Typically they were ordinary people (craftspeople, carters, etc.) who were at best extremely devout but almost always uneducated, and who remained on the fringes of hasidism and often slipped through the net.[36] In no way could they compete, however, with the hugely popular tsadikim in the mainstream, who also performed actions perceived as miracles, though this was not their main area of work.

[31] Even, *From the World of Hasidic Leaders* (Yid.), 254–5.
[32] Khayes, 'Death-Related Beliefs and Customs' (Yid.), 307.
[33] Sukher, 'With the Hasidim of Vizhnits' (Yid.), 250.
[34] Talko-Hryncewicz, *Zarys lecznictwa ludowego*, 76; *Segulot urefuot*, JTS, MS 9862, 94; Pulner, 'Obryadi i povirya', 108; Plaut, *Likutei ḥever ben ḥayim*, 7*a*. See Jakobovits, *Jewish Medical Ethics*, 42.
[35] Ada Rapoport-Albert takes issue, for example, with the views of Samuel Aba Horodecki in her entry 'Hasidism' in the online Encyclopedia of Jewish Women, on the Jewish Women's Archive website (accessed: 21 Nov. 2018).

Women seeking the help of a genuine tsadik either made pilgrimage to him personally or sent intermediaries—their husbands or fathers or a hasidic messenger for instance. In some situations they were unable to go themselves due to health reasons (for instance they were in labour) or their duties as housewife and mother. In any case, they were rarely granted access to the tsadik. In the literature, of course, there are many examples where such meetings did take place, predominantly in connection with a health issue. Rebbe Meir of Opatów (Apt), for example, granted an audience to a woman with a skin disease (she was guilty of violating the sabbath and therefore had been punished by God) and ordered her to give alms to a poor bride.[37] Usually, however, women had to be content with the *gabai* as go-between, who took the *kvitlekh* and a suitable 'soul ransom'.[38] Sometimes they would approach the tsadik's wife or another woman in his immediate circle. The wives and daughters of tsadikim are marginal figures in hasidic literature, but their role would probably be revealed to have been much more significant if it were possible to examine hasidism from the angle of ordinary women. The few stories that exist about them praise their modesty, piety, and erudition, and also mention miracles performed by them. It was said of the wife of Tsevi of Kamionka, for instance, that simply by crossing the threshold of the room in which a woman was giving birth she could ensure a successful delivery.[39] In any case, the same literature confirms the great engagement of tsadikim in helping women. Infertility, miscarriage, difficult births, and infant mortality were only some examples in an extensive catalogue of health issues which were addressed by hasidic leaders, largely at the request of Jewish women.[40]

It was a widespread conviction among the Jewish populace that physical possession by a dybbuk—the spirit of a deceased person—was a danger to which young women and girls were particularly vulnerable. This is confirmed by scholars of Jewish legends, who have demonstrated that female victims of dybbuks constitute a clear majority of all documented cases. In the hasidic literature this motif surfaces in contexts including betrothal and marriage.[41] One fairly typical case is the story of a lonely, impoverished

---

[36] See Mekler, *Fun rebns hoyf*, 236–41; Almi [Sheps], *A Reckoning and Summary* (Yid.), 47–8.

[37] Nigal, *The Hasidic Tale*, 108.

[38] See e.g. Dimond, 'Reminiscences and Historical Research' (Yid.), 10.

[39] Nigal, *The Hasidic Tale*, 123.      [40] Ibid. 113–21.

[41] See Elior, *Dybbuks and Jewish Women*; Chajes, *Between Worlds*. Possession by a dybbuk as a

orphan girl from Radom, who was possessed by the ghost of her mother. The tsadik of Radoszyce came to her aid and convened a *minyan* over the dead woman's grave with the purpose of placing a curse on her. This failed to produce the desired effect, but the dybbuk capitulated when the girl realized that she might still find a husband.[42] Unlike a *gilgul*, a lost soul which 'attached itself' to various beings and objects, the dybbuk attacked only humans, and could do only harm. It was said to assail women who left the house on Saturday evening without an apron, girls who were careless when pouring out domestic waste, and the deceased if left unguarded. Its appearance might be caused by an unfulfilled oath, in particular a betrothal. Symptoms of possession varied, from speaking in an altered voice to stubborn refusal to speak at all, from physical hyperactivity to total catatonia. The symptoms believed to indicate a dybbuk were also typical of insomnia, epilepsy, madness, and partial or total paralysis.

The only people who could exorcise a *gilgul* or a dybbuk were rabbis, tsadikim, and *ba'alei shem*. Mainstream rabbis were often unwilling to undertake exorcisms. At the beginning of the nineteenth century the author of the *Sefer haberit* unequivocally adopted a humoral interpretation of this phenomenon, identifying alleged cases of possession as insanity and melancholy. His comments, seasoned with acerbic criticism of superstition, were included in a late Yiddish-language edition of the work, and appear to have been a reflection of the rational opinion on this issue shared by much of the rabbinical elite.[43] Exorcism of dybbuks thus became the domain of hasidic leaders. The ritual usually took the form of an interrogation of the alien spirit by the tsadik, who would use threats, curses, or promises to persuade it to leave its victim's body. The body part through which the dybbuk left its host became dead; forcing it to leave through the throat was thus tantamount to risking the suffocation of the victim. It was widely believed that the best route was via the little finger on either hand (or sometimes the little toe). The dybbuk would then flee, smashing the window pane, which would have been prepared in advance with appropriate kabbalistic

manifestation of sexual drive and the links between this and views on hysteria have been studied by Yoram Bilu, the author of essays including 'Dybbuk-Possession as a Hysterical Symptom' (with Beit-Hallahmi) and 'The Taming of the Deviants', 41–72.

[42] Zuker, 'A Dybbuk' (Yid.), 273. An anthology of dybbuk stories has been compiled by Nigal (*'Dybbuk' Stories in Jewish Literature* (Heb.)). Jewish sources detail cases of possession of Jews, though there are also testimonies to dybbuk-possession of Christians. See Virshubski, 'The Dybbuk' (Yid.), 319–20.           [43] See Hurwitz, *Sefer haberit*, 51–9.

formulas.[44] Hasidic stories also register a variety of other methods of combating dybbuks. In one tale, a man possessed by a dybbuk was so persistent and impudent in his requests to Rebbe Yehezkel Shraga Halberstam of Sieniawa for help that the tsadik reportedly ordered him 'to go to all the devils', and this caused the dybbuk to leave his victim's body.[45] On another occasion David of Talne was approached for help by a man with 'glass legs' (he was afraid to bend his knees so as 'not to break the glass'). The tsadik bade his *gabai* conceal himself, and at his signal smash a glass. He then ordered the patient to sit down, and when the terrified man obeyed, he heard the sound of breaking glass and was cured.[46]

Lack of a cure from one tsadik left the patient free to seek help from another. Nonetheless, sources of all types emphasized the profound faith of the hasidim and their patience in awaiting deliverance. Abandoning one's own rebbe to seek help at another's court would be a repudiation of the bond that was the very essence of the mission of the movement's leaders as intermediaries. When one hasid of the tsadik of Rozwadów fell ill and in spite of the rebbe's promise could not get well, it was only with reluctance that he allowed himself to be persuaded to go to nearby Dzików, and the tsadik there succeeded in winning over heaven in his cause and freeing him from his illness.[47]

Given the wealth of strands in stories of the curative efforts of tsadikim, it is hardly surprising that the infiltration of elements of biomedicine, and to a limited extent also of alternative concepts (such as homeopathy), into the realm of popular Jewish belief provoked some friction. Doctors were not greatly trusted; they were seen as godless proponents of Enlightenment heresies who dressed in European fashion.[48] Their 'understanding' of illness thus also gave cause for doubt. It was said that *Di matseyves zaynen beste shvokhim farn dokter* (Gravestones are a doctor's best praise); *A dokter un a kvores-man zaynen shutfim* (The doctor and the gravedigger are in league); or, more bluntly, *A dokter iz a ganev* (A doctor is a thief). Many practitioners of biomedicine had become so acculturated that their return to contact with the Jewish community was as Christians, or at the least as

[44] Akalovich, 'Zamietki o yevrieiskoy narodnoy demonologii', 143–4; Segel, 'Chasydzi i chasydyzm', 681–2; Lew, 'O lecznictwie i przesądach', *Izraelita*, 42 (1896), p. 364. See Kotik, *My Memoirs* (Yid.), 148.          [45] Bakon, *The Rabbi of Sieniawa* (Yid.), 187.
[46] Mekler, *Fun rebns hoyf*, 136–7.     [47] Holender, 'A Kaddish for You, My Town' (Yid.), 44.
[48] The assimilated, doubting, or atheistic Jewish doctor was thought to be an incarnation of Satan himself. See e.g. Singer, 'The Gentleman from Cracow', 23–44.

advocates of the radical abandonment of tradition. This did not win them
many adherents. Antipathy towards hospitals and proponents of official
medicine increased during the cholera epidemic that ravaged eastern
Europe around 1900. Rumours even circled that there were forces of evil
behind the incomprehensible machinations of physicians, and that patients
in institutionalized healthcare establishments were being deliberately
poisoned.[49] Various sources reported the deliberate violation of sanitary
cordons by some members of Jewish communities,[50] attempts to resist both
the introduction of spittoons to synagogues and official orders to bleach
the gutters,[51] and the futility of proposals that fasting be abandoned.[52]
Sometimes the efficacy of biomedical procedures and therapies was overtly
called into question. In the novel *Anaf hayim*, the author, whose Orthodox
outlook strongly influenced the work, remarked that if during the cholera
epidemic *babske refues* and traditional *segulot* had been used instead of modern medications, there would only have been three victims more: the two
doctors and the pharmacist, who would have died of starvation.[53] The main
character in this book, one Hayim *royfe*, conducted a type of war against
learned physicians, and claimed superiority to them in view of his use of a
combination of simple natural remedies, prayer, and alms.[54]

The reserve with which biomedical assistance was treated reflected the
protracted process of familiarization with official medicine and negotiation
of its place on the scale of rationality, which remained founded on traditional views on health. Contemporary anthropology holds the view that
this process did not involve the sudden displacement of one system by
another, the overtaking of superstition by empiricism. A more accurate
description of it would be as a period of coexistence of alternatives, each of
which garnered a different degree of confidence and was employed in combination with the others by the same patient.[55] An interesting illustration of
this is the statement of the author of *Sefer haberit*, who used quotations
from the Bible to underline the rational dimension of doctors' recommendations: 'The words of doctors [who aver] that wine and spirits damage

[49] Lew, 'O lecznictwie i przesądach', *Izraelita*, 37, pp. 315–16; Perets, *One does not Die of
Cholera if One does not Want to* (Yid.), described in Chmielnicki, 'Y. L. Peretz's Popular Medical
Brochure' (Yid.), 150.
[50] Potocka, *Mój pamiętnik*, 167–9.          [51] Yunis, 'The Old Homeland' (Yid.), 92.
[52] Khazan, 'Wedding in the Cemetery' (Yid.), 384. See Plaut, *Likutei ḥever ben ḥayim*, 6b.
[53] Horowitz, *Anaf ḥayim*, 47.
[54] Ibid. 51.          [55] Pelto and Pelto, 'Studying Knowledge, Culture, Behavior', 151.

the eyes are written in the Torah: "His eyes are darker than wine" [Gen. 49: 12].'[56]

As has been mentioned above, religious law forbade the faithful to live in a town where there was no physician. The talmudic code *Kitsur shulḥan arukh* left no doubt that the right to practise medicine was enshrined in the Torah; indeed, it was a commandment, and anyone who was in possession of the necessary knowledge and skills but did not offer treatment would be liable for the deaths of those they did not treat.[57] At the same time, the sufferer should not solely wait for a miracle, as this could be interpreted as pride. The correct procedure was to contact the best possible doctor and retain hope and faith in God's healing power.[58] In fact, Ashkenazi Jews seem to have held the art of medicine in far higher esteem than the rabbis were prepared to admit. The motif of the prescription or pharmaceutical remedy as a way to cure the spirit instead of the body found a permanent place in Jewish ethical literature, and it figured in the writings of authors including Glückel of Hameln (1646–1724).[59] Towards the end of the nineteenth century a similar motif appeared in the popular volume *Ets ḥayim*, the Yiddish-language edition of the *Shenei luḥot haberit*, whose author claims to have borrowed the motif from Moses Cordovero.[60] It also found its way into hasidic literature: the Rymanów hasid Abraham Abele Kanarvogel included among the *segulot* gathered in his *Be'erot hamayim* the following description of a 'medication': 'Sweet preserves for weakness of spiritual forces. Take roots of humility, branches of enlightenment, herbs of the commandments, thorns of modesty, flowers of justice, creepers of reward; crush all this in a mortar of penitence, and make a dressing for above and below, and together with a stem of repentance and perfume of love, place over the heart.'[61] In the nineteenth century we find numerous instances of recommendations by hasidic leaders of 'miraculous' cures made according to the pharmaceutical art. The tsadik Simhah Bunem of Przysucha was once said to have received a hasid who had come to him with a request for the healing of a relative. Though the entire audience was punctuated by a series of remarkable happenings, the remedy recommended

---

[56] Hurwitz, *Sefer haberit hashalem*, 246.

[57] See Ganzfried, *Kitsur shulḥan arukh*, 192: 4. Grunwald, *Die Hygiene der Juden*, 184, 241, cited in Veynig, 'Doctors and Medicine in Jewish Sayings' (Yid.), 17.

[58] Ganzfried, *Kitsur shulḥan arukh*, 192: 3.  [59] *The Life of Glückel of Hameln*, 5–7.

[60] *Ets ḥayim*, 46.  [61] Kanarvogel, *Ta'amei mitsvot*, 18*b* (194).

by the tsadik was absolutely trivial; the hasid was to buy six zlotys' worth of sage from the pharmacy and make a tincture with it.[62] The Olesko rebbe cured a Christian woman of a headache by prescribing her an ointment which the pharmacist made up according to his recipe.[63] And one popular story tells of the tsadik of Wieledniki (now Velidnyky, Ukraine), who told infertility sufferers to buy a remedy from a stranger he had met on the dyke. This medicine was entirely conventional in form: the liquid in the little glass bottle, which could be purchased for three roubles, was to be poured over sugar and swallowed.[64] Regina Lilientalowa heard from her interviewees that a patient who had stored up particular merit in heaven might expect to be visited at night by one of the patriarchs, who would give them medicine on a spoon.[65] In Yiddish the word *refue* (remedy) became synonymous with a means of coping with problems. This metaphor would often be extended along its pharmaceutical axis, as in the saying that there was 'even less of [something material, such as apples, or traits such as courage] than of a medicine' (*afile oyf a refue nit*), or that something was a 'bitter remedy' (*a bitere refue*). On the other hand, traditional circles considered the direst plague of the modern world to be godlessness, which they were wont to liken to an 'infectious disease' (*onshtekende krankayt*).[66]

Jewish ethical writings from the period around 1900 did not deny the value of official medicine or the wisdom of doctors, although they still expressed attachment to premodern ideas about healing. Authors were cautious in their judgement, and stressed that the true source of healing is always God. They also drew attention to the limitations of biomedicine, which could not pretend to a full, universal understanding of human nature: 'There are virtually no professors in the world who are familiar with the entire human body in detail. Each one knows but a part of it. This one is an oculist, that one treats the ears and throat, this one specializes in skin diseases, that one in nerves, this one delivers babies, that one is a pediatrician. Though man appears to be but a small machine, after so many thousands of years, we still cannot learn him in full.'[67] Nonetheless, they did not question the overall efficacy of treatments supported by clinical experience. The popular *segulot urefuot* literature would attract new readers by advertis-

[62] Zamlung, *Eser zekhiyot*, 7. This anecdote gains flavour with the supplementary information that the rebbe was educated in pharmacy and supported himself by running a pharmacy outlet; see Dynner, *Men of Silk*, 28.       [63] Segel, 'Chasydzi i chasydyzm', 680.

[64] Rotner, *Sipurei nifla'ot*, 43–5.       [65] Lilientalowa, 'Wierzenia, przesądy i praktyki', 106.

[66] *Mekor dimah*, 35.       [67] Ibid. 19.

ing on the title pages that the content was sourced 'from great doctors' books'[68] or 'from a great physician, a doyen among physicians'.[69] Both printed works and manuscripts included kabbalistic remedies prescribed by great tsadikim side by side with medications attributed to proponents of conventional medicine. Indeed, the intermittent recurrence of names from the latter category in Orthodox Jewish writings seems even to have served the purpose of lending credibility to the recipes collected in them, like the phrase 'in the name of physicians', which is reminiscent of the 'canonical' formula 'in the name of the tsadikim' used to authenticate received tradition in hasidic texts.[70] The term *rofé mumkheh* or *rofé muvhak*, which in the early modern age denoted a university-educated doctor, was around 1900 used for biomedicine practitioners of authority, who might also be referred to as *Professoren*.[71]

Many sources report that people accustomed to treating themselves using traditional remedies and *segulot* would turn to proponents of official medicine only when it was too late. Gerszon Lewin recalled the case of a young woman who suffered from chlorosis (hypochromic anaemia) for two years, until the ailment intensified to such a degree that she was forced to visit a physician.[72] Although the talmudic wisdom that 'the best physicians go to hell'[73] was a much-repeated phrase, people did respect medical specialists, even if they were not Jewish.[74] In 1910 the 411 Jewish doctors in Galicia accounted for 29.9 per cent of all the physicians in the province,[75] while in Russia around the same time there were 1,077 Jewish doctors (just 6 per cent of all physicians in the empire).[76] In the nineteenth century some Orthodox Jews preferred to contact Christian practitioners, in order to avoid Jewish heretics at all costs. In time, however, practical considerations took precedence. A major problem when visiting non-Jewish doctors was

---

[68] *Refuot ha'am im darkhei yesharim*, 1.     [69] *Sefer refuot*, 1.

[70] One example of such treatment of biomedical authorities is to be found in Kanarvogel, *Be'erot hamayim*. See Tuszewicki, 'Chasydzi w Galicji', 49–83.

[71] Zimmels, *Magicians, Theologians and Doctors*, 33; Kanarvogel, *Ta'amei mitsvot*, 1.

[72] Lewin, 'Z pamiętnika lekarza', 234.     [73] BT *Kid.* 82a.

[74] B. Bernstein, *Memories and Personalities* (Yid.), 115.

[75] Friedman, 'Dzieje Żydów w Galicji', 406. In the immediate aftermath of the partition of Poland, the Austrian authorities attempted to restrict the work of Jewish doctors among Christians, and in Galicia twelve *jüdische Kreisärzte* (Jewish district doctors) were appointed, but as early as 1784 Joseph II abolished the separation of these offices, and also lifted the restrictions on Jewish physicians and barber-surgeons; see Bałaban, *Dzieje Żydów w Galicyi*, 31–2.

[76] Kossoy and Ohry, *The Feldshers*, 154–5.

the language barrier. This is clearly illustrated by an example from the town of Siemiatycze, where a young Polish doctor took over from his predecessor who had known a few words in Yiddish and could communicate with his patients. The new doctor was unwilling to make concessions to the minority language, and hence 'the Jewish women who came to him for treatment understood little of what he said to them'. This prompted the decision to have a Jewish physician brought to the town.[77]

It is also important to note that not only did hospitals and old people's homes exist in the Polish lands, but they were also gradually modernized and rebuilt according to the latest trends. However, at the turn of the twentieth century even state hospitals outsourced certain areas of their care, such as patient hygiene and meals, to Christian bodies. The traditional Jewish community remained suspicious of such confessional insitutions, and in particular avoided leaving their children in them.[78] As Edward Kossoy notes, in the late nineteenth century almost all the cities in the Kingdom of Poland with a population of over 20,000 had Jewish hospitals, which employed both qualified physicians and educated feldshers.[79] In Galicia there were nineteen such institutions in 1900, compared to thirteen just four years previously.[80] Christian hospitals either did not admit Jewish patients, or did not offer kosher meals or the facilities for them to perform their daily religious rituals. Although public hospitals in Galicia were obligated to accept all members of the population irrespective of their confession, it was not until 1874 that the National Diet passed an act enshrining the Jews' equal rights to treatment in the national hospital in Lwów.[81] In Wadowice the first Jewish patient was only admitted to hospital during an epidemic of typhoid fever in 1916. Seriously ill patients tended to be transported to Kraków, where there was a modern Jewish hospital.[82]

There was undoubtedly also a financial barrier blocking access to educated practitioners for the poorer strata of society. Gerszon Lewin compared his easy visits to the homes of the rich with difficult ones to 'paupers, where there is not even a place to lay one's hat, one has to make out the prescription on one's knee, and instead of collecting one's fee, one actually has

[77] Weissman, 'The Victory of the Jewish Doctor' (Yid.), 347.

[78] Herzog and Zborowski, Life Is with People, 355.

[79] Kossoy and Ohry, The Feldshers, 164.

[80] Franaszek, Zdrowie publiczne w Galicji, 153; Michalewicz, Żydowskie okręgi metrykalne, 178–80.                                                      [81] Franaszek, Zdrowie publiczne w Galicji, 49–50.

[82] Wiener-Ram, 'Our Town and Its Jews' (Heb.), 57–8.

to leave money for the medication'.[83] Nonetheless, given the numerous aid projects run by Jewish community organizations and the readiness of practitioners of biomedicine to treat poor patients free of charge, whether out of conviction or due to legal regulations, such contacts were far more frequent than the ratio of patient income to doctors' fees might suggest.[84] In extreme cases several patients from a town might pool their resources to pay for a doctor's travel and consulting fees.[85] At the same time, the sources document that many quacks, feldshers, and physicians did not take money from the poor, but treated such consultations as a *mitsvah*. It is hard to accept generalizations of this nature, however, especially in view of the knowledge that they all had to support themselves from this work. What is more, we also have testimonies indicating that payment was an important element of the treatment process from the point of view of the patient. As Lewin noted, one poor tailor preferred to pay for a visit rather than accept help free of charge. The grounds for this attitude are to be found in the talmudic warning: 'A physician who treats for nothing is worth nothing', which was taken extremely seriously.[86] The tailor took the comparison one step further, pointing out that if he were not paid for his sewing, he would not sew well either.[87]

The first contact with biomedicine was not necessarily through a physician. As mentioned above, at the beginning of the twentieth century it was often feldshers who brought in methods typical of modern medicine. Hasidic leaders, too, responded to the modernizing changes. And although in the earliest hasidic literature doctors tended to be depicted negatively in view of their moral failings, even the first leaders of the movement sometimes had positive things to say about them. The great Magid, Dov Ber of Mezeritch, was said to have believed that it was not medication that wrought the cure, but the doctors themselves, who had their own stars—angels responsible for their medications. There was an angel watching over every doctor, among them even the archangel Raphael.[88] The tsadikim themselves used the services of biomedical practitioners, and some of them, in the knowledge that they were authorities in the eyes of their adherents

[83] Lewin, 'Z pamiętnika lekarza', 232.
[84] See e.g. Więckowska, *Lekarze jako grupa zawodowa*, 11–28.
[85] Zeyerman, 'Medical Care' (Yid.), 124.
[86] BT *BK* 85a; Sperling, *Ta'amei haminhagim oyf ivri taytsh*, ii. 27.
[87] Lewin, 'Z pamiętnika lekarza', 233.
[88] Nigal, *The Hasidic Tale*, 177; Rothstein, *Tsadikim and Hasidim* (Yid.), 25–7.

and the hope of vast numbers of desperate men and women, employed the advances of science in their own work. We know of books written by Yehudah Yudl Rosenberg of Tarłów and Hayim Simhah Leiner of Radzyn and Ludmir (Volodymyr Volynskyi) that contain passages of varying lengths on biomedicine. Rosenberg also propagated homeopathic remedies widely, and cultivated contact with the proprietor of a pharmacy on Piotrkowska Street in Łódź.[89] Rebbe Israel Perlov (d.1921) of the Karlin-Stolin dynasty (founded in Karolin, today a district of Pińsk, now in Belarus) was a similar figure. The tradition of the movement has preserved the memory of the prescriptions he issued for his patients, who included Russian army officers, to have made up at the pharmacy. According to one story, the tsadik gave a man who had been suffering from headaches a prescription written in Polish. The hasid misunderstood his rebbe's intention and took the slip of paper to be an amulet. He tucked it inside his hat, and thenceforth enjoyed perfect health until his hat was blown away and lost in a violent storm.[90] In other reminiscences the 'women's tsadik' Reb Eliezer of Rzeszów made ointments which were well known throughout the area, under his own name: *Lozerls refues*.[91]

Around 1900 it was relatively common practice to visit the rebbe at his court for advice on how to proceed with respect to an illness, especially when lengthy or expensive treatment by biomedical specialists was expected. Ben-Zvi Bernstein of Przemyślany (now Peremyshlyany, Ukraine) recalls a case of a physician being called out to a patient in an emergency. He suspected diabetes, and ordained a urine sample for analysis to confirm the diagnosis. The patient's rebbe would not agree to this procedure, however, and the patient sought no further treatment.[92] On another occasion a highly respected hasid from Łódź paid a visit to the Aleksandrów tsadik when his son fell seriously ill. Although three physicians at a case conference deemed it vital that the boy be sent to Wrocław for treatment, before embarking on such a major logistical and financial venture his father decided to consult his spiritual master.[93] In hasidic narratives doctors were often cast in the role of actors in a divine plan, whose actions were monitored, controlled, and even directed by holy men. One tale told of an army

[89] Rosenberg, *Segulot urefuot*, 16; Robinson, 'The Tarler Rebbe of Łódź', 57.
[90] Ben-Amos and Noy (eds.), *Folktales of the Jews*, ii. 118–22.
[91] Weinstein, *Rzeszów: An Extended Poem* (Yid.), 75.
[92] B. Bernstein, *Memories and Personalities* (Yid.), 116.      [93] Zamlung, *Eser zekhiyot*, 72–3.

recruit who got sand in his eyes, doing more damage than he had expected. He took a variety of medications and *segulot*, but nothing helped. He went to see his rebbe, who told him to go to a Jewish doctor in another town and wait to be seen for a very small fee. And that is what happened. The doctor explained that he had had a dream about an old man (likely the tsadik) who had told him to go to that town.[94] Present-day hasidic communities still uphold the custom of asking their rebbe's advice on choosing or changing a biomedical practitioner.[95]

Another institution of seminal importance in terms of treatment alternatives was the pharmacy. This was not only an outlet selling medicines, but served in equal measure as an advisory point. Ruth Gay, in her description of the attitudes of Jewish immigrants in New York to one particular pharmacy owner, writes: 'He was the neighborhood pharmacist, which practically made him a doctor, which was as far as one's imagination could stretch.'[96] What set the pharmacy apart at least to some extent was the cleanliness and order that reigned in it. This so differentiated it from the world around it as to have found reflection in a Jewish saying: *A khazer ken nit lebn in an apteyk. A khazer muz lebn in blote* (A pig cannot live in a pharmacy. A pig has to live in mud).[97] Whether it was owned by a Jew or a Christian seems to have been largely irrelevant, though in the latter case it had the advantage of also being accessible on the sabbath.[98] The otherness of the pharmacy was by no means an impediment; on the contrary, it could reinforce imaginings of the therapeutic power of the remedies it sold. It was a space so different from the common 'Jewish street' that it could provoke associations with witchcraft: the pharmacy was 'the only store in which a kid with sidelocks would doff his cap and stand bare-headed. It had a smell of cleanliness and medicine. The sales assistants wore white coats, which looked—forgive the profanation—like the *kitls* worn at Yom Kippur . . . They said in *ḥeder* that the pharmacist was an apostate and had a cross branded on the back of his neck to prove it.'[99] People would some-

[94] Rotner, *Sipurei nifla'ot*, 54.

[95] See e.g. D. J. Rozen, 'Biomedicine, Religion and Ethnicity', 112–24.

[96] Gay, *Unfinished People*, 49.

[97] Beilin, 'Sprichwörter und Redensarten aus Russland', 39.

[98] Shlaferman, 'The Folklore, Customs, and Stories of Kazimierz' (Yid.), 171–2; regarding Christian pharmacies important to local Jewish communities, see also 'The Town' (Yid.), 19, 25; Wiener-Ram, 'Our Town and Its Jews' (Heb.), 58.

[99] Levita, 'A Stroll Around the Town' (Yid.), 172–3.

times grumble at the cost of medicine. At the beginning of the twentieth century the poorest people could count on support in this respect from aid organizations, such as the *bikur ḥolim* fraternities, whose members would either contribute to the cost of medications or distribute them entirely free of charge (and as they saw fit). The items they gave out were usually the most basic articles, such as cotton wool and iodine, as well as products vital during epidemics, such as carbolic acid.[100]

'Taking the waters' and spending time at health resorts was a custom that enjoyed considerable popularity among the Jewish populace. It is hard to pinpoint the moment when Jews began to take an interest in this area of medicine, but it was probably long before the advent of the regular Christian 'spa traffic' that they first recognized the therapeutic properties of thermal water. One former resident of the spa town of Strzyżów re-called: 'We had a beautiful river, beautiful surroundings . . . mineral springs which were said to heal the eyes and skin diseases.'[101] When in the nineteenth century spa resorts gained the endorsement of biomedical pro-fessionals, taking the waters became a fully legitimate method of convales-cence in the eyes of Jewish Orthodoxy. The custom was by no means a privilege of the wealthy; it filtered down to many ordinary people, who were able to afford a stay at a spa thanks to support from community organ-izations. Many poorer visitors would evade the spa taxes and stay with rela-tives, people from their own town, or in *pensions* whose proprietors agreed to host them as an act of charity or at a reduced rate.[102]

The presence of Jews added variety to the demographics of the resorts. In response to the influx of large numbers of visitors who observed Orthodox Jewish rules, kosher kitchens and canteens were opened, and synagogues and private prayer houses began to function in the area. The hasidim were among the most eye-catching visitors at spa resorts both in Poland and abroad. Particularly in the twentieth century, they stood out with their traditional appearance and attire and also in terms of their strict observance of the religious traditions. They came in great numbers, both the men, who constituted the force and core of the movement, and their families. The most important guests, however, were the tsadikim and

[100] Brikman, 'Jewish Charitable Institutions in the Town' (Yid.), 227; Slutski, 'Bobruysk (A Monograph)' (Yid.), 146; Khazan, 'Wedding in the Cemetery' (Yid.), 383.
[101] Klots, 'A Kaddish for You, My Shtetl' (Yid.), 292.
[102] See Epstein, 'Caring for the Soul's House', 192–8; Zadoff, *Next Year in Marienbad*.

their attendants. Their visits to Polish spa resorts have been immortalized in numerous photographs, which show them taking strolls or relaxing in parks. They almost always feature in these photographs in the company of their acolytes, which brings to mind images of royal courts, or of a master and his retinue.[103] A tsadik's stay at a spa was not a time of respite from his everyday role, however; on the contrary, a well-known leader would attract hordes of visitors, or simply people seeking help. The Austrian parliamentarian and social activist Josef Samuel Bloch (1850–1923) described in his memoirs a visit by the famous tsadik Hayim Halberstam of Nowy Sącz to the spa town of Iwonicz Zdrój. He held audiences for the hasidim, issued advice to the needy, and even healed a young girl who was possessed by a dybbuk.[104]

In summary, the attitudes of traditional Jews towards doctors and, more specifically, towards medicine founded on the biological sciences were not unequivocal. In the nineteenth century even those Ashkenazi communities most attached to tradition, despite voicing antipathy to change, accepted biomedicine as one option available to them in case of illness. And while they remained mistrustful of it and did not accept it as a superior authority, often refraining from taking further steps until their spiritual leaders had given their consent, neither hasidim nor the wider traditional Jewish community rejected contact with secular practitioners a priori; often they even sought justification in religious law for their actions.

The importance of the value of health, the multiplicity of treatment options available within the home and the immediate environment, and the initiative people demonstrated when seeking a cure—all these elements together produce an overall picture of Jewish folk medicine. This image is coloured in part by religious tradition, rooted in the sacred text of the Torah and its rabbinic and kabbalistic interpretations. This latter aspect may indeed be credited with lending the health-related beliefs and practices of the Jews many of the attributes which differentiated this community from its largely Christian and Slavic environment. Yet it was not this alone that was decisive in the Jews' perception of sickness and in their ultimate choice of remedies. As stated at the beginning of this section, no attempt to interpret folk therapeutic practices can be reduced to such

[103] Balakirsky Katz, 'Rebbishe Representation', 363–70.
[104] Bloch, *Erinnerungen aus meinem Leben*, 2.

a simple categorization. The same may be said of the question of the 'rationality' of folk medicine, which is a gateway to a broad field of multi-faceted anthropological and historical research.

# PART II

# A WORLD OF SIMILARITIES AND SIGNS

CHAPTER SIX

# MICROCOSM AND MACROCOSM

THERE IS A LONG AND RICH TRADITION of pragmatic explanations for the intricacies of folk medicine, though these explanations were usually shaped by a world-view and medical knowledge contemporary to the thinkers. Modern critics of old traditions either refused to accept what they perceived as 'folklore' or believed in the possibility of casting the premodern ideas in a form that could be useful in their own age. In many cases the motivation for such efforts was the desire to dig down to a 'rational core'—an objectively efficacious body of remedies. In others, however, these writings tended to be produced, or at least employed, as instruments of harsh criticism in the name of the struggle against ignorance and superstition. One issue of the periodical *Folksgezunt*, the press organ of the Society for the Protection of Jewish Health in Poland, published in Vilna (now Vilnius, Lithuania), ran an article on local health-related beliefs. Its author wrote: 'Given that the fundamental objective of this paper is prophylaxis, i.e. protection from illness, it is only fitting that it . . . devote a modicum of space to fighting all the various beliefs and superstitions which remain deeply ingrained in the minds of the Jewish masses.'[1] This did not mean, however, that the pioneers of ethnography, who counted some doctors among their number, were unaware of the syncretic character of folk practices. Izrael Fels, in a brief sketch on Jews' health-related beliefs, identified them as a composite of 'old superstitions . . . or the vestiges of early scientific medicine, or else the inventions of folk medicine'.[2] A similar opinion was voiced by Henryk Lew, who considered that 'homegrown treatments constitute a conglomerate of the notions, superstitions, and folk medicine of the peoples among whom the Jews have lived . . . and

[1] Tsart, 'Superstitions and Beliefs in Our Region' (Yid.), 51–2.
[2] Fels, 'Zabobony lekarskie u Żydów', 2.

the superstitions and medications of talmudic medicine, which . . . is based on Greek and Arab medicine'.[3]

The departure from the perception of folk beliefs and practices as either rational or irrational in favour of a search for the more profound structures organizing this sphere of culture revealed to scholars the vast significance of myth. It facilitated a better understanding of the 'fancies' forming a thin veneer that concealed a scale of opposing mythical forces— such as young and old, light and dark, and elements mediating between them—likened by Ludwik Stomma, whose interpretation of the culture of rural Poland was based on the theories of Claude Lévi-Strauss, to the periodic table of the chemical elements. Today we know that myth is a universal structure organizing our understanding of the world. Thinking in the categories of myth helps us to confront the unknown and systematize our perceived reality on the basis of our own logic. It also creates openings for actions employing magic with the intention of influencing the world and various aspects of it.

Nonetheless it is important not to lose sight of the notion of 'culture as the memory of history',[4] and to remember that this memory has tended to take most enduring form in the area of popular beliefs and practices. Between the wars the theory of the *gesunkenes Kulturgut* expounded by Hans Naumann was highly acclaimed by Jewish folklorists. This theory held that products of folklore are not original but reproductions of elements of high culture. As recently as the 1930s, perhaps under the influence of Naumann's involvement in the Nazi movement, Yehudah Leyb Cahan attempted to render these views with greater precision, pointing (in relation to songs) to at least three sources of folklore: the vernacular, the external, and the literary.[5] Whatever our attitude to these now outdated discussions, it is only fair to recognize that the medical concepts which predated the triumphal march of biomedicine did not disappear from the human consciousness with that advance. Motifs and symbols which once formed part of a culture become altered and their original meanings change, but they are rarely lost completely. Neither, then, should they be forgotten in reference to the conception of culture as a structuralistic 'table of the elements', the more so since in many cases their roots were similar to those of 'folk-type' convictions.

[3] Lew, 'O lecznictwie i przesądach', *Izraelita*, 37, p. 316.

[4] Kowalski, 'Wanda, Ofelia i inne topielice', 209–10.

[5] Cahan, ['Production and Reproduction in Folklore'] (Yid.), 222–7.

In his preface to *The Order of Things*, Michel Foucault drew attention to the profound changes in thought that began in the late seventeenth century, though they were founded not on the progress of reason but on change in the mode of reasoning. Until then, speculation about the mechanisms of the world and human anatomy was based on the coincidence of attributes noticed by observers of objects and phenomena. Mapping analogies and oppositions was one of the keystones of European culture. Before the revolution introduced by modern science, exploration of the world was based on seeking signs of similarity and deciphering the codes encrypted in the work of Creation. This was perhaps most fully expressed by Paracelsus (1493–1541), who explained herbalism using a theory of signatures bestowed by God on plants in order that humankind might distinguish them. The principles of *similia similibus curantur* and *contraria contrariis curantur*—treatment of like with either like or opposite—were key elements of this system. At the heart of all relations between beings was the bond between humans and the world; microcosm and macrocosm.[6] It was to be a long time before the transformations undergone by the culture of Europe's elites, which gathered pace during the Enlightenment, began to affect views on traditional medicine. The medical theories of earlier times constituted but one element of a broader system of beliefs that was bound up inextricably with the threads of myth, tradition, and religion.

The mores surrounding healthcare within a given folk culture cannot be understood without reference to the question of similarity. Foremost among the views on the aetiology of disease that functioned within the traditional Ashkenazi Jewish community until as recently as the 1930s was that based on the relationships between the matter and phenomena that made up the human body, on the one hand, and those which were commonly imagined to form part of the wider world on the other.[7] In Jewish thought the vision of a close bond between humanity and the cosmos emerged in the very earliest times, and recurred repeatedly in mystical and philosophical conceptions. The book of Genesis describes the creation of Adam from the dust of the earth, and this it employs as a justification for the origin of his name (Heb. *adamah*—earth). Rabbinic exegesis, which

---

[6] Foucault, *The Order of Things*, p. xxiv.

[7] The implications of several existing views of the world and humankind for views on the human body have been discussed in detail by Zbigniew Libera. His analysis of Indo-European mythology and Slavonic folk traditions in the volume *Mikrokosmos, makrokosmos i antropologia ciała* includes an extensive strand relating to Jewish culture.

developed its interpretation of the biblical narrative of the origins of the world over centuries, expounded on this strand in the talmudic treatises and the *midrashim*. It evolved a vision of the human body modelled from red clay (Heb. *adom*—the colour red) obtained by mixing the dust of the earth with water. This dust came either from the four corners of the earth or from its very centre, which was believed to be Mount Moriah, the place where God ordered Abraham to sacrifice his son Isaac, and where subsequently King Solomon erected the Temple of the Lord.[8]

The talmudic-era rabbis debated various aspects of the relationship between humanity and the world, but they did not tackle this issue in its entirety. One of the first examples of a systematized theory of the microcosm to be expounded in Jewish sources was the pronouncement of the second-century CE rabbi Yosé Hagelili cited in the minor treatise *Avot derabi natan*, which was edited between the seventh and ninth centuries. The medieval Jewish philosophers, most of whom came from Sephardi communities, speculated on the notions of microcosm and macrocosm in the spirit of Neoplatonism. One of these philosophers was Solomon Ibn Gevirol (b. *c.*1021), who, in his *Mekor ḥayim*, argued that humans should strive to come to an understanding of themselves and at the same time discover the purpose of their creation. The experience of the soul and knowledge about it were considered to open up possibilities for learning about both the world and God.[9] Joseph Ibn Saddik (d.1149), the author of the treatise *Ha'olam hakatan* (Small World), which was originally written in Arabic, came to similar conclusions. Moses Maimonides was likewise unable to discard entirely the microcosm theory, though he did demonstrate the inconsistencies at its core. He noted that the human heart, which is positioned centrally in respect of the other organs, not only powers them but is also supplied and protected by them, while in the universe there is no such interdependence between the Creator and his creation. What is more, human thought has a physical dimension and cannot be examined in isolation from corporeality, yet God not only does not have bodily form but actually exists outside matter.[10]

The quest for answers to the most fundamental questions via self-discovery and meditation on the essence of one's being was not alien to

[8] Schwartz, *Tree of Souls*, 127–8.
[9] Sirat, *A History of Jewish Philosophy in the Middle Ages*, 71.
[10] Haberman (ed.), *The Microcosm of Joseph Ibn Saddiq*, 23–6.

the Jewish mystics. The *Sefer yetsirah*, written in the first centuries of the Christian era, divided reality into three levels: the spatial (the universe), the temporal (the year), and the personal (the human soul). A human being, quickened by the soul, was a reflection of the world, in which life was dependent on God. Heaven was created from fire, earth from water, and the air maintained harmony by keeping the conflicted elements apart. The universal order thus imagined was reflected fully in the human anatomy (the head was fire, the chest air, and the belly water).[11] This became the main core of later kabbalistic thought. According to the Zohar, which was most probably written in the Middle Ages, humans represented a fusion of the upper world and the lower world. The human body was a model of creation deliberately chosen by God to reflect everything in existence in heaven and on earth. The concept of the primeval Adam (Adam Kadmon) as the embodiment of the ten divine manifestations (*sefirot*), which were at once the elemental parts of the first matter, was developed in Lurianic kabbalah. It was strongly influenced, however, by the idea of the infinity of God (*ein sof*): in order to be able to create his work, the Creator first had to undertake the task of self-contraction (*tsimtsum*). In the space thus created, and from the rays of his emanation, the first human came into being. In Adam Kadmon all the *sefirot* came together, and it was only at subsequent stages of Creation that they were blasted apart.

The hasidic literature, recorded in the lands of the first Polish Republic from the late eighteenth century, devoted considerable space to expounding on this conception of Isaac Luria's. It accepted in full his vision of the human as microcosm, as is evident from the writings of the first leaders of the movement.[12] Hasidic theoreticians often likened the Jewish community to the human body, in which every individual had an ordained role to play and was fulfilling the function ascribed to them. In this conception, the tsadik was portrayed as the head of the community, the 'eyes of the congregation', as some translations of the Bible have it (Lev. 4: 13), through whom the Shekhinah, the Divine Presence, could reach the less noble members of the flock. The central position of the hasidic leader was also reflected in the vision of the cosmos peculiar to this movement: the rebbe

[11] Kaplan, *Sefer Yetzirah*, 145–52.
[12] See Wertheim, *Law and Custom in Hasidism*; Lamm, *The Religious Thought of Hasidism*, 308–9. For more on the shared and differing views of Dov Ber of Mezeritch (Velyki Mezhyrichi, Ukraine) and Shneur Zalman of Liadi (Lyady, Belarus) on this matter, see Loewenthal, *Communicating the Infinite*, 52–3.

was seen as the *axis mundi*, and the biblical phrase *tsadik yesod olam* ('The righteous person is an everlasting foundation', Prov. 10: 25) was interpreted literally, as an indication that the tsadik was a pillar of the earth. In the stories of Nahman of Bratslav we find a depiction of the righteous individual as the mythical stone that formed the foundation for Creation.[13] In the eyes of the faithful, the seat of the hasidic leader was the new Jerusalem, the centre of the world. Within his immediate environment, objects, people, and rites took on the significance of elements of the Temple cult (his table corresponded to the altar; the tsadik himself to the high priest). References to this micro- and macrocosmic relationship also recur in popular tales about hasidic leaders. In some cases they show influences from midrashic literature and books of ethics published in Yiddish from the sixteenth century, such as the *Seyfer brantshpigl*. Naftali of Ropshitz (Ropczyce), for instance, who enjoyed a popular reputation as a pious man and a miracle-worker, likened the nature of woman, subordinated to the cyclicity of menstruation, to that of the moon, which grows and fills out for the first two weeks of its cycle and wanes over the latter two.[14]

These examples of conjecture by philosophers, rabbis, and kabbalists illustrate the historical and literary substrate for beliefs regarding the close bonds between humans and the world around them. In order to understand how these conceptions functioned within folk culture we must, in the first instance, look at the linguistic aspect and the way things were named. Of particular assistance in this domain are the findings of Russian cultural semioticians from Tartu and Moscow, which have been used in research into the culture of provincial Poland by scholars including Zbigniew Libera. Semiotics examines how individuals describe the reality around them using a diverse array of cultural codes. In explaining the structure and functioning of the world they use the ideas that are closest to them, among which are images of their own body. The anthropomorphic code thus created was adopted—and remains in use—in various languages to describe everyday objects and tools, on the basis of their more or less obvious similarity to the human body. Yiddish was no exception in this respect—and so a jug had a 'hand' (*hentl*), a needle had an 'ear' (*oyer*), a table was supported on 'feet' (*fis*), and so on. The lexicon of words connected with social institu-

<hr>

[13] Green, 'The Zaddiq as Axis Mundi', 327–47.
[14] Lifshits, *Segulot yisra'el*, 33*a*. See Riedel (ed.), *Moses Henochs Altschul-Jeruschalmi "Brantspigel"*, 8.

tions developed in a similar fashion. The person in charge of running the yeshiva or the community was its 'head' (*rosh-yeshive, rosh-kool*), and every organization, like any other body, had members (*mitglider*).

The various parts of the body ranked differently in status: the head, for instance, was perceived to be the seat of the intellect (an intelligent person might be said to have *a kop vi a minister*, lit. a head like a minister) and also the part of the body that was most to the fore (Yid. *berosh*, lit. forehead). An agile brain, that of a sharp, decisive person, was known as a 'Jewish head' (*yidisher kop*). The head should be as strong as iron (*ayzerner kop*), meaning that the person should have an excellent memory and be highly intelligent, unlike a peasant, who had a *goyisher kop*—that is, he was dull-witted and slow to understand. In one conjuration for headaches we find a modified quotation of Song of Songs 7: 6. The biblical verse says, 'The head upon you is like the Carmel [mountain], the locks of your head are like purple. A king is held captive in the tresses.' In the conjuration the words *kakarmel* (like the Carmel) were replaced with *kabarzel* (like iron).[15] Set in the head like precious stones were the eyes. Protecting someone or something dear 'like the eye in one's head' (*vi an oyg in kop*), or even 'like the pupil of one's eye' (*vi shvartsapl fun oyg*), was an expression of supreme solicitude. The arms and hands came a close second in terms of esteem. 'You shall enjoy the fruit of your labours [lit. your hands]; you shall be happy and you shall prosper', reads a verse in Psalm 128: 2, often cited in inscriptions on the tombstones of Jewish craftsmen. The hands performed all the tasks devised by the head, and to be without them was to be helpless and unable to act (Yid. *zitsn on hent*, lit. to sit without hands).[16] At the opposite end of this scale from the head were the buttocks. The low status of this part of the body was indicated by its very name (*tokhes*, bottom; cf. coll.: behind). It was associated with stupidity, and symbolized the opposite of thinking. *Hobn in tokhes* (to have something/someone in one's bottom) indicated a pithily expressed lack of interest, while *visn fun a tokhes tsu zogn* (to be capable of saying something with one's bottom) suggested a lack of even the most elementary knowledge. One vulgar saying referred to a talmudist not as a *talmid-khokhem* (learned sage) but as a *talmid-tokhes*, perhaps in view of the

---

[15] Goldberg and Eisenberg, *Sefer laḥashim usegulot*, 7b.

[16] An interesting collection of popular Yiddish expressions and sayings relating to the hands was gathered in the Minsk guberniya and published in the late 1920s. See Kvitni, 'Sayings Including "Hand"' (Yid.), 305–20.

fact that he spent his days not in physical labour but in 'kneading the bench' (*bank-kvetsher*).

While on the subject of the relative status of particular parts of the body, it is important to mention that Yiddish wishes of good health often included references to certain key parts, above all the head (*A lebn af dayn kop*; *A gezunt in dayn kop*; Life/health to your head[17]), the belly (*Zay gezunt, yasher koyekh, a gezunt in dayn boyekh*; Be healthy, may you go from strength to strength, good health for your belly), and the bones (*A derkvikung zol kumen af dayne beyner*; May strength come to your bones[18]). Similar principles were followed for imprecations; synonyms for 'head' were often used, including 'brain' and parts of the face (eye, ear, nose, tooth, mug, gob), while stomach, liver, or bowels might serve in place of 'belly'. These were the dominant words in Yiddish anatomy-related phraseology. One characteristic aspect of this area of language is that the topography of the upper and front parts of the body seems to have been of far greater interest to Jewish society than that of its lower and rear areas. One telling testimony to the 'dismissive' treatment of the lower parts of the body is the use of *fus* to denote essentially the whole leg (perhaps with the exclusion of the knees). The lower status of the nether regions of the body was also demonstrated in the ritual tying of a belt (*gartl*) around the waist before prayers, which represented a symbolic separation of the spiritual from the corporeal.

Drawing parallels between microcosm and macrocosm—using a cosmological code—is one of the ways in which humans describe the structure and sometimes the functioning of the body. *Der mentsh iz a kleyn veltl* (Man is a small world), went one Jewish proverb,[19] a world in himself (*a velt far zikh*). Understanding the cosmological code of a given community can contribute significantly to understanding the behaviour of its members in particular social contexts. Their observations of the world and the similarities they perceived between objects and people affected the methods and remedies used in their folk medicine practice. When a difficult birth was under way in a Jewish home, for instance, members of the household would perform all manner of actions mimicking pulling out, opening, delivering,

[17] Bastomski, *At the Source: Jewish Proverbs* (Yid.), 88.

[18] 'Minor Collections of Folklore' (Yid.), 203. Cf. Prov. 3: 8: 'It will be a cure for your body, a tonic for your bones.'

[19] Steinberg, *From the Fount of the Wisdom of the Jewish People* (Heb.), 12–13.

and so on, which, it was thought, would ease the suffering woman's pains and accelerate the arrival of her child. To this end, too, she would be symbolically 'liberated' from any bonds and ties binding her body, such as rings, necklaces, or bracelets. What is more, throughout the ninth month of a pregnancy, the prospective mother's husband should perform the *mitsvah* of taking the Torah scrolls out of the ark during the synagogue service.[20] Inside her house, too, doors, cupboards and drawers would be opened, with the intention that actions performed on inert objects should bring about a symbolic 'opening of the gates' through which the new human was to come into the world.[21]

Accessing such beliefs rooted in the relationship between the body and the world, however, can present a major problem for the scholar. Jewish folk culture places considerable demands on etymologists attempting to grasp its nature by exploring the provenance of the words it uses. The multilingualism of this community, which performed its religious rituals in Hebrew, spoke Yiddish for its everyday affairs, and maintained contacts with its immediate environment in the local language, causes considerable confusion in the area of its colloquial vocabulary. The task is further complicated by what are not always justified attempts to distil a purely Jewish essence from beliefs which undeniably had broader currency in a given geographical space and at a particular time.

In his book *Der oytser fun der yidisher shprakh*, Nokhem Stutshkov listed several words used to denote the body. Of these, *fleysh*, *kerper*, and *layb* are linked to the Germanic component of Yiddish, and *guf* to its Hebrew element.[22] These combined into semantic constituents expressing such notions as matter, corporeal reality (*gufniyes*, *gufish*, *kerperlekh*), fattiness, or obesity (*fleyshik*, *balaybt*, *baal-guf*). In colloquial understanding, the body was composed of two essential parts: the moist—flesh and blood—and the dry—skin and bones. The human being was 'flesh and blood' (*bosor vedom*); it was in these two elements that the spark of life was inherent. One expression of this conviction, for instance, was the biblical prohibition of eating life-blood (Gen. 9: 4). As mentioned in Chapter 1 above, a ruddy appearance, which was the external evidence of a fullness of flesh and blood, was the best sign of health in popular understanding. Withering

---

[20] Rosenberg, *Rafa'el hamalakh*, 62; *Segulot urefuot*, JTS, MS 9862, 82.
[21] See e.g. Yunis, 'The Old Homeland' (Yid.), 71.
[22] Stutshkov, *Thesaurus of the Yiddish Language* (Yid.), 175.

and wasting, by contrast, were the clearest symptoms of sickness and dying. A 'dry' person (*dar*) was lacking in flesh, he was a 'handful of bones' (*a hoyfn beyner*), or 'skin and bones' (*hoyt un beyner*). Naturally, both elements were necessary for the proper functioning of the body. Like their Slavic neighbours, the Jews saw in the human skeleton an analogy with the pillars supporting the structure of a house, and as such it should be as strong as iron (*ayzerne beyner*) or stones (a comparison further amplified by the rhyme between the words *shteyn* and *beyn*).

Bones were not the only elements of the anatomy that were associated with rocks and iron. Teeth ought also to be close to the folk ideal of *vayse perelekh* (white pearls). Like animals' canine teeth, they were seen as a kind of weapon—anyone born with teeth was reminiscent of a bloodthirsty vampire, so it was believed that they would grow up to be a murderer[23] or a witch (feeding on human flesh),[24] and when they died they would be buried differently from others—face down.[25] Conversely, a lack of teeth in young children was considered a symptom of their susceptibility to attack by the forces of evil; for this reason, great significance was attached to the teething period, and it was thought that until a child had all its teeth it should not be exposed to danger (for example to moonlight, or to its own reflection in a mirror),[26] kissed on the mouth, or lifted above one's head.[27] In the folk imagination there was also a link between lack of teeth and inability to talk. If a child was late to start talking, one of the remedies was to have a wise woman or *royfe* make incisions in its gums. Moreover, it was believed that until a child had its teeth it should not be given fish to eat, since 'fish have no voice'.[28] The loss of the milk teeth was the time for a ritual intended to ensure that the child grew healthy, strong new teeth. The milk tooth would be cast into the fire, and the stove (or, more often, the 'mouse'—an animal commonly associated with healthy teeth[29]) addressed with the words: 'Take

[23] Lilientalowa, *Dziecko żydowskie*, 30.

[24] Lew, 'O lecznictwie i przesądach', *Izraelita*, 38, p. 363. 'Of one born with teeth and a tail they say it will eat people, and may be killed. The sage told them: remove its teeth from its mouth, and its tail . . . and it will not be able to cause harm' (Judah Hehasid, *Sefer ḥasidim*, 136).

[25] Lilientalowa, 'Wierzenia, przesądy i praktyki', 109.

[26] See e.g. Pulner, 'Obryadi i povirya', 111; Sosnovik, 'Material on Jewish Folk Medicine in Belarus' (Yid.), 167; Fayvushinski, 'The Folklore of Pruzhana' (Yid.), 204.

[27] An-sky, *The Yiddish Ethnographic Programme* (Yid.), 48.

[28] Weissenberg, 'Kinderfreud und -leid bei den südrussischen Juden', 316.

[29] For this reason, for strong teeth it was recommended that one should eat bread nibbled by a mouse; Dan, 'Die Juden in der Bukowina', 178; Robinsohn, 'Tierglaube bei Juden Galiziens',

this tooth of bone, and give me a tooth of iron',[30] or 'give me a tooth of stone'.[31]

Analogies were likewise drawn between processes in nature, such as the sprouting of seeds or grains sown in the earth, and human growth and development. As already noted, according to the Midrash, the body of Adam had been formed from earth or clay mixed with water. This conviction was reinforced by the experience that even the soil could not live and bring forth life without moisture. In eastern Europe people would take their children out in the rain and take their caps and bonnets off to make them grow like young grass. One popular folk song called on God to send down rain specifically for the children: *Got, got, gib a regn, fun dayne kleyne kinder vegn*.[32] And, according to some sources, both May rain[33] and the herbs that grew after spring downpours were tried and tested hair-growth stimulants.[34] Likewise, the perspiration caused by running a fever at this time of year (*mayove kadokhes*) was considered gentle and good for the body.[35] Analogies were often drawn between humans and trees. When a young man was maturing it was said that his face became covered with boyish fluff, and by the time he was an old Jew he had a snow-white beard that 'spread out like the branches of a tree'. Humans shared two further characteristics with trees: their vertical posture and their height. A man of great stature was 'as tall as a tree' (*hoykh vi a boym*), while a large gathering would be referred to as a 'forest of people' (*a vald mit mentshn*), and of a child demonstrating similar traits to its parents it would be said that 'the apple

48; Sosnowik, 'Material on Jewish Folk Medicine in Belarus' (Yid.); Fayvushinski, 'The Folklore of Pruzhana' (Yid.), 203; 'Omens and Remedies' (Yid.), 285. Cf. Hovorka and Kronfeld (eds.), *Vergleichende Volksmedizin*, 856; Szukiewicz, 'Wierzenia i praktyki ludowe', 439.

[30] Sosnowik, 'Material on Jewish Folk Medicine in Belarus' (Yid.), 168; Grunwald, 'Aus unseren Sammlungen. II', 7; Lilientalowa, *Dziecko żydowskie*, 46. One form of protection from toothache was to wear a ring made from a bent nail taken from a horseshoe found by chance—perhaps in order to make the tooth as strong as iron. See Weissenberg, 'Krankheit und Tod bei den südrussischen Juden', 358; Sosnowik, 'Material on Jewish Folk Medicine in Belarus' (Yid.), 167.         [31] Yoffie, 'Popular Beliefs and Customs', 391.

[32] Ginzburg and Marek (eds.), *Yevrieiskaya narodnaya piesni v Rossiyi*, 90. See Elzet [Złotnik], 'Some Jewish Customs' (Heb.), 368; Weissenberg, 'Beiträge zur Volkskunde der Juden', 130. Lilientalowa, 'Wierzenia, przesądy i praktyki', 169; Buchbinder, 'Jewish Omens' (Yid.), 258.

[33] Veynig, 'Doctors and Medicine in Jewish Sayings' (Yid.), 21.

[34] Sosnowik, 'Material on Jewish Folk Medicine in Belarus' (Yid.), 165; cf. Hovorka and Kronfeld (eds.), *Vergleichende Volksmedizin*, 162.

[35] Nonetheless, proverbs indicate that the blessing of a May fever was one that people did try to avoid; see Pirozhnikov, *Yidishe shprikhverter*, 122; I. Bernstein, *Jewish Proverbs and Sayings* (Yid.), 231.

doesn't fall far from the tree' (*Dos epele falt nisht vayt fun beymele*). In the kabbalistic literature the following verse from the book of Deuteronomy (20: 19): 'Are trees of the field human to withdraw before you into the besieged city?' is being quoted to support this notion. Neither was it a coincidence that one of the most popular symbols in Jewish sepulchral art was a severed or broken tree stump.[36] The similarity between trees and humans was extended to a range of health-related convictions: like a tree, the human body could be felled, become infested with parasites, and become covered with growths such as *vortslen* (warts; this word in Yiddish is the same as the word for roots), *gersht* (styes; also the word for barley), and *royz* (erysipelas; also the word for rose). Pregnant women were warned not to step over cracked or fissured thresholds, or go near lumberjacks, for fear their child would be born with a hare lip.[37] By analogy, stepping over an axe would cause the child to be gap-toothed.[38] On occasion expectant mothers were also warned against stepping over bundles of kindling for fear of the umbilical cord becoming twisted around the child's neck and strangling it (like the hangman's noose, which was in turn suggested by the cord binding the kindling).[39]

The bond between the human body and the earth came to the fore in certain therapeutic practices. Earth (soil) was a remedy frequently employed in treating swelling, bruising, and pus-infected sites. Swollen legs would be soaked in water to which clay and salt had been added.[40] To relieve the pain of scalding, clay kneaded with Burow's solution would be laid on the affected area.[41] For nosebleeds, compresses of vinegar with an admixture of burnt brick were recommended.[42] One method of treating wounds is especially fascinating in this context, since it comprised both practical action and a magical incantation. It recommended that the patient

---

[36] See e.g. Trzciński, *Symbole i obrazy*, 53–80; Rozmus, *De Judeorum arte sepulcrali*, 157–86.

[37] Lilientalowa, 'Dziecko żydowskie', 143; Segel, 'Wierzenia i lecznictwo', 58; Bastomski, *At the Source: Jewish Proverbs* (Yid.), 109; Khayes, 'Death-Related Beliefs and Customs' (Yid.), 311. If the woman turned back, however, the child would be unharmed; Fayvushinski, 'The Folklore of Pruzhana' (Yid.), 202. Cf. Moszyński, *Kultura ludowa Słowian*, 284.

[38] Lew, 'O lecznictwie i przesądach', *Izraelita*, 38, p. 363.

[39] Pulner, 'Obryadi i povirya', 103.

[40] Sperling, *Ta'amei haminhagim oyf ivri taytsh*, ii. 107. Christian peasants reportedly copied local Jews and performed similar procedures, many of which had been recommended by tsadikim; From 'The Doctor and Domestic Remedies' (Yid.), 345.

[41] Rosenberg, *Der malekh refoel*, 25; Lilientalowa, *Dziecko żydowskie*, 66. Burow's solution is a remedy for swelling known and used since the nineteenth century.

[42] Rosenberg, *Der malekh refoel*, 16; Plaut, *Likutei ḥever ben ḥayim*, 8b; Cf. *Vade mecum*, 68–9.

sit on the ground and recite a conjuration in Yiddish which ran as follows: 'I exhort you [O wound] by heaven and earth with this conjuration, not to reach my blood or to swell, or to rankle, and that nothing bad should happen, in the name of the Lord, God of Israel, *amen selah netsaḥ netsaḥ va'ed.*'[43] It thus seems that a consequence of faith in the mythical ur-matter from which the body was made was the attribution to the earth of the ability to draw poisons out of the human body. In the folk imagination, the body and the earth could symbolically cohere, thus allowing the toxin to flow between them unhindered.

Some Jewish sources preserved conceptions of internal diseases that were based on the evaluation of similarities or oppositions noticed between symptoms, both those only felt by the sufferer and those visible to the naked eye, and other phenomena. According to Arthur Kleinman, misfortunes affecting the human body have multiple meanings and voices. The first and most immediate experience of them is influenced by the apparently 'natural' but actually culturally conditioned way in which a complaint is perceived and articulated, and also by the way it is woven into idiomatic expressions.[44] This is clearly illustrated in a story told by Sholem Aleichem about the curses used by his stepmother to call down upon him miseries such as 'swelling', 'breaking', and 'itching'. Each of these curses is a description of some physical sensation in the body. They do not have to be negative or disease-related experiences, but rather reflect phenomena observed in nature. The aspect of suffering, however, is adjoined to them within the context of the stepmother's curse.[45] Similar folk terminology was widespread in popular collections of remedies, which led to the emergence of multilingual patchwork phrases built of Hebrew, Yiddish, German, or even Slavic elements, such as *leshtekhenish baveten al yad 'luftfarshparung'* (For stabbing pains in the belly caused by 'flatulence').[46]

The vision of the human body as an organism that was affected by similar processes to those acting on plants and inanimate objects found reflection in popular terminology and anecdotes. But the consequences of this identification ran deeper, and became the grounds for speculation on symptoms and treatment methods. One prime example highlighting the extent of this issue is consumption (*sukhote*). The contemporary Yiddish literature,

[43] Rubinstein, *Zikhron ya'akov yosef*, 80a. See Goldberg and Eisenberg, *Sefer laḥashim usegulot*, 5a.

[44] Kleinman, *The Illness Narratives*, 10–18.

[45] Sholem Aleichem, *From the Fair*, 137–8.

[46] Rosenberg, *Rafa'el hamalakh*, 15.

like the Polish literature of the day, used this term almost exclusively to refer to tuberculosis. But the popular conception was that it denoted a sickness which caused rapid weight loss (the 'drying up' of the body), as reflected in one Yiddish synonym for it: *dur*, closely related to the German *dürr* (dry, brittle) and *Dürrsucht* (phthisis, physical atrophy, emaciation, cf. Pol. *dur brzuszny*—typhoid fever). These names were used interchange-ably; in the collection *Rafa'el hamalakh* they even feature in the same sentence.[47] Among the main methods of combating this wasting disease were baths, usually in combination with other types of action that often featured the motif of bread or dough, probably in view of its sacrificial character, or perhaps as a reflection of the fact that in the bread-making process dough rose and gained colour. One recommendation was to boil willow branches in 'silent water',[48] and then pour the brew into the kneading trough with a portion of leaven. After the sick child had been washed three times in this concoction, the water was to be poured out under the willow from which the branches had been taken, to the accompaniment of the following con-juration in Yiddish: 'Take this emaciation and wasting from the child X, son/daughter of Y.'[49] If the cause of the sickness was thought to be the fact that the patient had swallowed a hair or a feather, they would be given the fat of a dog spread on bread to eat, and bathed in water in which bagels had been boiled, with the addition of some hay and nine dough balls (made from flour taken from nine bakeries).[50] When the suspected cause was par-asites burrowing in the child's skin, a hot bath would be given and the para-sites scraped off the skin with a rough crust of bread.[51]

A young, energetic person with colour in their cheeks might be de-scribed as *blut un milkh*—blood and milk. In a reflection of this association, milk-based remedies were a second important element of consumption treatment among Jews. Possible ways in which milk might be served included still warm, fresh from the cow or goat; boiled with butter, wheat

[47] *Ḥoli dur hanikra gam ken 'sukhoti'* (ibid. 43).
[48] Yid. *shtilvaser, shtilshvaygende vaser*. 'Silent water' was drawn and brought into the house in silence (and usually at night) and had properties that were important for magical practices. This conviction has also been registered among Slavic peoples. See Levinski, 'Silent Water' (Heb.), 3–5.    [49] Rosenberg, *Rafa'el hamalakh*, 44.
[50] Lilientalowa, *Dziecko żydowskie*, 65. Cf. Biegeleisen, *Lecznictwo ludu polskiego*, 191. Some-times bathing in wheat bran (Lilientalowa, 'Dziecko żydowskie', 155) or in water with pierogi (Segel, 'Materyały do etnografii Żydów', 328) was also recommended.
[51] Sperling, *Ta'amei haminhagim oyf ivri taytsh*, ii. 111. For more on consumption and other wasting diseases in Slavonic folk medicine, see Paluch, 'Suchoty', 192–201.

flour, almonds, or honey; and taken on an empty stomach, or as *noytputer*, butter made by shaking a bottle of milk.[52]

The everyday observation of similarities to phenomena affecting the world of flora and fauna gave rise to the popular conviction of the presence of worms in the human body. The Polish populace—and in this respect the Jews were no different—believed that these could cause all kinds of sickness.[53] Worms not only fed on the digestive system, something of which there was widespread awareness, but also burrowed into the teeth and skin. Parasites were believed to be the cause of tooth decay; if teeth were not 'stone' or 'iron', like meat, they could easily fall prey to worms. Recommended remedies for toothache included sugar, salt, garlic, pepper (packed into the hole in the tooth), and vodka, including vodka previously poured over the above substances.[54] Smudging, a widely used technique that involved burning or roasting a plant, an object, or an animal organ to create a curative smoke, was also popular as a treatment for caries (using fool's parsley). All these remedies were believed to draw the worms out.[55] In terms of ectoparasites, one of the most dangerous, and which attacked children above all, was thought to be the *miteser*. An early version of this belief, and one that is known also from Polish and German ethnographic sources, held that these tiny mites burrowed into babies' skin (on their face and under their shoulder blades), in time causing wasting. In their removal, sugar or honey would be employed, which, in combination with hot baths, were thought to encourage them to 'stick their heads out', and they would then be 'decapitated' with a knife or other blade. By the early twentieth century these parasites were no longer known by the name derived from German folklore and early modern medicine. The only vestige of this word remained in the saying 'to eat as if one had a *miteser*',[56] denoting a child with a voracious appetite.[57]

Animals were also of considerable significance in folk medicine in view of the analogies perceived between the anatomy of certain species and that

[52] Lew, 'O lecznictwie i przesądach', *Izraelita*, 49, p. 476.

[53] Biegeleisen, *Lecznictwo ludu polskiego*, 4; Moszyński, *Kultura ludowa Słowian*, 181–2.

[54] *Refuot ha'am im darkhei yesharim*, 15; Lilientalowa, 'Dziecko żydowskie', 153; Rosenberg, *Rafa'el hamalakh*, 95; Sosnowik, 'Material on Jewish Folk Medicine in Belarus' (Yid.), 167; 'Various Medicaments for Toothache' (Yid.), 70; Shlaferman, 'The Folklore, Customs, and Stories of Kazimierz' (Yid.), 173; cf. *Apteka domowa i podróżna*, 9.

[55] Sosnowik, 'Material on Jewish Folk Medicine in Belarus' (Yid.), 168.

[56] The word *miteser* translates as 'fellow eater'; Lilientalowa, *Dziecko żydowskie*, 68.

[57] See Tuszewicki, 'O pasożytach wywołujących suchoty', 613–34.

of humans. People, however, realized that, despite the similarities, animals' organs or body parts often differed in their functioning from those of humans. This idea, in turn, was superimposed onto convictions regarding the characteristic traits attributed to various members of the animal kingdom. From antiquity, for instance, swallows had been considered keen-sighted, hens to be prone to blindness (hence: *zukhn vi a blinde hun a kerndl*;[58] cf. Pol. *trafić się jak ślepej kurze ziarno*—(of a benefit) to come to someone like a grain to a blind hen), and hares (or rabbits) to be prodigiously fertile. Medical recommendations in the traditional Jewish community in eastern Europe included numerous references to such convictions. Thus treatment advice for 'tissue on the eye' (macular pucker) was as follows: to gouge out the eye of a young swallow, and when its mother dressed the wound with grass (swallowwort), to cut off the young bird's head and burn it to ash. Next, a silver coin should be placed in the heap of ash and then laid on the affected site.[59] 'Chicken blindness' was an affliction that could be contracted by anyone who went out after dark to check whether their hen had laid an egg (hens were said to lose their sight in such circumstances) or who drank from a vessel from which a hen had also drunk.[60] Atrophy and infertility were treated using various parts of a hare's body, such as the stomach, heart, testicles, and fat.[61] Similar examples are legion, and the catalogue of potential ingredients of remedies encompassed not only body parts of the animal, but also objects with which it had come into contact and which were thus thought to assume its 'powers' in a symbolic sense. For instance, a hen's egg rolled over an infected or painful site was said to be able to absorb the sickness. According to Max Weinreich, in Belarus the egg would be rolled this way and that until the white grew opaque, which was believed to indicate that it had been 'saturated' with the sickness.[62] Henryk Lew believed that it was applied, by rubbing on children's eyes, both therapeutically and prophylactically.[63] The popular imagination was also inspired by

---

[58] Mark, 'A Collection of Folk Comparisons' (Yid.), 122.

[59] Rosenberg, *Der malekh refoel*, 10. This method was known to both ancient and early modern European medicine; see e.g. *Culpeper's Complete Herbal*, 43.

[60] Lilientalowa, 'Wierzenia, przesądy i praktyki', 166; 'Omens and Remedies' (Yid.), 279; Fayvushinski, 'The Folklore of Pruzhana' (Yid.), 200.

[61] See e.g. Goldberg and Eisenberg, *Sefer laḥashim usegulot*, 15b; *Segulot urefuot*, JTS, MS 9862, 23; Simner, *Zekhirah*, 53b; Ochana, *Mareh hayeladim*, 34b; Wilff, *Imrot shelomoh*, 97–8.

[62] See Weinreich's preface to Sosnowik, 'Material on Jewish Folk Medicine in Belarus' (Yid.), 172. See too Kotik, *My Memoirs* (Yid.), 219–20; Podbereski, 'Materyały do demonologii ludu Ukraińskiego', 68.          [63] Lew, 'O lecznictwie i przesądach', *Izraelita*, 41, p. 394.

different forms of animal behaviour, such as bird calls. Counting a cuckoo's cries as a method of foretelling how many years of life one had left is mentioned in a popular song about Sarah: *Zog mir feygele du mayn, vi lang vet mayn lebn zayn?* (Little bird of mine, tell me, how long will my life be?).[64]

Knowledge gleaned from observation of the animal world prompted people to exploit the habitual behaviour of animals in therapeutic practices. It was therefore recommended that in order to remove a flea from a human ear one should offer it some dog hair as an alternative,[65] and it was thought that certain types of worm could be tempted with a lettuce leaf.[66] On occasion, some other characteristic of an animal (such as its appearance) served as the basis for the remedy, and in this respect the role of animals differed little from that of mineral or vegetable substances. Raphael Patai noted that fish were considered a phallic symbol in view of their shape (an opinion supported by sources including the commentaries of Rashi), which contributed to their immense popularity as a fertility aid.[67] The same associations were probably behind the use of animal horns in remedies for male impotence caused by spells, in aids to conception, and in tinctures used to ease difficult births;[68] substances from horses or mares (or donkeys or jennies) were likewise given for similar conditions.[69]

Regarding the application of solid objects such as stones or nuts, note should be taken of the multidimensional approach to the question of similarity in the sphere of magic practices. The way in which they were used in the treatment process depended on the mental connection that existed between aspects of a given sickness—its name, symptoms, and impact on the patient's life—and the properties of the potential remedy or its ingredients. The simplest example illustrating this is that of 'whispering' shells, which were used in treating tinnitus.[70] Amulets from 'eagle stone'—a stone with one or more smaller stones inside it—were worn as protection against miscarriage. The Jewish populace tended to believe stones of this type to

---

[64] Pozniak and Laufer (eds.), *This Is How We Sang* (Yid.), 112–13; see e.g. Gustawicz, 'Podania, przesądy, gadki i nazwy ludowe', 144.   [65] Lilientalowa, *Choroby, lecznictwo*, fo. 139.
[66] Horowitz, *Anaf ḥayim*, 48.   [67] Patai, 'Jewish Folk-Cures for Barrenness, II', 208–10.
[68] Berger, *Imrei yisra'el*, 13a; Wilff, *Imrot shelomoh*, 101; Lukianovski, *Yad shalom*, 78–9; Lifshits, *Segulot yisra'el*, 78b–79a; Plaut, *Likutei ḥever ben ḥayim*, 7a; Patai, 'Jewish Folk-Cures for Barrenness, II', 216.
[69] Above all hair or fur and dung; see *Segulot vekameyot*, JTS, MS 10082, 3b; *Segulot urefuot*, JTS, MS 9862, 23, 79; Goldberg and Eisenberg, *Sefer laḥashim usegulot*, 15b; Rosenberg, *Rafa'el hamalakh*, 63; Wilff, *Imrot shelomoh*, 101; Plaut, *Likutei ḥever ben ḥayim*, 7a.
[70] Weissenberg, *Krankheit und Tod*, 358.

be *shternshis*, shooting stars. From the angle of folk medicine what is most important here is the similarity between the shape of the pregnant woman's belly and that of the stone. Just as teeth could be either as strong as stone or as soft and weak as meat, so a woman's womb might be strengthened by virtue of her wearing a 'stone' amulet.[71] Jewish sources treat this remedy very seriously, and rabbinic authorities wrote extensively about its benefits in cases when miscarriage was a threat; the *Kitsur shulḥan arukh* permitted it to be worn on the sabbath.[72] In fact, there are a considerable number of conflicting testimonies surrounding the issue of exactly what *shternshis* was. Some maintained that it was bluish in colour;[73] others said that it was red,[74] and identified it as ruby[75] or topaz.[76] Another example of a similar talisman was a double nut: by eating one of these a woman might expect its dominant characteristic—its duality—to be passed on to her foetus; that is, she would have twins.[77] Foremost among stones with unique properties was a magnetic stone, which was used to help sustain pregnancies, and towards the end to move the baby down and thus facilitate its entrance into the world.[78]

It was plants that were of the greatest importance in folk healing, however. Certain afflictions had 'botanic' names related to their appearance, such as styes ('barley') or localized redness caused by burst blood vessels ('raspberry'), and the similarity this represented was justification enough for the firm conviction that they had a similar incubation period to the vegetation period of their vegetal namesakes. The method for curing a stye almost invariably required the use of a real grain of barley, which, according

[71] A brief description of the use of *shternshis* is given in Hurwitz, *Sefer haberit* (Yid.), 22. Many other sources aver that *shternshis* is the 'eagle stone' known since the days of Dioscorides; see e.g. Shlaferman, 'The Folklore, Customs, and Stories of Kazimierz' (Yid.), 173; Klein, *A Time To Be Born*, 38. This is also how it is identified in Preuss, *Biblisch-talmudische Medizin*, 446.

[72] Ganzfried, *Kitsur shulḥan arukh*, 84: 19.

[73] Lilientalowa, 'Zjawiska przyrody w wyobrażeniu', 62; ead., *Dziecko żydowskie*, 20; ead., 'Kult ciał niebieskich u starożytnych Hebrajczyków', 15.

[74] See Opatoshu, *A Day in Regensburg* (Yid.), 76–7.

[75] Klein, *A Time To Be Born*, 41–2; Trachtenberg, *Jewish Magic and Superstition*, 137.

[76] In this interpretation the biblical name *tarshish* was to have become distorted into *shternshis*; Pulner, 'Obryadi i povirya', 102.

[77] An-sky, *The Yiddish Ethnographic Programme* (Yid.), 20. It was also believed that a woman would give birth to twins if she ate a double apple or any other 'double' fruit; Lilientalowa, 'Wierzenia, przesądy i praktyki', 158. Double fruits or vegetables were also sometimes considered aids to conception; 'Omens and Remedies' (Yid.), 294.

[78] Wilff, *Imrot shelomoh*, 97; Lilientalowa, 'Wierzenia, przesądy i praktyki', 163; *Segulot urefuot*, JTS, MS 9862, 65.

to some sources, had to be stolen.[79] The procedure would be performed either before sunrise or after sunset, and it involved three repetitions of a dialogue 'refuting' the existence of the complaint and touching or circling the affected site with the barley or other cereal (sometimes with nine grains), which would subsequently be carefully buried or thrown into someone else's garden.[80]

A second reason for the ubiquity of plants as remedies was the fact that there was a broad selection of them readily available. They were used to make a variety of juices, tinctures, and preserves, which would be given at the first suggestion of illness. Although folk medicine is usually associated with herbs gathered by the healers themselves, for the period around 1900 this assumption would give a very inaccurate picture. Aside from plants grown in gardens, others were also used which could only be sourced by going further afield—into pastureland, woodland, or down to the river, for instance. It should not come as a surprise, then, that a considerable proportion of such ingredients was purchased, whether from traders (many of them non-Jews) or in stores selling imported goods, in perfumeries, or in pharmacies.

The use of various types of seeds (sunflower, flax, or poppy seeds, to be swallowed) for the treatment of infertility suggests a link with the concepts of multiplicity and giving birth.[81] The matrimonial handbook *Imrot shelomoh* likened a woman's womb to the soil, in which seed had to be sown, and drew attention to the talmudic mention of male and female seed.[82] There is also the ambiguous phonetic similarity of the words *mon* (poppy) and *man* (husband), which may have amplified interest in poppy seeds as a remedy 'for children'. Among the plant remedies used by the Jews were some of a relatively obvious apotropaic character (garlic, onion, common rue, and asafoetida, or devil's dung), but in many cases it seems impossible to identify an unequivocal reason for the choice of particular herbal medicines. Many of them had been in widespread use in European culture since ancient times. To induce menstrual bleeding, for instance, which could be tantamount to aborting a foetus, the herb savin juniper, already known to Dioscorides, was recommended (steeped and drunk like tea),[83] as, possibly,

---

[79] Fels, 'Zabobony lekarskie u Żydów', 5.          [80] Lilientalowa, 'Dziecko żydowskie', 154.
[81] *Segulot urefuot*, Bibliotheca Rosenthaliana, HS. ROS. 444, 4*b*; Silverman-Weinreich, 'Beliefs' (Yid.), 33.                               [82] BT *Nid.* 31*a*; Wilff, *Imrot shelomoh*, 63.
[83] Rosenberg, *Rafa'el hamalakh*, 31. Cf. Dioscorides, *De materia medica*, 102.

were substances obtained from the cherry tree.[84] A vast quantity of preparations of this type was used in early modern medicine, and even in biomedicine. Thus the advised remedy for swollen legs was to rub them with
tincture of wormwood,[85] and coughs were treated with marsh mallow
syrup.[86] Jewish sources often published similar recipes with annotations
claiming as their sources tsadikim, doctors, or pharmacists.

Although herbs were not considered particularly powerful as remedies
in themselves, their strength could be amplified by means of a variety of
manipulations—gathering the herbs at a particular time of day (for example
at dawn) or of the year (in the spring; at the flowering of cereal crops;[87] for
bilberries in the week of the reading of the 'Korah' Torah portion—at the
turn of June and July[88]), or in specific places (in a cemetery, by a boundary
stone)—or by their having been in contact with objects of great magical
potency (such as sacred texts), and so on. Indeed, sometimes it was only
these latter circumstances that rendered a given plant useful as a remedy
at all. Other product types, for example of mineral or animal origin, underwent similar transformations in the folk imagination. The importance
attached to the place where they were acquired is illustrated in the following recommendations regarding dust, powder, or soil. Dust collected from
underneath the threshold or ashes from the stove took on magical properties in view of the position of these features within the house, and in the
latter case undoubtedly also due to the stove's assumption of the characteristics of fire.[89] Gathered from beneath the feet of a rabbi reciting the Ami-

---

[84] Jewish sources mention especially cherry bark in this context; see *Segulot urefuot*, Bibliotheca Rosenthaliana, HS. ROS. 444, 6*a*; Plaut, *Likutei ḥever ben ḥayim*, 8*b*; Petrovsky-Shtern,
*The Golden Age Shtetl*, 213. Bark brews were used to induce menstruation by ethnic populations
including Belarusian women; cf. Wereńko, 'Przyczynek do lecznictwa ludowego', 111.
Dioscorides mentions juice of the Chamaedaphne fruit (round and red, identified as cherries),
which, in combination with wine, was said to help expel menstrual blood; *De materia medica*,
696.

[85] *Segulot urefuot*, Bibliotheca Rosenthaliana, HS. ROS. 444, 14*a*. Cf. Haur, *Ekonomika
lekarska*, 203; *Vade mecum*, 68.

[86] Sperling, *Ta'amei haminhagim oyf ivri taytsh*, ii. 116; Lilientalowa, 'Dziecko żydowskie',
153; Cf. *Vade mecum*, 76.

[87] Reuben ben Abraham, *Sefer derekh yesharah*, 81*a*; *Segulot urefuot*, JTS, MS 9862, 18.

[88] Num. 16: 1–18: 32. Berries were said to have grown in the place where Korah was swallowed up by the earth; Ben-Ezra, 'Customs' (Yid.), 172. One Jewish proverb interpreted the
name of this biblical figure as an acronym: *Az es geyt a sidre koyrekh, kumt oyf: karshn, retekh,
khreyn* (When the Korah passage comes, cherries, radishes, and horseradish grow); I. Bernstein, *Jewish Proverbs and Sayings* (Yid.), 248.

[89] According to various testimonies, earth from under the threshold offered protection from

dah prayer in the synagogue, dust invited unequivocal associations with the piety of prayer and, drunk with water, could be used to treat infertility.[90] Soil from a cemetery bore connotations of death and the other world, and was perceived to be a bearer of attributes of both this world and the next. It might be considered particularly useful if it came from the grave of a pious person; such figures would often be petitioned for intercession in heaven.[91] One source recommended as a cure for insomnia was the application to the patient's temples of compresses made from earth from beneath three walls of their own house,[92] perhaps in the belief that the earth had absorbed one of the traditional attributes of stone—silence—and that the magic number three would lend additional power to this remedy.[93]

Another important factor that could influence the effect of a substance intended as therapeutic was the time of day at which it was gathered. This was the case for many plants and also for 'silent water', all of which required a pre-dawn foray, but also for some objects that had been used in festive rituals (for instance an *etrog* or willow twigs for *hoshanot*, which were subsequently utilized for medicinal purposes). The time at which a therapeutic procedure was conducted might also be of significance; this might depend on several factors, not all of which were magical—for example a draught might have to be taken first thing in the morning, on an empty stomach. The therapeutic properties of a given remedy might be connected with the amount to be taken (a handful, or a specific quantity related to the numbers three, seven, or nine) or with the way in which it was obtained. Objects used in magic rituals had to be purchased without haggling, for the first price offered. Perhaps this meant that they were perceived to be closer to 'nature' (raw, or new); the same may have been true of items that were stolen or found by accident rather than looked for. In the popular imagination finding an object by chance might ensure that it retained its original properties, which were vital for ensuring its therapeutic efficacy. Another factor of

---

charms (Lilientalowa, *Dziecko żydowskie*, 49), difficult childbirth (Lifshits, *Berit avot*, 3*a*), and convulsions (Berger, *Imrei yisra'el*, 9*b*). Earth from under the stove—in earlier sources referred to by the German word *Backenofen* (Plaut, *Likutei ḥever ben ḥayim*, 8*b*)—was also an ingredient of one panacea.

[90] Rotner, *Sipurei nifla'ot*, 13.

[91] *Segulot urefuot*, Bibliotheca Rosenthaliana, HS. ROS. 444, 7*a*.

[92] *Refuot ha'am im darkhei yesharim*, 13.

[93] As the saying went, *Dray mol iz tsu gezunt* (Three times is for health); Einhorn, 'Folk Proverbs' (Heb.), 406.

particular significance for the potency of all manner of remedies was the magic formulas accompanying their application.[94] The fact that there were so many variables makes the chain of cause and effect in the therapeutic process seem extremely complex. This, compounded by the laconic character of some ethnographic sources, can render the rediscovery of the meanings behind the actions performed impossible. The various circumstances were nonetheless rarely entirely detached from the prevailing vision of cosmic order and its reflection in the structure and functions of the human body.

[94] See Libera, *Medycyna ludowa*, 51; Wasilewski, 'Po śmierci wędrować', 80–1.

# CHAPTER SEVEN

# HUMORAL PATHOLOGY

THE LINKS between the microcosm and macrocosm that are evident in so many aspects of folk beliefs and therapeutic practices formed a natural reservoir for theories which evolved in various parts of the world. In Mediterranean culture, for centuries a prominent theory was that of humoral pathology, which had emerged in ancient Greece. It was a vision of the four elements—air, water, fire, and earth—as the foundation for the Hippocratic model of the four humours—blood, phlegm, yellow bile, and black bile—and the correspondent catalogue of four types of remedy: warming, moistening, drying, and cooling. Humoral pathology, rather than seeking the roots of illness in some disobedience to divine will, focused on nature. According to Hippocrates (c.460–377 BCE) and his school, the fundamental cause of physical indisposition lay in the body itself. This represented a radical break with theurgic medicine, which was controlled by priestly circles. It held that states of illness developed as a result of an imbalance in the natural proportions of internal fluids, and their treatment was based on restoring the right proportions. In this system both prognoses and recommended therapies—which were based primarily on natural substances, whether in their simplest form or processed in some way, and also on procedures designed to eliminate excess humours—were closely linked to cosmology. In other words, they were linked to the way in which the experience of the macrocosm was transposed into action taken in respect of its reflection in the human body.

The emergence of this explicitly rational interpretation of the art of medicine was made possible by the intellectual ferment of the ancient Greek world. Developed by Alexandrian and Roman physicians, and supported by the authority of philosophers and thinkers, it came to form the foundation of European medicine. In time, it became fused with the culture of the people of that continent to such an extent that teasing its strands apart from the tangle of symbols and meanings surrounding it today is extremely difficult. Throughout the Middle Ages and the early modern age the conviction that the elements of which the wider world is composed are also the formative components of the human body and have a definitive role in character formation spread beyond the intellectual elites. In Ashkenaz it was expressed on the pages of ethical works and halakhic literature, not to mention medical manuals both printed and handwritten.[1] The Talmud rarely made overt reference to humoral theory, though one direct link to it may be perceived in the sentence: 'At the head of all sickness am I, Blood' (BT *BB* 58*b*), and there are a few other similar passages. Explicit references to opinions of physicians who subscribed to the humoral theory were far more numerous, however. Outside the Talmud, too, humoral theory put down strong roots in Jewish culture and remained a presence over the ages. It is traceable in early *midrashim*, probably inspired by ancient philosophy. The name Adam was explicated as a compound formed from the initials of the words *efer* (dust), *dam* (blood), and *marah* (bile). These were believed to be the component elements of the human body, and disturbance of the harmony between them could have serious consequences.[2] It is worth adding that rabbinic, and later also hasidic, homiletics perceived a connection between the theory of the elements, God, and the human body. The *Ta'amei haminhagim*, a book of customs, citing the opus of one of the early hasidic leaders, Barukh of Międzybóż (grandson of the Ba'al Shem Tov), gave the following explanation for the meaning of the words *refuah shelemah min hashamayim*—the customary good wish addressed to a sick person:

The reason why in praying for a cure we are asking God to send down *full healing from heaven*. Why do we not formulate other requests in the same way? Because humans were created from four elements: earth, wind, fire, and water. And the fact that someone, God forbid, falls ill is due to an imbalance of these elements. One becomes dominant over another and there is no peace between them. For we read: 'God called the expanse Sky' [Gen. 1: 8] . . . Rashi says: The sky [*shamayim*] is fire [*esh*] and water [*mayim*]. Even fire and water are in opposition to each other, for water quenches fire, so God brought peace between them and made them into sky. And this is why we ask for full healing [*refuah shelemah*], as he made peace [*shalom*] in heaven. In this way we are adding 'from the sky' [*min hashamayim*].[3]

[1] Zimmels, *Magicians, Theologians and Doctors*, 78–80.
[2] Graves and Patai, *Hebrew Myths. The Book of Genesis*, 60–1.
[3] Sperling, *Ta'amei haminhagim oyf ivri taytsh*, ii. 14–15.

*Altsding darf zayn mit a mos* (Everything should be in moderation),[4] it was said in Yiddish, in an expression of the belief that equilibrium in all things was of key importance in every aspect of life. In traditional Jewish society the belief that sickness was a visible sign of an imbalance in the inner harmony of the body remained widespread until the twentieth century. The theory of human temperaments presented in the Mishnah (*Avot* 5: 11) divided them into four types: the person who is easy to anger and easy to calm; the one who is hard to anger but also hard to calm; the one who is hard to anger and easy to calm (this is the pious person); and the type who is easy to anger and hard to calm (the evil person). The nineteenth-century Moravian rabbi Joachim Pollak, in his book *Mekor ḥayim*, explains the talmudic division of the temperaments in full accord with the theory of the humours, attributing to each type one of the following names in Yiddish: *zangviniker, melankholiker, flegmatiker*, and *kholerishe*.[5] These concepts became integrated into popular culture and entered the vernacular language. A woman suffering from mood swings would be dubbed a *more-shkhoyrenitse*, because the Yiddish word *more-shkhoyre* (Heb. *marah sheḥorah*, black bile) was the equivalent of the Greek term *melankholia*. Descriptions of someone's actions as phlegmatic (*flegmatish*), or of a person as a *kholer-nik*, became firmly lodged in Yiddish phraseology.

In both Jewish medicine and rabbinic literature, views on the elements, the humours, and the temperaments were concordant with the dominant conceptions across Europe and in the Middle East. As Hagit Matras, a researcher of the *segulot urefuot* books published among the Ashkenazim, has noted, the visions of the world these works reflect combined to form an image of a hierarchized, co-ordinated system. This was to a large extent a consequence of the perception of human beings as a representation of the cosmos on a micro scale, and more precisely of the humoral vision of humanity developed by Hippocrates and Galen (*c.*130–*c.*210 CE).[6] The presence of the humoral theory in Jewish folk beliefs around 1900 may not have been, as Izrael Fels claimed, merely a 'vestige' of early scientific medicine.[7] In fact, until the most recent times it was a significant element of most popular publications cited in traditional health and medical manuals

---

[4] Einhorn, 'Folk Proverbs' (Heb.), 345.

[5] Pollak, *Mekor ḥayim*, 92a. Pollak's book is a commentary on Isaac Arama's fifteenth-century philosophical treatise, *Akedat yitsḥak*.

[6] Matras, 'Wholeness and Holiness in Sifrei Segulot', 99.          [7] See p. 103 above.

in both Hebrew and Yiddish. It was in evidence in the medical treatises of authors including the perennial authority Moses Maimonides. It was analysed in popular encyclopaedias such as the medieval *Shevilei emunah* and the early modern *Ma'aseh tuvyah*. When the author of one vademecum published in Hungary in the late nineteenth century tackled the problem of verrucas (Heb. *yavelet*), it was the *Shevilei emunah* that he cited in his description: 'The verruca, in Arabic *talula*, and in Latin *verruca*, is a secondary body on the skin, in particular the hands and feet. And there are two types thereof: the soft and painful, of white phlegm, and the hard, this from black bile.'[8] Humoral pathology was the foremost interpretation of human physiology until the Enlightenment (*Sefer haberit*), and remained a presence on many levels for a long time thereafter. Aaron Bernstein (1812–84) wrote about the temperaments in German in his *Naturwissenschaftliche Volksbücher*, which were translated into Yiddish and published at the beginning of the twentieth century.[9]

With the rise of biomedicine, memory of the origins of many views and practices derived from humoral pathology faded. Nonetheless, like the temperaments, they remained a presence in colloquial phraseology. Blood was considered to be the most important component of the human body; as mentioned above, without it the body would dry out and die. Blood was seen not only as the seat of the soul, but also as the medium of kinship (*blut iz nit keyn vaser*, blood is not water).[10] It reflected the most powerful and intimate experiences, from friendship (*blutfraynd*) to hatred (*blutfaynt*). The source of blood was thought to be the heart, where, according to the humoral interpretation of anatomy expounded in *Sefer haberit*, it underwent fermentation.[11] The same organ was also credited with a connection to feelings, wisdom ('He whose heart is wise accepts commands'; Prov. 10: 8), and memory ('Keep them in your mind' (Heb. *betokh levavekha*, lit. inside your heart); Prov. 4: 21). A person who could keep their immediate urges and desires in check was described as 'cold-blooded' (*kaltblutik*), as opposed to someone who followed the voice of their heart (*heysblutik*). In terms of health, this humour was said to be indicative of vitality, give the body colour, and fill it to overflowing with energy. An anaemic person would be said to be suffering from 'poverty of blood' (*blutoremkayt*); a healthy person

---

[8] Lifshits, *Segulot yisra'el*, 50b.

[9] A. Bernstein, *Bernstein's Popular Books on the Natural Sciences* (Yid.), xii. 47–55.

[10] I. Bernstein, *Jewish Proverbs and Sayings* (Yid.), 31; Stutshkov, *Thesaurus of the Yiddish Language* (Yid.), 175.        [11] Hurwitz, *Sefer haberit* (Yid.), 48–9.

was 'full-blooded' (*fulblutik*). Many patients, however, were diagnosed not so much with a lack of blood as with 'bad blood' (*shlekhte blut*). Ridding the body of such blood was believed to be the first step on the road to recovery.

Until the end of the nineteenth century, bloodletting procedures were hugely popular across almost every stratum of Jewish society. These took a variety of forms, from opening veins and wet cupping (*gehakte bankes*)—application of cupping glasses to skin into which shallow incisions had previously been made—to the use of leeches (*piyavkes, eglen*). The circumstances in which these procedures would be performed varied according to the interpretation of the cause of the 'bad blood'. It was sometimes thought to have been caused by poisoning, for instance as a result of a bite from a rabid dog[12] or a snake.[13] In other situations, bloodletting might be used for headaches[14] or eye pains,[15] which might be due to poor diet or natural humour fermentation processes. According to folk medicine, blood quality might also be affected by factors such as the season, the weather, and the influence of astral bodies. All this often prompted people to have the above procedures performed as part of their regular prophylactic care. The author of *Sefer haberit* wrote about the practice of opening haemorrhoids (*meridn*),[16] which was considered to be a highly beneficial procedure, and anyone whose haemorrhoids had not opened naturally by the age of around 28 was thought to have no option but to visit a physician for leeches. Nonetheless, Jewish sources also contain significant quantities of information on remedies for assuaging or curing haemorrhoids. These remedies were mostly natural in character, comprising baths and various types of topical ointment (containing, for instance, egg whites and alum).[17]

Aside from procedures usually associated with the barber-surgeon or feldsher's line of work, folk culture also had a large arsenal of other

[12] Rosenberg, *Der malekh refoel*, 28.
[13] Rosenberg, *Rafa'el hamalakh*, 47; id., *Der malekh refoel*, 27.
[14] *Segulot urefuot*, Bibliotheca Rosenthaliana, HS. ROS. 444, 9*b*; *Refuot ha'am im darkhei yesharim*, 5.  [15] *Refuot ha'am im darkhei yesharim*, 11.
[16] Haemorrhoids were so common among Polish Jews that there was even a Yiddish saying, *A yidishe yerushe iz gildene oder* (Haemorrhoids are a Jew's inheritance). See Cahan, *The Jew on Himself and Others* (Yid.), 11; M. P., 'Jüdische Sprichwörter und Redensarten aus Öst.-Ungarn', 43. Cf. Ger. *goldene Adern*, Pol. *złota żyła* (the golden vein); Jerzy Klus, *Neues Taschenwörterbuch deutsch–polnisch und polnisch–deutsch*, 290. A few prescriptions for *di gildene oder* are to be found in publications including the pamphlet *Sha'ar efrayim* (26*b*–27*a*) and Barukh of Shklov, *Derekh yesharah*, 5*b*.
[17] Hurwitz, *Sefer haberit hashalem*, 161; see also Rosenberg, *Rafa'el hamalakh*, 38–9; *Segulot urefuot*, JTS, MS 9862, 73, 89, 106. Cf. Haur, *Ekonomika lekarska*, 212.

methods designed to draw the sickness out of the body along with the blood. Chickenpox (*pokn*), for instance, was widely considered to be an ailment caused by 'bad blood'. It was thought that a toxin had entered the child's body while it was still in the womb, or as a result of its mother's having nursed it during menstruation; indeed, this latter was held to be the main reason why this illness affected anyone at all.[18] The appearance of scabs on the patient's skin was nonetheless not only a symptom but also proof that the body had cleansed itself of the excess bad blood; thus such breakouts on the skin were not seen as negative, and patients were consoled that they would make them feel better. The saying that *a make iz gut* (a boil is good) even has a place in the treasury of Yiddish proverbs, albeit usually with the rueful addendum: *bay yenem untern orem* (under someone else's armpit).[19] The received advice was not to apply anything to them so as not to redirect the sickness 'back inside' and thereby cause the patient's condition to worsen.[20]

Notions of the pores of the skin as a natural exit route for corrupted humour had far-reaching consequences. In order to aid the removal of toxins, the patient had to be kept warm and given warming beverages (such as honey boiled up with ginger[21]). Interesting testimony to the firm belief of Jews that sudation (sweating) was one of the most important symptoms of recovery is found in a number of hasidic short stories, such as the one about the illness of the tsadik Mordecai ('Motl') Twersky[22] and another about the tsadik of Radzymin, who ordered walnut shells to be placed on the temples of a woman with typhus: 'After a quarter of an hour, she began to sweat, and was restored to health, to live out another nineteen years.'[23] The most common cause of aggravation of a sickness and its consequent 'escape' back inside the patient's body was catching a chill. The recommendation was that the sufferer be covered up and protected from the cold, the windows were to be shuttered, and no cold drinks should be given.[24] Similar steps were taken in the treatment not only of chickenpox and measles (Yid. *mozlen*),[25] but also of other conditions presenting with

---

[18] See e.g. Hurwitz, *Sefer haberit hashalem*, 160–1; Zimmels, *Magicians, Theologians and Doctors*, 80.          [19] I. Bernstein, *Jewish Proverbs and Sayings* (Yid.), 160.

[20] Lew, 'O lecznictwie i przesądach', *Izraelita*, 42 (1897), p. 406.          [21] Ibid. 407.

[22] *Atarat tsadikim*, 14–15.          [23] M. A. Bergman, *Ma'asiyot nora'im*, 32–3.

[24] *Segulot urefuot*, Bibliotheca Rosenthaliana, HS. ROS. 444, 3*b*; Schneersohn, *Sefer refuot*, 27; Shifman, 'Dangerous Beliefs about Measles' (Yid.), 31–2.

[25] These two diseases were often treated using the same methods, and were described in the

a fever. According to a Jewish doctor from Wołożyn (now Valozhyn, Belarus), who collected folk curios in the course of his work in the field, it was common practice to avoid changing the patient's sheets, underwear, and clothing; and washing them with clean water (even wiping their face), and even the use of cold compresses, would be forbidden. There was no question of opening the window or giving the patient a bath. By way of prophylaxis, children would ideally not be allowed outside on cold days and were kept instead in stuffy rooms with the intention of protecting them from catching colds.[26] Similar precautions were taken in the room where a woman lay in confinement; moreover, her bed linen would not be changed for four weeks (until her next ritual immersion).[27] The foul air in such rooms was thought to be evidence of the presence of the forces of evil and the struggle against sickness as a demonic being.

The application of all manner of substances with the intention of 'bringing out' crusty pustules, or simply of removing the spoiled blood from the body, was no less widespread. Two recommendations are particularly striking: bloodletting from the vena cava, or at least wet cupping, or giving mare's milk to drink; this latter was also used as a body rub, particularly on the areas around the throat and heart, and as eye drops.[28] While the first of these methods seems to be a clear legacy of the traditions of early medicine, the second is reminiscent of many similar 'wise women's remedies'. Nonetheless, it is worth remembering that in the folk imagination horses were categorized as draught animals and attributed high sexual potency. Therefore contact with them, even in an indirect form, was thought to intensify sexual urges, which were assiduously stifled by the traditional community. As in the Middle Ages, people with an insatiable libido were seen in this environment as corrupt, and were often depicted as boil-ridden and worm-infected. Walking over the place where a horse had rolled in heat, and even watching one do so, was believed to cause scaly skin, warts, or scabies

sources together as *pokn un mozlen*. See e.g. Rosenberg, *Rafa'el hamalakh*, 74–5; *Segulot urefuot*, Bibliotheca Rosenthaliana, HS. ROS. 444, 3*a*.

[26] Tsart, 'Superstitions and Beliefs in Our Region' (Yid.), 51–2. Also worthy of note is the description of the poor tailor's home and the transformation of his rooms after the death of the patient in Gerszon Lewin, 'Z pamiętnika lekarza', 231–4.

[27] Segel, 'Wierzenia i lecznictwo', 58.

[28] *Segulot urefuot*, Bibliotheca Rosenthaliana, HS. ROS. 444, 3*a–b*; Rosenberg, *Rafa'el hamalakh*, 74; 'Omens and Remedies' (Yid.), 289. Cf. Talko-Hryncewicz, *Zarys lecznictwa ludowego*, 124–5; Wereńko, 'Przyczynek do lecznictwa ludowego', 184.

('horse scabies', *ferdishe krets*)—visible evidence of sexual corruption.[29] Indeed, even freckles were thought to be caused in this way, and the recommended treatment for them was mare's milk mixed with birch sap.[30] This choice of remedy was thus directly linked to the principle of humoral harmony. The purpose of the milk was to accelerate the scabbing process, which was thought to guarantee rapid removal of the 'bad blood' and restoration of humoral homoeostasis.

Headaches, in the popular view, were caused by rushes of blood and/or mucus, and thus, couched in the terminology of humoral theory, by an excess of blood or an excess of phlegm. The former of these two causes, as numerous examples show, might be alleviated by bloodletting or other forms of haemorrhage. Several independent sources advised the application of leeches behind the ears in such circumstances.[31] For the same reason no attempt was made to staunch light nosebleeds unless they seemed to present a threat; the reasoning given was that 'it is good for the head if blood leaves via the nose from time to time'.[32] The recommended action to combat the second of the causes of headaches was to provoke the sneeze reflex using a *fonfa*, a piece of paper rolled up into a tube with snuff inside,[33] or to inhale the smoke from burning feathers.[34] If this failed to produce the desired effect, a sudatory method would be applied, such as compresses of oats boiled in wine vinegar (to the forehead in case of a head cold, or on the abdomen if it was a 'chill of the innards').[35] The author of *Sefer haberit* also devoted some space to the issue of excess moisture in the body. Firstly, he noted, phlegm gathers in the mouth and can be expelled by spitting. It also collects in the brain, whence most of it is able to leave the body via the nose. Moisture on the brain which cannot be drained through the nose, however,

[29] Lilientalowa, 'Wierzenia, przesądy i praktyki', 165; Fayvushinski, 'The Folklore of Pruzhana' (Yid.), 203. Rashes were also associated with dogs and cats, especially when they were in season. The books *Brantshpigl* and *Zekhirah* warn against allowing children to go barefoot in the months of Tevet and Shevat (January–February), the cat mating season, as this would result in their contracting incurable *katsn-shporn* on their feet. See Simner, *Zekhirah*, 26a; 'Katzensporn: Eine Umfrage', 77–8, 139, 168–9, 206–7, 227–8, 252, 296.

[30] Segel, 'Materyały do etnografii Żydów', 327. Cf. Haur, *Ekonomika lekarska*, 215.

[31] Likewise in the case of eye pain; *Refuot ha'am im darkhei yesharim*, 5, 11; *Segulot urefuot*, Bibliotheca Rosenthaliana, HS. ROS. 444, 9b.

[32] Lilientalowa, *Choroby, lecznictwo*, fo. 92.

[33] Lew, 'O lecznictwie i przesądach', *Izraelita*, 46, p. 446; id., *Izraelita*, 49, p. 475.

[34] Rosenberg, *Der malekh refoel*, 54; Lilientalowa, *Dziecko żydowskie*, 66.

[35] Rosenberg, *Rafa'el hamalakh*, 87; Lew, 'Lecznictwo i przesądy', *Izraelita*, 47, p. 493.

causes growths, sores, or mange on the head or the body.[36] Other sources extend the scale of dangers further still. Phlegm draining down from the inside of the head onto the gums, for instance, was thought to soften them, thus rendering them more susceptible to attack by worms.[37]

While the conviction that 'it is impossible to live without bile'[38] was widespread, an excess of this humour, as of any other, could cause illness. Ethnographic material reveals the belief among the traditional community that the liver was the seat of anger, while laughter came from the spleen.[39] The latter organ was of course also the source of melancholic states and mood swings, which were caused by a plethora of black bile. The former, on the other hand, by producing green bile (Yid. *grine gal*), generated outbursts of anger. Someone who was placid and rarely grew angry was said to have a 'white liver'[40] or to 'have no bile in him'.[41] Mothers were warned not to nurse their babies when upset or angry, for in such a mood their milk would be full of bile, and thus harmful.[42] One of the simplest methods of eliminating an excess of this humour was to induce vomiting. As the saying went: *Opbrekhn un opshprekhn iz a volvele refue* (Throwing up and driving out are cheap remedies).[43] Many of the recommended methods for inducing vomiting involved the consumption of something revolting: a jaundice sufferer, for instance, might be given dried pig,[44] cockerel,[45] or goose[46] droppings to drink. The same need to remove excess bile from the body also contributed to the popularity of the broad array of purgatives that could be given in case of ill health, in particular castor oil,[47] used in the treatment of cholerine,[48] diphtheria,[49] or even stomach ache.[50] The same

[36] Hurwitz, *Sefer haberit* (Yid.), 48.     [37] *Refuot ha'am im darkhei yesharim*, 15.
[38] 'Useful Proverbs' (Yid.), *Yidishe shprakh*, 10, p. 60.
[39] Lilientalowa, 'Wierzenia, przesądy i praktyki', 170.
[40] i.e. their liver was filled not with bile but with the white humour, phlegm; thus they were phlegmatic; see Landau, 'Sprichwörter und Redensarten', 347.
[41] Stutshkov, *Thesaurus of the Yiddish Language* (Yid.), 655.
[42] Lew, 'O lecznictwie i przesądach', *Izraelita*, 40, p. 382.
[43] Veynig, 'Doctors and Medicine in Jewish Sayings' (Yid.), 20.
[44] J. Ashkenazi, *Tsene urene fun harav hekhasid*, 3; Lilientalowa, *Choroby, lecznictwo*, fo. 89v.
[45] *Segulot urefuot*, Bibliotheca Rosenthaliana, HS. ROS. 444, 8b.
[46] Halpern, *Toledot adam*, 33; *Segulot urefuot*, Bibliotheca Rosenthaliana, HS. ROS. 444, 14a; Lew, 'Lecznictwo i przesądy', *Izraelita*, 48, p. 505; Goldberg and Eisenberg, *Sefer laḥashim usegulot*, 19a.     [47] Lilientalowa, *Choroby, lecznictwo*, fo. 119.
[48] Rosenberg, *Der malekh refoel*, 51.     [49] Rosenberg, *Rafa'el hamalakh*, 14.
[50] Lilientalowa, 'Dziecko żydowskie', 155; Shlaferman, 'The Folklore, Customs, and Stories of Kazimierz' (Yid.), 172.

was true with regard to the use of enemas in cases of poisoning,[51] typhoid fever,[52] rickets,[53] and many other ailments.

Excess bile was considered to be the main cause of jaundice (Yid. *gelzukht*, the green sickness). The Talmud itself (BT *Shab.* 33*a*) avers that this disease was a sign of groundless hatred (i.e. anger). The colour of the sufferer's eyes and skin made a huge impression on the popular imagination and prompted widespread use of remedies from the categories of both *similia similibus curantur* and *contraria contrariis curantur*, many of them familiar across Europe. These included wearing items made of gold or red beads,[54] and laying a tench (a fish with golden-coloured scales), cut in half, on the patient's abdomen,[55] to name but two. Another of the most widely used methods of tackling the illness, pressing a pigeon of the appropriate sex to the patient's navel, was somewhat reminiscent of these two methods, though more closely linked to humoral theory: its anus was to be pressed to the patient's body so that it could 'draw in' the unnecessary humour. This was possible in light of the belief, in currency since antiquity, that the pigeon had no bile, as evidenced by its benign disposition.[56]

According to the *Sefer haberit*, which draws more directly on early medical wisdom than many other writings on health found in ethnographic collections, excess bile blocking the cerebral veins caused madness. This piece of ethical literature, steeped in kabbalah, also combined warnings against feeding children or pregnant and nursing women animal hearts, livers (which 'block the head'), spleens (the child 'would constantly be laughing'), or brains ('it will make their nose run') with the theory of *gilgulim* and the dangers of the animal soul transmigrating and becoming 'attached' to the human soul with the ingestion of its blood. Nonetheless, Jerzy S. Wasilewski would seem to be right in suggesting that these restrictions

[51] Rosenberg, *Der malekh refoel*, 34–5.

[52] Sperling, *Ta'amei haminhagim oyf ivri taytsh*, ii. 108.        [53] Ibid. 110.

[54] Lew, 'Lecznictwo i przesądy', *Izraelita*, 48, p. 505; Segel, 'Materyały do etnografii Żydów', 328; id., 'Wierzenia i lecznictwo', 55; Weissenberg, 'Das neugeborene Kind', 85.

[55] Lew, 'Lecznictwo i przesądy', *Izraelita*, 48, p. 505; Rosenberg, *Rafa'el hamalakh*, 21. Cf. Talko-Hryncewicz, *Zarys lecznictwa ludowego*, 181; Haur, *Ekonomika lekarska*, 199.

[56] *Segulot urefuot*, Bibliotheca Rosenthaliana, HS. ROS. 444, 14*a*; Segel, 'Materyały do etnografii Żydów', 328; Berger, *Imrei yisra'el*, 13*a*; Rosenberg, *Rafa'el hamalakh*, 21; id., *Der malekh refoel*, 37. Cf. Andrzej of Kobylin, *Gadki o składności członków człowieczych*, 54. A far more detailed historical analysis of this practice was undertaken more recently by Fred Rosner, who unfortunately passed over the humoral aspect and focused on the objective (in)efficacy of the remedy. See Rosner, 'Pigeons as a Remedy for Jaundice', 59–68.

were anchored in a fear of upsetting the homoeostasis of the humours.[57] In many cases only the comparison of diverse sources, including foreign-language medical literature predating the biomedicine era, can help to comprehend the relationship between diseases and the array of highly enigmatic remedies. The collection *Rafa'el hamalakh*, and Lilientalowa too, perhaps in reference to it, confirm the custom of giving parsley infusion as a diuretic, while Dov Ber Schneersohn's book of remedies contains a note to the effect that the same preparation helps to break down blockages caused by an excess of phlegm.[58] Lilientalowa, the pioneer of Jewish ethnography, also noted that couples would urinate before sexual inter-course in an attempt to purify their blood and prevent scrofulosis, while again, authorities of early medicine (among them the Polish *Medical Economics*) attributed the cause of this disease to overproduction of phlegm.[59]

One fascinating instance of interdependence perceived by Jewish folk culture was that between the human body and the frog, which was held to be capable of casting curses and causing illness,[60] in particular swellings and growths of various kinds on the skin. Ethnographic sources reflect the conviction that certain illnesses could owe their origin to a frog having found its way into the patient's body. 'A frog under the tongue' (*a frosh unter der tsung*), for example, was said to be the cause of swelling in the lower half of the oral cavity.[61] At the same time, frogs functioned in the popular imagination as creatures able to suck out various types of fluids. Their use in therapeutic practices involved pressing them onto the affected site, and the best evidence that healing was in progress was the death of the frog.[62]

---

[57] Sperling, *Ta'amei haminhagim oyf ivri taytsh*, ii. 10. See Wasilewski, 'Tabu, zakaz magiczny, nieczystość', 7–45. These warnings appear, often in highly laconic form, in writings including the Talmud (*Hor.* 13b), the medieval *Sefer ḥasidim*, and the early modern *Shenei luḥot haberit*. According to one testimony from Gorodets in Belarus, the heart of a slaughtered calf would be given to its mother on a slice of bread so that she would forget about it and not miss it; Ben-Ezra, 'Customs' (Yid.), 175.

[58] Rosenberg, *Rafa'el hamalakh*, 96; id., *Der malekh refoel*, 14; Lilientalowa, *Dziecko żydowskie*, 69; Schneersohn, *Sefer refuot*, 15.          [59] Lilientalowa, *Dziecko żydowskie*, 20–1.

[60] If one came across a frog 'cursing' on the threshold, or stepped on one, one should repeat the words: 'Salt in your eyes, pepper in your nose' three times; Yunis, 'The Old Homeland' (Yid.), 70. See Lilientalowa, *Obrzędy pogrzebowe*, 182; 'Omens and Remedies' (Yid.), 283; Fayvushinski, 'The Folklore of Pruzhana' (Yid.), 200; Ayznbund, *The Jews of Nesvizh* (Yid.), 194.

[61] Schneersohn, *Sefer refuot*, 16. The standard recommendation for combating this complaint was to rub the affected area with radish, which was also used to treat other types of swelling; see Segel, 'Materyały do etnografii Żydów', 327.

[62] See e.g. Libera, *Medycyna ludowa*, 132.

The popular 'toad stone' (*crapaudina*), after being boiled in milk and laid on a bite (for example from a rabid dog), could draw the poison out.[63] The *Rafa'el hamalakh* advised that for swellings[64] and distended bellies[65] an ointment be made up from frogs boiled in oil, though Lilientalowa has this same remedy as a cure for rheumatoid arthritis (or rheumatic pain).[66] Yet other sources mention frog-based ointments for warts and ulcers, and these were used by both Jews[67] and the Slavic population;[68] a further use of this creature, for jaundice, was to press a lacerated specimen to the patient's neck.[69] It is possible that the same association gave grounds for the emergence of speculation on the use of frog powder to staunch blood (during menstruation, nosebleeds, or from circumcision wounds;[70] this seems likely given that the primary haemostatic method used by the *mohel* was *metsitsah*—suction).

While humoral pathology had developed as a branch of natural philosophy, closely bound up with Aristotelian views and augmenting the arsenal of rationalist theories, as it filtered down into folk culture it began to interact with magic and religion, even offering grounds for speculation on the extrasensory world, angels, and so on. The populace tied it into their own system of myths sufficiently strongly that vestiges of it are to be found in conjurations for charms and, more generally, in a range of actions intended to combat demons. In one incantation published in *Toledot adam*, the prophet Elijah addressed the malevolent planet Kokhav (Mercury): 'I adjure thee in the Name of the Lord of Hosts, who created heaven and earth, the sea and the wind and fire and dust.'[71] In another version, used to lift 'charms and other sicknesses', he called on them not to wreak harm 'either by sight, or by speech, or by silence, through the medium of any of the four ERME elements [*esh, ruaḥ, mayim, efer*—fire, wind, water, earth],

[63] Wereńko, 'Przyczynek do lecznictwa ludowego', 189; Cf. *Compendium medicum auctum*, 115 and 504.    [64] Rosenberg, *Rafa'el hamalakh*, 15; id., *Der malekh refoel*, 41.
[65] Rosenberg, *Rafa'el hamalakh*, 70.
[66] Lilientalowa, 'Wierzenia, przesądy i praktyki', 172.
[67] *Segulot urefuot*, Bibliotheca Rosenthaliana, HS. ROS. 444, 14a.
[68] Warts were thought to be caused by 'water spat out by a frog'; see Biegeleisen, *Lecznictwo ludu polskiego*, 2. Perhaps for the same reason early modern medicine recommended the application of frogspawn as a remedy for freckles; see *Apteka domowa i podróżna*, 10.
[69] Lew, 'Lecznictwo i przesądy', *Izraelita*, 48, p. 505.
[70] Halpern, *Toledot adam*, 8–9; Rosenberg, *Rafa'el hamalakh*, 25; *Segulot urefuot*, Bibliotheca Rosenthaliana, HS. ROS. 444, 6a; Plaut, *Likutei ḥever ben ḥayim*, 8b; Lifshits, *Berit avot*, 96b.
[71] Halpern, *Toledot adam*, 15; *Segulot vekameyot*, JTS, MS 10082, 4a; Ochana, *Mareh hayeladim*, 39b; Plaut, *Likutei ḥever ben ḥayim*, 6b.

or any unclean forces'.[72] Establishing the boundary between Hippocratic
and Galenic medicine and folk culture with any precision is rendered all
the more difficult by the fact that many of the notions which operated in
both worlds were easy to reconcile. It is worth noting that ancient experts
did not refute the therapeutic and especially prophylactic significance of
amulets. Thus on occasion we will find reference in Jewish ethnographic
sources to methods of this nature that were known even in antiquity. One
was that of carrying a spider in a walnut shell as protection from fever,[73]
or peony root to guard against convulsions.[74] An extremely common conviction was that of the demonic aetiology of disease, recovery from which
demanded the expulsion, by force or request, of the evil spirit from the
body of the unfortunate sufferer—steps which were akin to healing procedures based on the theory of humours. Further examples of similar con-
currences will be given in subsequent chapters.

[72] *Segulot urefuot*, Bibliotheca Rosenthaliana, HS. ROS. 444, 6b–7a.

[73] See e.g. Rosenberg, *Rafa'el hamalakh*, 84; Rechtman, *Jewish Ethnography and Folklore*
(Yid.), 304. Cf. *Sposób domowy leczenia tak ludzi jak bydląt*, 18; Haur, *Ekonomika lekarska*, 13.
Similar practices were described in the seventeenth century by Robert Burton in his *Anatomy of
Melancholy* (p. 459) as a method used by his mother, but are also to be found in the works of
Dioscorides (*De materia medica*, 205).

[74] Dioscorides, *De materia medica*, 529–30. See Ch. 11 below.

# CHAPTER EIGHT

# ASTROLOGY

A SIDE FROM HUMORAL PATHOLOGY, another field of great significance for therapeutics was astrology, much debated by the rabbis.[1]
The Bible exhorted Israel not to fear 'portents in the sky' that caused the
pagans to tremble (Jer. 10: 2), though it did admit the possibility of good
omens appearing in the heavens, an example of which is the messianic
prophecy 'A star rises from Jacob' (Num. 24: 17). Later Jewish literature
made open references to discussions linking human vicissitudes with the
influences of astral bodies. The Greek terms *astrologos* and *astrologia* appear
in the Jerusalem Talmud. Likewise, the Babylonian Talmud, while using a
different vocabulary, also contained passages about 'stargazers'.[2] The signs
of the zodiac became an important element of Jewish culture. Deliberations on them have been found in the Dead Sea scrolls,[3] and they feature in
some of the earliest kabbalistic texts (such as *Sefer yetsirah*),[4] while zodiacal
images may be seen in synagogue art, in eastern Europe as elsewhere.[5]

The spiritual leaders of Israel emphasized that, unlike other nations,
the Jewish people did not have a constellation of its own (*ein mazal le-
yisra'el*),[6] though they did not refute convictions of the influence of the
stars. While they rejected the speculations of astrologers of other nations
and doubted the accuracy of their predictions, the actual idea of astral
influences recurred frequently in their own writings.[7] The context in which
it was mostly found was that of bons mots by various talmudic rabbis, not
always directly connected with the subject under discussion. Rava, for
instance, commented that '[the length of our] life, having children, and
our source of income are not dependent on our merits but on our star'.[8]

[1] See Leicht, 'The Planets, the Jews and the Beginnings of "Jewish Astrology"', 271–88.
[2] Altmann, 'Astrology', 616–17.
[3] See Jacobus, '4Q318: A Jewish Zodiac Calendar at Qumran?', 365–95.
[4] Kaplan, *Sefer Yetzirah*, 209–10.
[5] Trzciński, 'Zachowane wystroje malarskie bóżnic w Polsce', 81–2.
[6] BT *Shab.* 156a, which in the popular wisdom translated as *A yid hot nisht keyn mazl* (A Jew
has no luck).     [7] Altmann, 'Astrology', 616–20.     [8] BT *MK* 28a.

His words suggest an attempt to use astrology to overcome the contradiction between human experience and the ethics of divine reward, which held that all of these blessings should accrue to the righteous. In this regard folk culture differentiated between the sexes according to their societal roles, as expressed in the following proverb: *Parnose iz inem mans mazl, kinder zaynen inem vaybs mazl* (The source of income is in the constellation of the husband, and children are in the constellation of the wife).[9] Another passage of the Talmud contains the musings of Samuel on the subject of suitable times for bloodletting. Among his comments is a warning against carrying out such procedures on Tuesdays, owing to the convergence of even-numbered hours and the rule of the planet Mars, which was associated with death and the spilling of blood.[10] A more detailed explication of talmudic astrology is to be found in the words of Rabbi Hanina. He believed that the planetary system influences human wisdom and wealth, and that the workings of the constellations are most visible at the moment of a person's birth. People born under the influence of the Sun (Hamah) would be handsome and genuine in their actions, those born under the influence of Venus (Noga) rich and promiscuous, those under the influence of Mercury (Kokhav) wise and blessed with a good memory, those under the influence of the Moon (Levanah) would suffer and enrich themselves on the suffering of others, those born under the influence of Saturn (Shabetai) had no hope of achieving their plans, those under Jupiter (Tsedek) would be righteous, and those born under the influence of Mars (Ma'adim) were destined to spill blood.[11] The talmudic sages had a rival system of predictions to classic astrology, based on the biblical description of creation, according to which anyone born on the second day was said to be of a difficult disposition, for it was on that day that the 'waters were parted'.

The words of the early rabbis had a strong influence on the speculations of the medieval astrologers and their successors. Knowledge of basic astrological concepts was crucial to an understanding of many aspects of Jewish culture, above all the calendar and the rabbinic discussions surrounding it. It is telling that Rashi, the author of the most fundamental commentary on the Talmud, cited astrological texts. In his exegesis of passages on the subject of the planets he made use of the text of the *Ḥakhmoni*,

⁹ I. Bernstein, *Jewish Proverbs and Sayings* (Yid.), 205; Stutshkov, *Thesaurus of the Yiddish Language* (Yid.), 652.          ¹⁰ BT *Shab.* 129*b*.          ¹¹ BT *Shab.* 156*a*.

a work by the Italian physician Shabetai Donnolo (d. *c.*982).[12] The early modern ethical literature also made reference to astrological topics. It emphasized the special role of the Jews as the chosen people, surrounded by divine protection. It also employed the study of the stars to reinforce desirable forms of behaviour; only those who strove for closeness to God could be free of astral influences—for only in so doing could one be assured that everything one encountered was from the Creator. Anyone who did not follow a sanctified path laid themselves open to the workings of the stars.[13]

The strong attachment to astrological notions rooted in antiquity is hardly surprising, given that they were a constant presence in that field of Jewish literature which explicated the functioning of the world. Neither the much-read early modern encyclopaedia *Ma'aseh tuvyah* nor the Enlightenment-era *Sefer haberit* (which was also published in a popular Yiddish translation) accepted the Copernican model of the universe. The authors of both works preferred a middle way, and proposed as true theories that did not undermine the general thrust of the speculations of the ancients. They illustrated the influence of the heavenly bodies on human physiology by applying the theory of the four elements: every person's nature is dominated by one or other of the elements, but is also under the protection of one of the planets. Thus a person born under the rule of Saturn and endowed with a nature in which air was the dominant element would be fortunate, respected, just, and wise. If earth was the dominant element in his nature, however, he would prove to be false, vengeful, and belligerent.[14] The author of *Sefer haberit* also devoted considerable space to the signs of the zodiac,[15] as well as to the related subject of alchemy (the seven metals),[16] while some of his comments were of a more general character: for instance, he noted that in the Jewish month of Adar (February–March) the sun was said to be detrimental due to the high level of moisture in the body.[17]

[12] Donnolo's book is essentially a commentary on the kabbalistic *Sefer yetsirah*; see Leicht, 'The Reception of Astrology in Medieval Ashkenazi Culture', 205–10.
[13] Danzig, *Hokhmat adam*, 219.
[14] Hurwitz, *Sefer haberit* (Yid.), 76–7.        [15] Ibid. 67.        [16] Ibid. 16.
[17] Ibid. 73. As the Jewish saying goes, *Rosh-khoydesh oder lozt men zikh tsu der oder* (On the first day of Adar one should open a vein); I. Bernstein, *Jewish Proverbs and Sayings* (Yid.), 5. The name of the month of Adar was also explained as an acronym of the words *Ani d' rofekha* ('I the Lord am your healer' (Exod. 15: 26); *d'* is a common Hebrew abbreviation for God's name); Y. Tsherniak, 'Linguistic Folklore in Yiddish' (Heb.), 104.

There are two important sources from the period around 1900 which devote passages to the influence of the planets: A. I. Sperling's *Ta'amei ha-minhagim* and the medical manual *Rafa'el hamalakh* by Y. Y. Rosenberg. These publications contain tables also known to wider European astrology, showing the various planets (for example Saturn, the Sun, the Moon, Mars) along with the times of day and night when they were thought to rule.[18] And while the latter treated the subject rather sparsely, placing it in its entirety in the context of the rules for making amulets and the connection between the time of day or night, the ruling star, and the relevant name of God, Sperling's book contains far more interesting information. Firstly, the primary source on which he drew was 'our sages', that is, the talmudic-era rabbis—there was no doubt, therefore, that his ideas were not heretical. Secondly, he interpreted the power of the heavenly bodies as an emanation of divine might. It was the Creator who assigned the planets their roles, and it was on his authority alone that any interference in the established order might occur. Humanity, and in particular devout Jews, were not at the mercy of the stars as long as they cultivated good relations with God. Thirdly—and particularly interestingly in the context of the Slavic population's perception of the Jews as 'planetarians' (*płanetnicy*)[19]—a knowledge of the times at which each planet ruled also helped to forecast the weather. It was believed that if the new moon appeared at a time when Saturn ruled, the month would be a cold one, and if Mars was the ruling planet the first half of the month would be dry and the second half wet. Its appearance at the sun's ruling hour heralded a warm, dry spell in summer or a frosty one if it was winter. Venus meant an average month, with around a week of rain, and so on.[20] The tables showing the influences of the seven planets were quite popular, even affecting some religious practices. As Yosef Margoshes noted, Galician hasidim would not say the blessings over wine on the eve of

[18] The system of ascribing certain hours of the day to the seven planets was known to Hellenistic astrologers, including Vettius Valens (d. *c.*175 CE). Also related to this system was belief in the patronage by the various planets of particular days of the week (e.g. Saturn governed Saturday, the Sun Sunday, the Moon Monday, Mars Tuesday). Many European languages have retained vestiges of this belief in the names of the days of the week—see e.g. the French *mardi* (Tuesday), *mercredi* (Wednesday), etc. See Leicht, 'The Planets', 277–9.

[19] 'Planetarian' refers to people able to influence atmospheric phenomena—to produce clouds, storms, hail, etc.

[20] Sperling, *Ta'amei haminhagim oyf ivri taytsh*, ii. 122–4. See Belova, 'Narodnaya magiya', 113.

the sabbath between six and seven in the evening, as this was the hour of the
malevolent Saturn.[21]

The ethnographic material amassed by the pioneers in this field leaves
no doubt as to the prevalence of astrology-related beliefs derived from the
speculations of ancient and medieval philosophers. The conviction that
the seven planets influenced human life and health, in particular at the hour
of one's birth, had put down deep roots in the popular consciousness.[22]
*Mazl tov!* was the customary congratulatory formula on any joyous occasion, such as births or weddings, and the Hebrew word *mazal* (star, constellation) in Yiddish came to be synonymous with good fortune. Good
wishes for anyone embarking on a new venture would express the hope
that it would be launched 'in the right hour' (*in a mazldiker sho*). Anyone
considered habitually lucky would be known as a *bar-mazl* (lit. the son of
a [good] star), while someone unlucky, ill-fated, was dubbed a *shlimazl* (cf.
Ger. *schlimm*, bad) or a person with a 'dark star' (*fintster mazl*). The panoply
of Jewish curses included this expressive example: *Dayn mazl zol dir laykhtn
vi di levone in soyf-khoydesh* (May your star shine like the moon at the end
of the month),[23] which was obviously intended to wish the hapless addressee ill luck. Other proverbs in Yiddish suggest that every child is born with
its own star (*Itlekhs kind vert geboyrn mit zayn mazl*), and that their parents
can pass on to them everything except a good star (*Eltern kenen alts gebn, nor
nit keyn mazl*).[24]

The traditional Jewish community cultivated the conviction that a premature infant would have a chance of survival as long as it was born in the
seventh month (*zibele*). Aside from the symbolic meaning of the number
seven, which in Jewish religious literature signified the completion of a full
cycle, the influence of the heavenly bodies also played a role in this belief.
Each month of a pregnancy was governed by one of the planets, and it was
in the seventh month, during the rule of the moon, that the formation of
the foetus was completed. Thus a child born at this time was treated as a
normal infant, and in the case of a boy the circumcision ceremony would be
performed, even if the appointed day fell on the sabbath. No such violation
of the rules of the day of rest was permissible if the child was born in the

[21] Margoshes, *Memories from My Life* (Yid.), 84. On the subject of drinking water between
the third sabbath meal and the *melave malke*, see Lipiets, *Sefer matamim*, 124.

[22] Lilientalowa, *Dziecko żydowskie*, 28–9.

[23] I. Bernstein, *Jewish Proverbs and Sayings* (Yid.), 157; Lilientalowa, 'Kult ciał niebieskich', 6.

[24] Stutshkov, *Thesaurus of the Yiddish Language* (Yid.), 171.

eighth month of pregnancy, which was under the influence of the planet Saturn. *Akhtele*, as such babies were known, were given minimal chances of survival,[25] and even if they did live, they were to remain under close observation over subsequent years. It was believed that they were vulnerable even until the age of 20 to all kinds of dangers that had their roots in the prenatal period.[26] If the child did display health issues, it would sometimes be referred to as a *mapil-kind*, a miscarried child.[27] In order not to put their offspring at risk, women in the seventh and ninth months of pregnancy would perform a ritual purification from sins and the effects of enchantment by immersing themselves in the *mikveh* three times. They did not do this in the eighth month, however.[28] Likewise, it was recommended that the family pray for a successful delivery, except in the eighth month.[29] Performance of the circumcision rite precisely on the eighth day from birth allowed each of the planets to exert its influence on the newborn child over the preceding seven days. This done, the sign of the covenant would liberate the Jew from the influence of the stars.[30]

As was the case in other cultures, the Jews perceived a link between the movements of the heavenly bodies (interpreted as waning and waxing) and the comparable phenomena of dying and returning to life that they observed in nature. In the folk imagination such parallels could not be —and never were—without consequence for human health. Occurrences or progressions such as setting (of the sun or moon), fading, or falling (*fargeyn, farloshn vern, faln*) were generally associated with weakening, and even with imminent death.[31] All types of eclipse were considered harbingers of inevitable punishment for sins.[32] In the folk imagination the image of the sky was enriched by the conviction that everybody had a light, or lamp, up there which was extinguished with their death (sometimes it would go out suddenly, causing an untimely, unexpected death at a young age).[33] It was believed that anyone who saw a fading or shooting star in the morning would die that same year.[34] In order to avert this threat, one had

[25] This notion was known even to Hippocrates and Galen; see Jakobovits, *Jewish Medical Ethics*, 317; Metzler, *Disability in Medieval Europe*, 83–4.
[26] BT *Yev.* 80*a–b*.     [27] B. Y. Rozen, 'A Collection of Idiomatic Expressions' (Yid.), 73.
[28] Lilientalowa, *Dziecko żydowskie*, 25–6; Fels, 'Zabobony lekarskie u Żydów', 3.
[29] *Ets ḥayim*, 96–7.     [30] Wilff, *Imrot shelomoh*, 105.
[31] See Khayes, 'Death-Related Beliefs and Customs' (Yid.), 284.
[32] Lilientalowa, 'Kult ciał niebieskich', 8, 12.
[33] Zelkovitsh, 'Death and Its Accompanying Moments' (Yid.), 155–6.
[34] Segel, 'Wierzenia i lecznictwo', 60.

to exclaim three times 'Not mine!', 'Not my star!', or 'I am not yours, you are not mine!',[35] simultaneously plucking a hair from one's head. On seeing a brightly shining star, one should say: 'This one is mine.'[36]

This belief about fading stars was probably connected with another that was widespread in many ethnic groups in eastern Europe. According to Jewish sources one should not point at the sky, the moon, or the stars, and anyone who did so without taking remedial measures, such as biting the finger that pointed, or treading on it with their heel, would have to face unpleasant health-related consequences.[37] Warnings of this nature in the folk culture of the Jews often had biblical roots; the taboo of pointing at the morning star, for example, was connected to its role in ending the duel between Jacob and the angel (Gen. 32: 27).[38] Sources on the ethnography of the Slavs likewise evince the conviction of a clear cause-and-effect relationship between finger-pointing and fading or falling astral bodies.[39] The custom cited in the previous paragraph of hailing a star as one's own would also appear to be an important vestige in this respect; perhaps it, too, was once accompanied by similar prohibitions whose meaning became lost to later generations.

The aspect of cyclicity was the dominant factor in the perception of the moon. This seems the more understandable in light of the fact that the rhythm of traditional Jewish life was strongly subordinated to the religiously sanctioned system of measuring time. The Jewish calendar was based on the phases of the moon. The Yiddish word for 'month', *khoydesh*, derived from the Hebrew *ḥodesh*, meant renewal (of the moon). A half-moon would be referred to as *moyled* (nascent). The general word used to denote the moon—*levone* (Heb. *levanah*, white)—brought to mind associations with the silver or pale colour of its face. In Yiddish, as in English, the moon was the trope used to convey the idea of something much desired but unattainable, and would be referred to as a plate or disc (*a telerl fun himl*). In comparisons it featured as a synonym of beauty (*sheyn vi di likhtike levone in*

---

[35] Ibid. 51; Khayes, 'Death-Related Beliefs and Customs' (Yid.), 299.

[36] Fels, 'Zabobony lekarskie u Żydów', 4. This belief probably became generalized over time; according to some informants, any wishes made on seeing a fading or shooting star had the potential to come true, whatever their character; see Khayes, 'Death-Related Beliefs and Customs' (Yid.), 299.

[37] Lilientalowa, 'Zjawiska przyrody w wyobrażeniu', 58; ead., *Święta żydowskie*, ii. 15–16. See Wuttke, *Der deutsche Volksaberglauben der Gegenwart*, 13.

[38] Lilientalowa, 'Kult ciał niebieskich', 13.

[39] Lebeda, 'Gwiazdy', 24–6.

*khotse khoydesh*, as beautiful as a bright full moon), but also invited associations of paleness and death (*blas vi di levone*, as pale as the moon). In biblical literature there was one more name for the moon: *yare'aḥ*, which was used both for the celestial body and in equal measure for the period of its cycle (month). This word did not occur in the vernacular language of the Ashkenazi diaspora, however.

The beginning of a new month, because of the appearance of the new moon, was perceived as a time of growth, rebirth, and plenty. The rabbis believed in an inverse correlation of the cyclical phases of the moon with the regular process of the waxing and waning of severity in divine judgement.[40] The moment of renewal was awaited in an atmosphere of contemplation, and particular religious practices were recommended: 'Day 28 is very good and recommended for fasting; likewise days 29 and 30, that is, observance of the eve of Rosh Hodesh. And it is important not to forget almsgiving, which is particularly auspicious at this time, and to redouble one's studies.'[41] The eve of the new month was known as 'minor Yom Kippur'. Aside from fasting, another characteristic feature of this day was the liturgy, which was similar to that around the Day of Atonement, and which included propitiatory prayers and confession of sins. Some folk customs also made reference to Yom Kippur, above all the practice of women making candles and taking them to the synagogue as a votive offering for the health of their children.[42] Rosh Hodesh (lit. the head of the month) itself was festive in character. In ancient Israel the *shofar* would be blown in the Temple, and the Halel—the cycle of thanksgiving psalms customarily read at festivals—was recited. In more recent times fasting was not allowed (except in the case of need for redemption from a nightmare),[43] neither were other ascetic practices, though religious law did allow work on that day. Women celebrated Rosh Hodesh even more ceremonially, by refraining from doing handicrafts. According to the ethical literature, this custom was in commemoration of the Jewish women's opposition to the sin of idolatry during the casting of the golden calf (Exod. 32).[44]

[40] Sperling, *Ta'amei haminhagim umekorei hadinim*, 417–18.

[41] Lifshits, *Segulot yisra'el*, 57*b*.

[42] Simner, *Zekhirah*, 103; Lilientalowa, *Dziecko żydowskie*, 74. See Chapter 10 below.

[43] On waking in the morning, a person frightened by the signs in their dream could undertake a special fast. This *tones-kholem*, or 'dream fast', took precedence even over the festive mood of the sabbath or other feasts; see BT *Ta'an.* 12*b*, *Ber.* 31*b*. There were also many folk methods for nullifying bad dreams.                    [44] *Ets ḥayim*, 112.

The first day of the month was considered lucky. Whatever happened on Rosh Hodesh, it was said, would continue throughout the month.[45] One way of ensuring for oneself a long life was purportedly to add the biblical quote about the longevity of Abraham (Gen. 24: 1) to the end of one's prayers on that day, together with a petition for long life to the Almighty, 'in whose hands [rest] the souls of all beings'.[46] This was the preferred day for weddings and house moves in the Jewish community,[47] and anyone born on Rosh Hodesh would have a reputation for being lucky. The leading medieval Ashkenazi Pietist, Judah Hehasid, introduced a prohibition on cutting hair (including the beard) and nails at the time of the new moon, though some people claimed that this was in fact the best time to wash and trim children's hair.[48]

With the waxing of the moon came the opportunity for the return of lost energy and vitality. Herbs gathered at this time, especially in the spring months (for example Iyar), were said to have particularly strong therapeutic powers.[49] For the same reason it was best to take medication, get married, or embark upon a course of study in the first half of the month, when the disc was growing.[50] At the new moon one could attempt to rid oneself of warts by saying: 'Let what I see grow; let what I touch go.'[51] Toothache might be assuaged by looking at the moon and reciting the dialogue between the prophet Elijah and the suffering Job,[52] or the incantation in Yiddish: 'The moon in the sky, I on Earth, the stone in the depths of the sea, the bear in the depths of the forest; until the one meets the other, let this toothache not return to me; amen, selah, netsah va'ed.'[53] The same might also be cured using Slavic incantations, which were popular among

[45] Grunwald, 'Aus unseren Sammlungen. Teil I', 71.

[46] Rosenberg, Rafa'el hamalakh, 14.        [47] Lilientalowa, 'Kult ciał niebieskich', 5–6.

[48] Grunwald, 'Aus unseren Sammlungen. Teil I', 81; Lilientalowa, 'Kult ciał niebieskich, 7. See Judah Hehasid, Sefer hasidim, 23–4.

[49] Schneersohn, Sefer refuot, 23. Cf. Paluch, Świat roślin w tradycyjnych praktykach leczniczych, 160.

[50] Grunwald, 'Aus unseren Sammlungen. Teil I', 71; Wilff, Imrot shelomoh, 52–3, 58.

[51] Lilientalowa, 'Zjawiska przyrody', 60; ead., 'Kult ciał niebieskich', 6. A recommended remedy for skin lesions was to splash the face with water on seeing the new moon; see Lilientalowa, 'Wierzenia, przesądy i praktyki', 174; ead., 'Kult wody', 12.

[52] Rosenberg, Rafa'el hamalakh, 109, Sperling, Ta'amei haminhagim umekorei hadinim, 588.

[53] The Yiddish conjuration resonates with the echo of the ritual of the blessing of the moon; see Rosenberg, Rafa'el hamalakh, 109; Avida [Złotnik], 'Incantations and Remedies in Arabic and Yiddish' (Heb.), 7; Lilientalowa, Choroby, lecznictwo, fos. 101, 142; Heller, Medicaments and Remedies (Heb.), 33.

the Jews, or their direct equivalents in Yiddish. 'Moon, moon, golden horn, to your growth, and to my health. Moon, moon, do dead teeth hurt? They do not', the person treating the ailment would say in Ruthenian, after which the patient would respond three times, 'Neither let them hurt me.'[54] A woman suffering from eight warts would take two white sticks and whittle four notches into each of them, then go out at the half-moon to a parting of roads and throw them behind her, saying in Ruthenian the words: 'Young moon, when you go behind the wood, take my eight [warts] with you.'[55]

As the moon waned, disintegration progressed in all manner of materials. As the *Sefer haberit* emphasized, at this time of the month clothes soaking in water would rot, trees with severed roots would wither up, and picked fruit would go bad.[56] Similar processes affected not only the human body but also the diseases inhabiting it. An especially large number of treatments for warts and ulcers have been preserved that are linked to the gradual waning of the moon, with which the breakdown of the growths was also associated. In one cure for abscesses, the affected spot should be rubbed with a handkerchief when the moon was on the wane, and then the handkerchief thrown over the shoulder.[57] Other sources mentioned smearing warts with tar or rubbing them with sand at the full moon (while reciting the conjuration: 'Just as I don't know where they're from, may I not know where they're gone').[58] Some methods of treating toothache were also to be used at this particular time of the month. A manuscript ascribed to the Magid of Chernobyl (Mordecai Twersky) contains one conjuration in Ruthenian, which ends with a Jewish formula casting out pain 'in the name of the God of Israel' in the wake of the departing moon.[59] The waning of the moon was also the appropriate time to do battle with parasites. On the eve of Rosh Hodesh Jewish women would give their children *verem-tsukerlekh*, homemade concoctions to flush out worms, which were thought to burrow in the digestive tract and to be vulnerable at this

[54] Maggid, 'Inoyazichniye zagavori u ruskikh yevrieyev', 587–8; Goldberg and Eisenberg, *Sefer laḥashim usegulot*, 8a. These authors also record another variant of this incantation, 8b. Cf. Talko-Hryncewicz, *Zarys lecznictwa ludowego*, 358.

[55] U. Weinreich, 'Beliefs: Remedies for Warts' (Yid.), 62. According to other versions, the notches were made in a broom handle or some other long stick, which on being lost would bring about the disappearance of the warts; see Segel, 'Materyały do etnografii Żydów', 325; Tarlau, 'Volksmedizinisches aus dem jüdischen Russland', 144.

[56] Hurwitz, *Sefer haberit* (Yid.), 81.    [57] Grunwald, 'Aus unseren Sammlungen. Teil I', 90.

[58] U. Weinreich, 'Beliefs: Remedies for Warts' (Yid.), 62–3. Cf. Biegeleisen, *Lecznictwo ludu polskiego*, 127.    [59] 'Items' (Heb.), 381.

particular time, probably as there was no moon. These were usually the seeds of herbs, generally considered to be anthelmintic (*veremkroyt, vemut*), dipped in honey or sugar or boiled up with prunes. Sometimes these remedies would also contain cow or horse dung mixed with water, possibly in order to intensify their purgative properties.[60]

Certain therapeutic practices could not be carried out if there was no moon: the Talmud advised against bloodletting during the first three days of the month, for instance.[61] This seems understandable in light of the belief, articulated in sources including *Sefer haberit*, that the cold, damp light of the moon brings grass out of the ground and increases the amount of marrow in human bones and blood in the veins.[62]

Worth mentioning in this context is the interesting custom of blessing or sanctifying the new moon (*kidesh-levone*). In the vernacular the name of the ritual became distorted in a curious way: it was known as *khidesh-levone*, using the periphrastic verb *mekhadesh zayn*, 'to renew'. From the rabbinic standpoint this twist was unacceptable, since 'renewal of the moon is something only the Lord God is capable of doing'.[63] Nonetheless, the language of the people doggedly reflected the belief in an interdependence between prayer and the waxing of the new moon. Religious Jews tried to perform this ritual some time between the third day of the month, when the new moon appeared in the sky, and the fifteenth (kabbalistic tradition mandated waiting until the seventh day). Talmudic treatises underscored the unique significance of the blessings recited,[64] as they likened the moon to the Shekhinah, the reflected glory of God, and even to God himself. The sanctification was performed standing, in a group, in the open air, at the end of the sabbath. The fulfilment of the *mitsvah* depended on the visibility of the moon in the sky. In addition to the main text of the prayer,[65] the blessing of God the Creator and ruler of nature in Psalm 148: 1–6 was also recited, and this was usually followed by dancing and joyful leaping, in more recent times possibly replaced by standing on tiptoe. The participants would address the moon directly with the words: 'Just as I dance

[60] Sperling, *Ta'amei haminhagim oyf ivri taytsh*, ii. 110; Rosenberg, *Rafa'el hamalakh*, 98 (*yikneh ba'apteyk 'pastilkes' letola'im*); id., *Der malekh refoel*, 63 (as an epilepsy remedy); Elzet [Złotnik], 'Some Jewish Customs' (Heb.), 368; Lilientalowa, 'Kult ciał niebieskich', 6; ead., *Dziecko żydowskie*, 58; Silverman-Weinreich, 'Beliefs' (Yid.), 33; Farber, 'Folk Healing' (Yid.), 180.          [61] BT *Shab.* 129*b*.

[62] Hurwitz, *Sefer haberit* (Yid.), 81; Lilientalowa, 'Kult ciał niebieskich', 6.

[63] Liberman, 'Discussion' (Yid.), 309.          [64] BT *San.* 42*a*.          [65] BT *San.* 41*b*–42*a*.

before you but cannot touch you, so may all my enemies be unable to touch me', repeated three times, followed by repetition of the phrase 'David, king of Israel, lives forever', the greeting of the moon with the words *shalom aleikhem* (peace be with you), and recitation of certain other passages from the Scriptures and the Talmud. The part of the ritual which referred to protection from misfortune was usually understood literally: whoever performed the sanctification would not have to fear death in the coming month.[66] According to one popular story, the words 'as I dance' would protect the traveller from attack by bandits.[67] Many sources also cite as a remedy for toothache the addition to this phrase of the words 'and my tooth shall not hurt', which embellishment was attributed to the tsadik Israel Friedman of Rużyn (now Ruzhin, Ukraine).[68] Other anecdotes, invoking Naftali of Ropczyce, advocated where necessary the addition to the prayer of words said to be able to cure one's wife of irregular menstruation.[69] Women themselves, however, were excluded from the ritual, and tradition warned them that listening in on the *kidesh-levone*, and even merely looking at the moon when pregnant, could cause complications in delivery.[70] Only rarely was it said that conception could be aided by the woman looking into water on which the moon had gazed.[71]

Some customs reflect the profound respect in which both Jews and their Slavic neighbours held the moon. Ethnographers have noted that, according to the folk imagination, household waste should not be thrown away in places exposed to moonlight (this was detrimental to women's periods), and one should never point at the moon in the sky.[72] Exposing oneself to the effects of its light likewise posed a danger to one's health. While gazing at its glow might sometimes alleviate toothache[73] or pain in the eyes,[74] other testimonies warned that after half an hour this would inevitably cause

---

[66] Sperling, *Ta'amei haminhagim oyf ivri taytsh*, i. 42; Lilientalowa, 'Zjawiska przyrody', 58; ead., 'Kult ciał niebieskich', 1. The statement that those who had performed the sanctification did not need to fear death was included in the *sidur* (prayer book), at the end of the Kidush Levanah section (e.g. *Sidur keminhag polin*, 189*b*).      [67] *Ets ḥayim*, 116; Lipiets, *Sefer matamim*, 93.
[68] Sperling, *Ta'amei haminhagim oyf ivri taytsh*, ii. 101; Lilientalowa, 'Kult ciał niebieskich', 5. See Herzog and Zborowski, *Life Is with People*, 316.      [69] Lifshits, *Segulot yisra'el*, 33*a*.
[70] Lilientalowa, 'Kult ciał niebieskich', 2; Pulner, 'Obryadi i povirya', 111.
[71] Lilientalowa, *Coitus, ciąża, poród*, fo. 10.
[72] Segel, 'Wierzenia i lecznictwo', 50; id., 'Materiały do etnografii Żydów', 325; Lilientalowa, *Święta żydowskie*, 15; Fayvushinski, 'The Folklore of Pruzhana' (Yid.), 201. Cf. e.g. Wuttke, *Der deutsche Volksaberglauben*, 13; Zawiliński, 'Przesądy i zabobony z ust ludu w różnych okolicach zebrane', 254.
[73] Lilientalowa, 'Kult ciał niebieskich', 5.      [74] Rosenberg, *Der malekh refoel*, 9.

blindness, and after an hour even death.[75] Sleeping or urinating in the light of the full moon, and even looking directly at the silver disc, were all bound to lead to somnambulism or melancholy in the common opinion. If a pregnant woman were to fall asleep in a moonlit spot and her belly were accidentally to become uncovered, her child would also be a sleepwalker, or would suffer from *levone-shayn* (sparks in the corners of the eyes).[76] Unborn children and infants were especially susceptible to the effects of moonlight. Sexual intercourse by even the palest light of the moon might result in the child conceived by that act suffering from convulsions.[77] For this reason great care was taken to ensure that the windows of bedrooms, particularly those occupied by women who had just given birth, were heavily curtained with no chinks. Every effort was also made not to leave nappies hung up to dry in places exposed to moonlight (others specified the yard or attic in this respect, and a duration of three months from the child's birth). The child wearing them would otherwise be at risk of enchantment by Lilith, or of some other type of ailment (poor sleep, fretfulness, and so on).[78]

At this point it might be useful to devote a little extra space to two interesting cases of sickness believed to be caused by the moon. The first was said to have its source in the foetal period, when the hapless victim of the disastrous effect of exposure to moonlight was turned into a monster termed a *monkalb* or *munkalb* (moon calf). This was a belief which had its roots in the folk culture of the Germanic peoples, though it reached the Polish lands at a relatively early date, in the late sixteenth century.[79] According to several sources, the *monkalb*, though born from a normal relationship between a man and a woman, had some of the physical features of

[75] Lilientalowa, 'Kult ciał niebieskich', 8; Khayes, 'Death-Related Beliefs and Customs' (Yid.), 299.

[76] Lilientalowa, 'Kult ciał niebieskich', 1; Segel, 'Wierzenia i lecznictwo', 53; id., 'Materiały do etnografii Żydów', 319. Lew does not mention the name *levone-shayn*, but he does refer to eye infections in infants caused by light shining in through the window; 'O lecznictwie i przesądach', *Izraelita*, 41 (1897), 394. A slightly different name is cited in the eighteenth-century collection of Tsevi Hirsh Khotsh, which refers to the condition *levone-bashaynt*; see Khotsh, *Segulot urefuot*, 7–8.

[77] Wilff, *Imrot shelomoh*, 40; Auerbach, *Shomer yisra'el*, 29.

[78] Segel, 'Wierzenia i lecznictwo', 57; Lew, 'O lecznictwie i przesądach', *Izraelita*, 40, p. 381; Lilientalowa, 'Dziecko żydowskie', 148; Fayvushinski, 'The Folklore of Pruzhana' (Yid.), 203; Meler, *Besorot tovot*, 50. Cf. Biegeleisen, *Matka i dziecko*, 143.

[79] Information on this belief appears in the legal verdict of Rabbi Samuel ben Fayvish of Przemyśl (sixteenth–seventeenth centuries), *Teshuvot haga'on rabi shemuel mipremesla*, 254.

a calf or a piglet. Such a child would be born if the husband urinated in the moonlight prior to having intercourse with his wife. The child's monstrous appearance was not all, however; it was said to be a particular danger to its mother, whom it had the potential to kill with its squeal.[80] Around 1800 the term *Monkalb* was still being included in midwifery manuals (such as *Grundlegung zur Hebammenkunst für die Wehmütter und für Frauen, die Wehmütter werden wollen*, Flensburg-Leipzig, 1793), medical texts, and encyclopaedias. In the literature this was the name given to molar pregnancy, which was for the initial period of gestation indistinguishable from a normal pregnancy but which ended in the miscarriage of an amorphous mass (the mole).[81] Later Yiddish literature used the word to denote cases of miscarriage which revealed foetal defects. Isaac Joel Linetski scathingly derided the 'ignorance' of the hasidim in his description of a debate on the sanctity of a rebbetsin's pregnancy: 'Did not the great Reb Hile say of the old rebbetsin when she was pregnant that she was carrying two Torah scrolls [meaning two sons, twins] . . . And did she not give birth to a girl and a *monkalb*? Well, there it is.'[82] In common parlance and folklore the term continued to mean a monster, a freak, which is reflected in sources including the stories of Sholem Aleichem.[83]

   The second example of physical abnormality in a child caused by the moon's light was *vasermun*, described by Lilientalowa in several places as 'moon water'. The catalogue of symptoms of this condition included diarrhoea, dull, glazed eyes, and yellowish skin. She cited a number of examples of remedies said to cure this ailment, involving washing or spraying the body of the affected child with water prepared in specific ways.[84] It is also important to note in this context that the notion of the *vasermun* or *vaserman*, meaning 'drowned man' (or water sprite), functioned in the folklore of the German–Slavic borderlands.[85] Moonlight was associated with damp

   [80] Rosenberg, *Der malekh refoel*, 15; Lilientalowa, 'Kult ciał niebieskich', 1; ead., *Dziecko żydowskie*, 20. Cf. Grimm, *Deutsche Mythologie*, 1111.
   [81] Lat. *Mola hydatidosa*; see Bandtkie, *Nowy słownik kieszonkowy polsko-niemiecko-francuzki*, 498.                                              [82] Linetski, *The Hasidic Boy* (Yid.), 98.
   [83] *A farzeenish, a vishkrobik, a monkalb, an opkumenish far fremde zind!* (The spectre, the imbecile, the monster, punishment for the sins of others!); Sholem Aleichem, 'The Creature' (Yid.), 179. Stutshkov cites the word *monkalb* as a synonym for expressions such as *farzeenish*, *briye meshune*, and *monster*, i.e. negatively charged descriptions of individuals considered abnormal; see *Thesaurus of the Yiddish Language* (Yid.), 574.
   [84] Lilientalowa, *Dziecko żydowskie*, 39–40; ead., 'Kult ciał niebieskich', 1.
   [85] Dźwigoł, *Polskie ludowe słownictwo mitologiczne*, 175.

and chilliness, and these, in turn, were immediately identifiable as the sali-
ent characteristics of water. What is more, in Slavic tradition the moon
was a key element of stories about drowned characters coming back to
life, something certainly not alien to Jewish folklore. Indeed, some of the
symptoms of *vasermun* call to mind aspects of the appearance of victims
of drowning. Any doubts as to the similarity between death by drowning
and *vasermun* are unequivocally allayed by a quote published in 1906 in
Max Grunwald's *Mitteilungen*, which was sourced from the collection *Sefer
refuot*, compiled in the Pale of Settlement. This contains a description of
an illness known as 'the drowned man or the moon' (*fun vaserman un
fun levone*), which produced the following symptoms in the affected child:
glazed eyes, diarrhoea, and excessive thirst. The presumed cause of this
ailment was the child's having looked into water, or 'the moon looking at
[the child]'. The remedy, according to the same source, entailed 'washing
off the drowned man' (*do gis ikh op dem vaserman fun dem kind*).[86]

The effects of the sun's rays were perceived to be the exact opposite.
Although a considerable proportion of the Jewish populace spent their days
indoors, in densely built-up urban areas, working as craftspeople or studying the sacred books, their culture consistently upheld an image of the sun
as the source of warmth and life. Children, whose lot—to be corralled in
the dark, stuffy rooms of the *ḥeder* from morning till night—was bemoaned
by the propagators of the Haskalah, would greet the sun with the following
rhyme (recorded in Borszczów):

> Zun, zun, geyt oyf,
> Moyshe rabeynu ruft dikh oyf!
> Dort vestu esn broyt mit zalts,
> Do vestu esn broyt mit shmalts,
> Dort vestu lign oyf der hoyler bank,
> Do vestu lign in betgevant.[87]

> Sun, sun, rise,
> Our teacher Moses calls you!
> There you'll get bread and salt to eat,
> Here you'll have bread and dripping to eat,
> There you'll lie on a bare bench,
> Here you'll lie in a feather bed.

[86] Grunwald, 'Aus Hausapotheke und Hexenküche II (Forts.)', 145. See Khotsh, *Segulot urefuot*, 8; David ben Aryeh Leib, *Sod hashem*, 33.
[87] 'Reminiscences: A Little Bit of Everything' (Yid.), 48–9.

The importance of the sun for physical and mental health was not unknown to the Jews. The halakhic compendium *Kitsur shulḥan arukh* contains the advice that homes should be well lit with direct sunlight in order to ensure good eyesight, a recommendation which would have been of particular significance to those who spent most of their day reading. A house should therefore have windows giving onto the east, south, and west.[88] Naturally, the sun's rays could also have a specifically therapeutic effect, which was intimated by both biblical quotes and talmudic advice.[89] Ruth Gay, recalling the life of Jewish immigrants on the Lower East Side, commented that 'air and sun were the great panaceas and healers of New York tenement life. They prevented bed bugs; they forestalled tuberculosis; they brought good health'.[90] Folk wisdom recommended spending time in the sun, which could 'bring out' (i.e. remove) the cold—as its Hebrew name (*ḥamah*, hot) indicates—for those with a fever[91] and for children suffering from 'the English disease' (rickets).[92] The tsadik Moses Teitelbaum of Sátoraljaújhely, who was for a time the rabbi in Sieniawa on the river San, believed, in accordance with a quote from the book of the prophet Malachi, that 'a sun of victory shall arise [with healing in its wings]' (Mal. 3: 20), meaning that warming oneself in the sun's rays could be therapeutic.[93] At the same time, too much sun could prove harmful. Several sources warned against exposure to it, especially in the summer months, Tamuz and Av,[94] and also in the month of Adar.[95] Aside from heatstroke, for which the recommended treatment was cold compresses and drinks,[96] particular subgroups of the population could also be vulnerable to various other onerous consequences of exposure to the sun. Girls would be warned not to go out into the sun because they might get freckles (*zunenshprenklekh*)— and this would inevitably reduce their chances of finding a good match.[97]

As in the case of the moon, there were a variety of therapeutic practices linked to the cyclicity of the sun's appearance in the sky. The folk imagination was particularly inspired by two aspects of this phenomenon:

[88] Ganzfried, *Kitsur shulḥan arukh*, 32: 27.
[89] 'But for you who revere My name, a sun of victory shall arise to bring healing' (Mal. 3: 20); 'As the day progresses, sickness is lifted' (BT *BB* 16*b*).
[90] Gay, *Unfinished People*, 44–5.    [91] Lew, 'Lecznictwo i przesądy', *Izraelita*, 50, p. 530.
[92] Such children might be buried in the sand, exposed to the hot sun up to their shoulders; Lilientalowa, *Dziecko żydowskie*, 65–6.    [93] Roker, *Toledot anshei shem*, 101–2.
[94] Sperling, *Ta'amei haminhagim oyf ivri taytsh*, ii. 33.    [95] Hurwitz, *Sefer haberit* (Yid.), 73.
[96] Rosenberg, *Der malekh refoel*, 46.    [97] Bergner, *In the Long Winter Nights* (Yid.), 28.

sunrise and sunset. These formed a clear, natural point of distinction between night and day, which gave important guidance to those undertaking various forms of treatment. This is why the sources cite so many examples of rituals and other actions that had to be performed specifically either before or after dawn or dusk. The same applied to designating the times of day at which medications were to be taken. If one was embarking on a journey or arriving in a town, the time to do so was at sunrise.[98] Looking into running water in which the first rays of the morning sun were reflected was considered to be a good way of relieving eye pain.[99] One conjuration for snakebites, published in the periodical *Yevreiskaya Starina*, contains the words: 'When the sun sets, so you too will die.'[100] This brings to mind the mechanism of waiting for a sickness to leave the body with the disappearance or setting of a heavenly body as seen in the discussion of motifs connected with the moon.

Ashkenazi communities observed the rite of sanctification of the sun (*kidesh-hakhome*), which was based on the Talmud, *Berakhot* 59b. This involved the ceremonial recitation once every twenty-eight years of the words: 'Blessed are you Lord, our God, King of the World, Maker of the work of Creation.' The ritual was held in the open air on a sunny day. Reuven Ayzland remembers that in Radomyśl Wielki preparations for the first day of the new solar cycle entailed intense study of the Mishnah, and the day itself was considered to be particularly auspicious for obtaining blessings, with great feasts organized to mark the occasion. According to one testimony from Kolbuszowa, a rabbi from the hasidic dynasty of Komarno who was staying in the town apparently made it possible for the local Jews to perform the ritual blessing by scattering the clouds that were blocking the sun. While this action secured for him the friendship of the residents, they nonetheless suspected him of witchcraft, and scrutinized him when he visited the *mikveh* to check whether he was wearing a cross around his neck.[101]

It is pertinent to add that the sun, moon, and stars (and sometimes also the seven planets) featured extremely frequently in the texts of Jewish con-

---

[98] Lilientalowa, 'Zjawiska przyrody', 58; ead., 'Kult ciał niebieskich', 12; Benet, *Sheloshah sefarim niftaḥim*, 76b. Cf. BT *BK* 60b.

[99] Lilientalowa, *Dziecko żydowskie*, 62; ead., 'Kult wody', 11; Rosenberg, *Rafa'el hamalakh*, 74.

[100] Maggid, 'Inoyazichniye zagavori', 584.

[101] Ayzland, 'In the City of Torah Scrolls' (Yid.), 400–1; Ferderber-Zalts, 'Of Events and People' (Yid.), 356–7. Cf. Lilientalowa, 'Kult ciał niebieskich', 12.

jurations. They were mentioned above all in incantations, alongside the attributes of God and religious paraphernalia endowed with an aura of sanctity. One prime example, which was known in a number of variations across eastern Europe, is this conjuration in Yiddish, sent in to An-sky from Vitebsk:

In the Name of the God of Israel, send down your archangel Raphael to me, that he might heal my son X/daughter Y of all his/her sickness and pain, whatever sickness it might be. I command, by the Almighty God and all His command-ments, the sun and the moon, and by the angels living in heaven with the Lord our God, and by the stars in the sky, by nine generations and by nine Torah scrolls, by the Ten Commandments and the ten *ofanim*, this weakness to leave my sick son X/daughter Y.[102]

The heavenly bodies might also be invoked in Jewish therapeutic magic in reference to Joshua's miracle of calming the sun and the moon (Josh. 10: 12–13). This was the case in one incantation for stemming nosebleeds, for instance.[103] Elsewhere, as some eighteenth-century manuscripts testify, conjurations were cast on evil forces to prevent their having dominion under any constellation (*mazalot*) or any of the seven planets, either by day or by night. Conditions including *koltun* (*Plica polonica*, or Polish plait) were treated in Hebrew in this way.[104] Naturally, the number of incantations in which heavenly bodies featured or played a role of any sort may have been far higher than what we find in our sources, particularly given the numer-ous borrowings from non-Jewish languages.

The turning of the seasons was no less special. Many Jewish authors from the Middle Ages onwards believed these periods to be times when the forces of evil were particularly active. This matter was the subject of heated debate among the religious authorities of virtually all medieval centres of the diaspora, from Hai Gaon (939–1038), through the Sephardi rabbis, to the leader of the Ashkenazi pietists, Judah Hehasid.[105] It was also present in Jewish culture in the Polish lands around 1900. The Galician rabbi

---

[102] An-sky, 'Charm Reversals and Conjurations' (Yid.), 167; Rechtman, *Jewish Ethnography and Folklore* (Yid.), 297. Some scholars believe this model of driving out sickness to be at least as old as the Ashkenazi diaspora. Evidence of it can certainly be traced back to late medieval (thirteenth-century) incantations; see Shulman, *The Ashkenazi Jewish Language* (Yid.), 213.

[103] An-sky, 'Charm Reversals and Conjurations' (Yid.), 165.

[104] *Segulot vekameyot*, JTS, MS 10082, 6*a*.

[105] Ta-Shma, 'The Ban on Drinking Water' (Heb.), 21–32; Bar-Ami [Segel], 'Thekuphah', *Izraelita*, 35, pp. 409–10, and *Izraelita*, 36, p. 421.

A. I. Sperling, in his *Ta'amei haminhagim*, warned his readers not to drink water at these transitional times because it was contaminated with blood, which was said to be harmful and cause swelling. As justification for his advice he cited the relevant passages from the Torah, though at second hand, from a fourteenth-century treatise by David Abudraham.[106] The 'changeover' days fell in the months of Nisan (the spring equinox—for it was at this time that the waters of Egypt were turned into blood), Tamuz (the summer solstice—when blood spurted from the rock struck by Moses), Tishrei (the autumn equinox—when Abraham was to have killed Isaac, and his knife caused a trickle of blood to run down Isaac's neck), and Tevet (the winter solstice—when the blood of the daughter of Jephthah of Gilead was shed). According to another interpretation, which features in the writings of Abraham Ibn Ezra as an 'old wives' tale' but in Sperling's collection is on a par with others, it was at these times that the heavenly guardians (archangels) changed guard, and the world and its people (thus possibly also water) were left for a while untended. The poisoned water was no longer potable and it had to be poured away.[107] Lilientalowa also cites this view as one that existed among Polish Jews. Her sources claimed that the forces of evil added the poisonous blood not only to drinks but also to certain foods, such as schmaltz, meat, and eggs (where the indication of the presence of the poison was a red blemish on the yolk).[108] Some authorities suggested that cooked, dipped, and salted foods were a particular risk. Another variation on this conviction had as the rotational guardians the four wives of Jacob: Bilhah, Rachel, Zilpah, and Leah. The choice of these particular biblical figures was justified not only by the number of seasons of the year. Firstly, the first mothers of the people of Israel were the obvious protectors of their descendants from the nefarious doings of Lilith, the mother of demons, whose menstrual blood it was that poisoned the water at these changeover times. Secondly, the initials of their names in Hebrew form the word *barzel*, iron. Like fire, objects made from iron were thought to be particularly effective in the fight against demons. For this reason the easiest way of protecting water and food at *tekufot* was to place a piece

[106] See *Abudraham*, 168.       [107] Sperling, *Ta'amei haminhagim oyf ivri taytsh*, i. 94.
[108] Lilientalowa, 'Wierzenia, przesądy i praktyki', 149–50. According to some medieval Ashkenazi rabbis it was not demons but the angel of death himself who poisoned the water at these times; see Ta-Shma, 'The Ban on Drinking Water' (Heb.), 26; Grunwald, 'Aus unseren Sammlungen. Teil I', 97.

of metal (for example a nail) in the vessels in which they were stored;[109] it did not have to be physically touching the food, merely to rest in the vessel. Moreover, water made ready for the performance of a *mitsvah* (such as the production of matzah or washing a corpse) would not become contaminated.

To summarize this examination of the extent to which elements of early medicine and astrology remained current in the traditional Jewish therapeutic model, it is important to stress that these areas of lore are not easy to tease apart from the wider theme of this book. They did not constitute an arcane sphere of knowledge accessible only to the initiated: educated physicians or 'stargazers'. On the contrary, they were reflected in procedures followed by both tsadikim and healers, men and women, and frequently recurred in both medical manuals and colloquial expressions. In other words, they were an intrinsic aspect of views on the rules governing the world that dominated thought in Jewish society until the early twentieth century.

There were several reasons for this. The visions of humoral pathology and of the influence of the heavenly bodies had largely evolved out of human speculation surrounding the links between the body and both the animate and inanimate elements of the environment. The traditional Jewish communities of eastern Europe constructed their own conceptions of the aetiology and treatment of disease on the basis of the same roots, and while these tended to be dependent to a large extent on the sphere of myth, in many respects they were concordant with the suppositions of the early philosophers (for example in terms of the key dimensions of homeostasis or attempts to 'draw' the sickness out of the patient's body). The fact that the beliefs of the ancients unfailingly found support among the religious authorities should not be ignored. They were regularly reproduced not only in publications on medicine but also in the words of figures who were the pillars of both rabbinic Judaism and hasidism, and in the ethical literature. Eventually they became part of the canon of knowledge acquired by members of the Jewish community as they grew up; while both *ḥeder* and yeshiva students were inspired by visions of the world to come, they were, of course, also interested in the temporal world. Since the path to discovery

---

[109] Hirshovitsh, *Minhagei yeshurun*, 261; Sperling, *Ta'amei haminhagim oyf ivri taytsh*, i. 94; Grunwald, 'Aus unseren Sammlungen. Teil I', 97; id., 'Aus Hausapotheke und Hexenküche III', 217.

of the rules governing it led through the treacherous terrain of philosophy (which concealed above all the hazard of free thinking), and they did not have access to literature in foreign languages, they turned to works of ethics. These tended to explain the functioning of the world and the human body with reference to the theory of the four elements, humoral pathology, astrology, and so on. One such young man was the future writer Isaac Bashevis Singer: 'As I knew none of the languages of the *goyim*, I sought knowledge in Yiddish and the sacred tongue. But [secular] books in Yiddish and Hebrew were considered *treif* in our community. I discovered science via the *Shevilei emunah* and the *Sefer haberit*. I also devoured the *Moreh nevukhim* [Maimonides] and the *Kuzari* [Judah Halevi], but I found it hard to understand them.'[110]

[110] Y. Varshavski [Isaac Bashevis Singer], 'Of the Old and New Homelands' (Yid.).

# PART III

# REDEMPTION AND FESTIVALS

# CHAPTER NINE

# SIN AND REDEMPTION

$A$N OVERVIEW of the relevant literature written over the past few decades invites the conclusion that scholars of folk medicine have tended to take far greater interest in the material, practical aspects of therapies (such as herbalism) than in their spiritual dimension.[1] Certain cultural facts—in particular those rooted in religious tradition (whether Jewish or Christian)—may indeed have sometimes been passed over as too obvious. On occasion categorized expressly as religious, they became marginalized and disappeared from the horizon of ethnographers studying medical culture. Another reason why this area of research has been ignored is the greater accessibility and clarity of source material relating to the physical side of therapeutics; yet another the declared hope of finding rational justification for the therapies recorded by collectors of folklore. Yet it would be almost impossible to imagine folk medical practices as unrelated to religion and demonology. The two worlds were closely entwined, each incomplete and unexplainable without the other. Until quite recently, visions of the might of divine judgement and the wiles of the forces of evil were a contingent element of the majority of human endeavours, and seemed no less real than concepts such as fever or diphtheria. Thus any attempt to describe east European Jews' understanding of their world must take a broad enough view to include fields dismissed by biomedicine and science as superstition and assiduously suppressed over the past two centuries.

Within traditional Jewish society, as in other east European communities, reality was not confined to the physical. The existence of an extrasensory dimension perceptible only to a select few through visions and other mystical experiences, often in the context of unusual, even perilous, circumstances, was not called into question. This was a dimension that would

---

[1] In recently published studies, matters relating to religiosity and demonology are either absent altogether (e.g. Jeszke, *Lecznictwo ludowe w Wielkopolsce*) or constitute no more than a marginal strand (e.g. Jaguś, *Lecznictwo ludowe w Królestwie Polskim*).

be revealed in full after the Rubicon of life and death was crossed, and it was believed to encompass both this world, along with all its incorporeal inhabitants (demons, errant souls, etc.), and the world to come. These two spheres—the visible and the invisible—though governed by separate laws, were nonetheless bound up in a tightly woven mesh of interdependencies. Not only did they influence each other in matters including human health, but they were also, to an extent, reflections of each other. This in turn meant that the list of potential dangers—and with it the catalogue of therapeutic alternatives—was inexhaustible, the rational and magical dimensions of folk medicine eminently reconcilable, and ancient texts and beliefs constantly current as sources providing rationalization for the occurrences people witnessed.

Although life was an unending round of struggles with the reverses of fate, folk culture cultivated a memory of mythical times in which the human body had been free of all weakness. According to the Talmud, old age had not existed until the time of Abraham, and sickness had been unknown before the days of Jacob. It had only come into the world as a result of his prayers: knowing that the earlier patriarchs had departed this life with just a sneeze, without suffering or agony, Jacob implored God to give him a warning of his impending death, because he wanted to bid his sons farewell. The Lord therefore sent down an illness on him as a visible sign of his imminent demise. The book of Genesis reads: 'Joseph was told, "Your father is ill"' (Gen. 48: 1). Sneezing remained as a warning, and the *de rigueur* response was *Tsu gezunt!* (To your health!).[2] Even in the late nineteenth century Jewish sources were still perpetuating a popular vision of the dawn of humanity in which Adam and Eve did not suffer from any illness because their bodies were covered with rough, horny skin, which they later lost due to sin. This was a recurrent motif in the context of illness and dying. It was the reason why Eve's actions were the point of reference in justifying the warning that a pregnant woman who stepped on scattered finger- or toenail clippings was bound to miscarry.[3] A patient who stared at their own fingernails was believed to be at death's door,[4] and a common saying was 'Look at your nails and you'll soon stop smirking.'[5] Nail clip-

---

[2] BT *BM* 87a; Lew, 'Z ludoznawstwa', *Izraelita*, 18, p. 196.
[3] Lipiets, *Sefer matamim*, 83; Wilff, *Imrot shelomoh*, 100; Buchbinder, 'Jewish Omens' (Yid.), 250.          [4] Lilientalowa, 'Wierzenia, przesądy i praktyki', 106.
[5] See Khayes, 'Death-Related Beliefs and Customs' (Yid.), 308.

pings would not be thrown away but inserted into a door panel or window frame, or between slats on a desk, thrown behind a bookcase in the *beit hamidrash* (study hall), or—preferably—burned or buried. Tradition had it that anyone who failed to do this would be vulnerable to attack by demons. Their nail clippings would even testify against them at the last judgement.[6]

The concept of sin (*zind*, *khet*) in the culture of east European Jews essentially consisted in violation of the system of prohibitive and imperative commandments issued to Israel by God during the revelation at Mount Sinai. Sin was interpreted as rebellion against the authority of the Law in dealings with other people and relations with the Creator, to whom the Jewish nation was bound by the Abrahamic covenant. According to tradition, which was reinforced by a wealth of ethical and kabbalistic sources, people had free will and tended to act on their own decisions, though they might have a particular penchant for either good or bad deeds (*yetser hatov* and *yetser hara*, respectively, the latter sometimes identified with Satan). They had to face the consequences of their actions, and in the ethical sphere these were invariably connected with their health. For the assiduous performance of *mitsvot* the Creator showered his faithful with all manner of blessings: 'The Holy Blessed One gives you light in your eyes and hearing in your ears and legs with which to walk . . . and all this he gives for free', one religious book printed in Yiddish explained. 'And if sometimes he does not reward you after a *mitsvah* is performed . . . He had already endowed you with goodness before you performed it.'[7] In contrast to rewards, punishments were always sent down *post factum*. Nonetheless, there could be no doubt that they would come. The inevitability of judgement was experienced even by biblical greats such as the prophetess Miriam, sister of Moses, whom God punished with leprosy for disobedience to his will (Num. 12: 9–10).[8] This will, closely connected to the physical side of human life, could be weighed and measured, and successive generations of rabbis devoted themselves to doing just that.

The Talmud is the earliest source to mention the number of commandments recorded in the Torah: the 365 prohibitions were reflected in the number of days in the solar calendar, while the 248 imperatives were

---

[6] Grunwald, 'Aus unseren Sammlungen. Teil I', 81; Lilientalowa, 'Przesądy żydowskie', 279; Ch., 'Materiały do etnografii Żydów polskich', 437; Yoffie, 'Popular Beliefs and Customs', 379.

[7] *Ets ḥayim*, 9.

[8] According to the ethical literature Miriam was punished for *lashon hara* (derogatory speech), i.e. defamation of her brother; see T. H. Koydanover, *Kav hayashar*, 157.

echoed in the number of limbs, tendons, and bones in the human body.[9] The rabbinic authorities were not in unanimous agreement as to their enumeration, and Moses Maimonides (*Sefer hamitsvot*) played a decisive role in influencing later Judaism in this respect. In any examination of Jewish tradition it is hard to ignore the importance in ethical ruminations of the connection between violation of the commandments and the body. Each one of the 613 *mitsvot* was believed to correspond to particular parts of the human anatomy. While the exact number and position of the bones were associated with the positive Torah commandments, the 365 prohibitions were held to be equivalent to the number of veins. This vision of the human body as inextricably enmeshed in a web of divine commandments remained dominant in the spiritual culture of the Jews until contemporary times. A prime example of its significance for folk therapeutics is the words of the Ba'al Shem Tov, the founder of hasidism, to his doctor after he had undergone a successful course of treatment: 'You approached the sick man corporeally and I approached him spiritually. A man has 248 members in his body and 365 veins. Corresponding to them are 248 positive and 365 negative commandments. If a man commits one crime, God forbid, the corresponding member or vein begins to fail. If he contravenes many interdictions, many veins fail. The blood no longer flows in them and the person is in danger.'[10]

The notion of sickness as punishment recurs several times in the Talmud, including in the well-known proverb that no one will cut their finger if it has not been ordained in heaven.[11] However, the use of divine justice as an explanation for misfortune did not necessarily preclude other types of aetiology. The causes of ailments, like their very nature, were interpreted using a combination of conceptions drawn from various, often mutually contradictory, traditions. Many sources state explicitly that supernatural and natural explanations were enmeshed, even in the most prosaic of cases. As we study Jewish medical practices it should come as no surprise that in case of mechanical injuries, in particular external ones, recourse in the first instance was to ancient surgical practices. Wounds would be dressed with cobwebs and bread.[12] In the Belarusian town of Horodets, anyone who got

[9] BT *Mak.* 23*b*.    [10] Ben-Amos and Mintz, *In Praise of the Baal Shem Tov*, 178.
[11] BT *Ḥul.* 7*b*; Nüsel, 'Sprichwörter und Redensarten aus Posen', 67.
[12] Halpern, *Toledot adam*, 34; *Segulot urefuot*, JTS, MS 9862, 56 and 58; Lilientalowa, 'Dziecko żydowskie', 153; Farber, 'Folk Healing' (Yid.), 180; Shlaferman, 'The Folklore, Customs, and Stories of Kazimierz' (Yid.), 172; Silverman-Weinreich, 'Beliefs' (Yid.), 33.

sand in their eye would go to a man named Isaac Aaron, who would lick the affected site.[13] The recommended course of action for a broken limb was to splint it, rub it with bear fat and milk, and avoid movement.[14] And yet behind each of these complaints there was also a supernatural explanation. The *Ta'amei haminhagim*, a book of customs published in Galicia which drew on the medieval *Sefer ḥasidim*, exhorted its readers not to seek the cause of indisposition in unhealthy food or even in a beating by rogues, but to be aware that everything comes from the Creator.[15] The author of *Kav hayashar*, citing the Zohar, argued that just as a guttering candle should be shaken to revive the flame, so a sinful person whose soul was dimmed through iniquity would be visited by suffering from God.[16] Authors from slightly later periods drew attention to the perils of frequenting places full of bandits or one's foes, or entering buildings with structural faults— in such environments, they said, people's sins would come back to haunt them.[17]

The talmudic catalogue of iniquities engendering divine punishment was extremely broad. Among the sinners who could expect their days to be numbered were scholars who were called up to read the Torah but declined, or were given wine to bless but refused to do so, and those who sinned in pride.[18] The rabbis also enumerated specific examples of sins that could bring about the death of women and unscholarly men, whose spiritual imperfection was, in the clerical opinion, beyond doubt. Death in childbirth, for instance, awaited women who failed to observe the commandments concerning ritual impurity, taking *ḥalah*, or lighting the sabbath candles, but also those who washed their children on the sabbath or demonstrated ignorance of ritual matters.[19] Naturally, the list of sins detailed in the Talmud was not exhaustive, and successive centuries of exegesis lengthened it considerably. The motif of punishment was a perennial

[13] Farber, 'Folk Healing' (Yid.), 178; Neumann, 'Our Town' (Yid.), 423. See Lilientalowa, *Dziecko żydowskie*, 62.

[14] Plaut, *Likutei ḥever ben ḥayim*, 9b. Fractures and certain other injuries to the limbs (such as gunshot wounds or shards of glass in the hand) would also be treated by holding the injured body part in the entrails of an animal (sometimes one that had been slaughtered for the sabbath); see *Segulot urefuot*, JTS, MS 9862, 30; Rotner, *Sipurei nifla'ot*, 3; Maimon, *An Autobiography*, 37.

[15] Sperling, *Ta'amei haminhagim oyf ivri taytsh*, ii. 41.   [16] Ibid. 141.   [17] *Ets ḥayim*, 29.

[18] BT *Ber.* 55a. Other sources added also those who failed to rise to their feet on seeing the Torah being taken out of the ark in the synagogue. See Auerbach, *Shomer yisra'el*, 7.

[19] BT *Shab.* 32a.

subject of study in rabbinic Orthodoxy and hasidism alike. According to one anthology of tales of the miracles wrought by tsadikim, a man might become infertile if he beat his wife[20] or if he failed to make good a sin he had committed against his neighbour.[21]

The Jews living in eastern Europe believed that there were seven things which made life shorter: anger and envy, greed and pride, gossip, debauchery,[22] and idleness.[23] Anyone who lived to a ripe old age—*arikhes yomim* (lit. long years)—was considered fortunate and blessed, however. 'The span of our life is seventy years', the psalmist wrote (Ps. 90: 10), and this conviction put down deep roots in the popular consciousness, which recast the sentiment in its own idiom: *Biz zibetsik yor lernt men zikh seykhl un men shtarbt fort a nar* (You spend your first seventy years learning common sense, but you die a fool anyway).[24] The traditional Jew feared 'counting the days of his life', which was tantamount to tempting fate (or the forces of evil, or the angel of death). Any sin, any transgression of the will of the Creator or of one's neighbour, when judged, would shorten one's time on earth. Nonetheless, it was believed that evil could be outsmarted. Even a person who took pride in their age would merely say: *Ikh bin alt vi mayn kleyner finger* (I'm as old as my little finger). If the subject of age was broached, for prudence's sake they would say they were younger than they actually were, or add the caveat *biz hundert un tsvantsik* ([May I live] up to 120).[25] Anyone who lived longer than seventy springs considered their longevity a reward for their earthly merits and rejoiced in the years granted them by God (*geshenkte yor*). At that age they would start counting from zero again, and, on reaching their eighty-third year, could claim to have reached the age of second *bar mitsvah*.[26] Anyone who did not live to be 70, however, was widely believed to have contravened the divine will.

Those who died prematurely were thought to have to live out the rest of their years in another incarnation.[27] This is one example of the kabbalistic concept of the transmigration of souls (Heb. *gilgul hanefesh*), which,

---

[20] Rotner, *Sipurei nifla'ot*, 11–12.                                    [21] Ibid. 14–15.

[22] The term *zenut* might also encompass various types of forbidden sexual activity (adultery, intercourse during menstruation, homosexual acts, etc.) in the Jewish tradition.

[23] Bastomski, *At the Source: Jewish Proverbs* (Yid.), 8.

[24] Einhorn, 'Folk Proverbs' (Heb.), 343.          [25] Lilientalowa, 'The Evil Eye' (Yid.), 249.

[26] Bin Wolf, 'Memories from My Father's House' (Heb.), 149.

[27] Khayes, 'Death-Related Beliefs and Customs' (Yid.), 285; Lilientalowa, 'Życie pozagrobowe i świat przyszły w wyobrażeniu ludu żydowskiego', 351.

ignored by most rabbis until the sixteenth century, was systematized by the proponents of Lurianic kabbalah (in works including *Sha'ar hagilgulim*). Along with other concepts propagated by the mystics of Safed, over the ensuing centuries this idea spread throughout the culture of Ashkenazi Jews, becoming fused with the myths dominant among the peoples of eastern Europe. If a *gilgul*, as the migrating soul was known, had only a few years to live out, or was not burdened by excessive sin, it might be reborn in the body of a sickly infant and die again shortly thereafter. For this reason babies would not be named after anyone who had died prematurely.[28] And unlike adults, children would have years added to their age if asked, so that they might sooner 'reach' an age considered safe.[29] The majority of dead souls, however, roamed the world or took on a form appropriate to their sins: those who had not kept kosher would return bound to leaves (whipped by the wind and forced to bear immense suffering); informers would come back fused to mute stones; those who had shirked ritual ablutions were tied to rocks in a river; people who had sinned through pride were reborn as dogs, apostates as pigs, and so on. Sinners' souls might be saved by the actions of the living, in particular those of especial virtue, such as hasidic leaders.[30] The tsadik Mordecai Twersky of Chernobyl was said to select the willow branches for his Sukkot *lulav* in such a way as to redeem only the worthy souls from among those who had been condemned to *gilgul*.[31] His son, David of Talne, offered the following interpretation of the importance of eating fish during the first sabbath meal: souls were drawn to fish because in this way they might find their way onto a tsadik's table, and if a righteous man fulfilled one of the sabbath commandments (eating fish) through their agency, they would be redeemed.[32]

In the popular understanding the bond between the human soul and body was so strong that even the smallest flaw in the former would immediately manifest in the latter. Material form reflected spiritual faults, which

[28] Fels, 'Zabobony lekarskie u Żydów', 4; Weissenberg, 'Das neugeborene Kind', 87.

[29] Lilientalowa, 'The Evil Eye' (Yid.), 249.

[30] Akalovich, 'Zametki o yevrieiskoy narodnoy demonologii', 138–43. This was how hasidism interpreted and reprocessed in its own way the story of the kabbalist Isaac Luria; see T. H. Koydanover, *Kav hayashar*, 12–13.

[31] Mekler, *Fun rebns hoyf*, 259–60. It was for this reason—in view of the sinful souls inhabiting them—that it was forbidden to break off lilac branches and eat elderberries (Yid. *meshugene grayplekh*, crazy berries); see Segel, 'Wierzenia i lecznictwo', 50; 'Omens and Remedies' (Yid.), 295–6.                                                   [32] Mekler, *Fun rebns hoyf*, 91–3.

was particularly evident in the case of debauchery. Acne breakouts on the face or back were known in Polish as *zachciewajka* (lust rash), because they were thought to be a symptom of strong sexual urges. This name passed into Yiddish (*zakhtsianke*),[33] despite the fact that there were far more colourful synonyms to choose from: *ahave-rabe-prishtshes* (great love spots),[34] *yetser-hore-blotern* (evil desire abscesses),[35] *tayve-kretslekh* (urge scabies),[36] or *froyengenitung* (lust for women).[37] Similarly, physical ailments were said to be detrimental to the moral sphere. An infertile person was thought to be heartless, as evidenced by the saying: *A bezdietnik iz a bezhartsnik.*[38] The designation of a person with disabilities as *farkriplt* (crippled) or as a *ba'al mum* (deformed) could refer to both spheres of their existence—the physical and the spiritual—in equal measure. There are a number of expressions in Yiddish reflecting the belief in this equivalence: 'a *ba'al-mum* is always twisted',[39] 'every *ba'al-mum* is evil',[40] or 'deficient in body and twisted in soul'.[41] These popular convictions took on particular significance in times of plague. The selection from among the disabled of a 'bride' and 'groom' to perform the ritual of a 'black wedding' was not based solely on the concept, expounded in the ethical literature, of *hakhnasat kalah*—an act of charity consisting in endowing a poor girl with a dowry and finding her a husband. The 'black wedding' was undertaken by the community to protect itself against an epidemic, which, in the nineteenth century, primarily meant cholera. Since it focused on marrying a pair of 'unfortunates', the rabbis interpreted it as a way to supplicate for God's mercy through the *mitsvah* performed by the entire shtetl.[42] Without refuting this interpretation, it is important to note the apotropaic aspect of the custom: disabled people were held up to the forces of evil as a mirror of their own 'twisted'

[33] 'Letter Box' (Yid.), *Folksgezunt*, 3 (1925), 99. Cf. Kolberg, *Dzieła wszystkie*, 165.

[34] Yofe and Mark (eds.), *Great Dictionary of the Yiddish Language* (Yid.), i. 49; Stutshkov, *Thesaurus of the Yiddish Language* (Yid.), 420.      [35] 'Letter Box' (Yid.), *Folksgezunt*, 11 (1926), 258.

[36] Ibid. 3–4 (1924), 88.                     [37] Ibid. 5–6 (1923), 35.

[38] 'Useful Proverbs' (Yid.), *Yidishe shprakh*, 14, p. 62. Aside from heartlessness, another character flaw directly associated with childlessness was miserliness. See Nagelberg, 'Sagen galizischer Juden', 257; Golenpol, *Lexicon of Hebrew Folklore* (Heb.), 17.

[39] 'Useful Proverbs' (Yid.), *Yidishe shprakh*, 11, p. 55.

[40] Stutshkov, *Thesaurus of the Yiddish Language* (Yid.), 407–13.

[41] 'Useful Proverbs' (Yid.), *Yidishe shprakh*, 11, p. 55.

[42] Veynig, '*Mageyfe* Weddings' (Yid.), 30. Cf. Moszyński, *Kultura ludowa Słowian*, 624–6. For more on the subject of the 'black wedding' ritual as protection from cholera, see e.g. Veynig, 'Medicaments and Remedies among the Jews' (Yid.), 25–31; Węgrzynek, '"Shvartze khasene": Black Wedding among Polish Jews', 55–68.

countenances. There was believed to be something demonic about those with disabilities; people with one eye, for instance, were said to find it easy to cast the evil eye. Indeed, for this reason it was not considered wise to make fun of the disabled, or to count the blemishes on people with spots, boils or warts; it was believed that in doing so one might bring the disease on oneself.[43]

Sickness presented an opportunity to purify oneself from sins. Like ascetic practices, it was a situation that could bring about the moral improvement of the sufferer. It was said: *A make un a tsore iz beser vi a magid un a muser-seyfer* (Wounds and misfortunes are better than a preacher and a holy book).[44] One author wrote: 'As a father punishes his child so that it will be good and pious, so too does the Holy Blessed One. Let every person know that God does not send them anything ill, but when he does send misfortune, it is all for their own good, that they might expiate their misdemeanours and reduce their punishment in the world to come.'[45] Recovery from a serious illness was a clear sign to the community that the person who had been cured had found the Creator's grace. People were convinced that if the sufferer had not purified themselves from their sin, they would not have recovered. 'Blessed be He who heals the sick' was the customary greeting on seeing a friend who had recently been restored to health.[46] Recovered patients themselves should thank heaven for being spared by reciting the 'Gomel' blessing. The connection between physical indisposition and asceticism was also strongly reinforced in hasidic texts. According to the tsadik Isaac of Niesuchojeże (Neskhizh), at the divine judgement bodily sufferings would be counted as merits:

Once, when I was having an *aliyat neshamah* [elevation of the soul] to the world above, a man was brought to judgement. His merits and his sins were weighed up, but the former were insufficient to tip the scales. He was condemned to hell. As he was being handed over to the angel that was to take him to hell, [another] great and terrible angel came up and spoke thus: 'I have exculpation for him.' And he brought out huge sacks full of sufferings that [the man] had borne in his lifetime, and of which the angel himself was made. These tipped the scales, and the verdict was changed to paradise.[47]

[43] Lilientalowa, 'Wierzenia, przesądy i praktyki', 159; ead., *Dziecko żydowskie*, 64. Even making an involuntary count of warts was said to attract them to oneself: ead., *Choroby, lecznictwo*, fo. 79.   [44] 'Useful Proverbs' (Yid.), *Yidishe shprakh*, 14, p. 62.
[45] *Ets ḥayim*, 14.   [46] Veynig, 'Doctors and Medicine in Jewish Sayings' (Yid.), 17.
[47] Moshkovitsh (ed.), *Otsar hasipurim*, 26.

The image of the heavenly tribunal portrayed here reflects the popular interpretation of the teaching on reward and punishment. It recurs repeatedly in both rabbinic and kabbalistic works and in collections amassed by the pioneers of ethnography. A proper understanding of this lore helps to comprehend many of the customs whose purpose was to safeguard the human body. The Jews of eastern Europe believed that God, who, as the ruler of the world, was constantly passing judgement on it, was characterized by two main attributes: *midat hadin*, the quality of justice, and *midat harahamim*, the quality of mercy. According to Rashi, the work of Creation as it had begun, based solely on the former quality, proved unsustainable, and so the Creator combined this stern justice with mercy, just as 'he created heaven and earth'. In the sphere of health, sickness or other forms of physical indisposition could be an expression of *midat hadin*, just punishment for sins committed, while *midat harahamim* brought relief from suffering, the alleviation of symptoms, or even full recovery. Folk mythology painted an expressive picture of judgement, with sins and offences against God and one's neighbours on one arm of the scales, and conscientious fulfilment of the commandments, good deeds, and other merits on the other. This latter category (*zkhus*), which counted towards a verdict in one's favour, encompassed in equal measure one's own deeds and those of one's ancestors (*zkhus-oves*). It also included the intercession of devout, pious individuals, who, like the souls of one's parents and grandparents, could act as one's advocates before the heavenly tribunal. As mentioned, however, it might also manifest as actions performed as elements of other rites (for example the sabbath feast). The law of inheritance likewise extended to sins, though to a lesser degree. On Mount Sinai God told Moses that he would punish children for the sins of their parents to the fourth generation (Exod. 20: 5). Thus the reason for the death of a child was believed to be the immorality of its parents, and on occasion even of the whole community. Similarly, the death of a parent was believed to be due to the sins of their offspring.[48]

The heavenly tribunal comprised prosecutory figures (*kateyger*, from the Greek *kategoros*), often identified with Satan, and the defence (*sneyger*, from the Greek *synegoros*, but also *meylets-yoysher*), which role was played by the archangel Michael.[49] The presiding judge, of course, was the Creator, who, in the face of death, was always referred to as Dayan Emet—Judge of

---

[48] Zelkovitsh, 'Death and Its Accompanying Moments' (Yid.), 155.          [49] Dan. 10: 13–21.

Truth. This tribunal operated outside time, and its verdicts were sometimes passed simultaneously to events occurring in this life.[50] It influenced a person's lot in life and the fate of their soul after death in equal measure. People rarely perceived positive verdicts; they were far more likely to be afflicted by indictments (*gzar*). *A nar iz a gzar*, it was said, which may be translated as: 'A fool is a divine decree.'

Regardless of the outcome of the weighing, the judgement of the Judge of Truth was associated with the attribute of justice. If the verdict was unfavourable there was always the possibility that it might be suspended or reversed if the Creator shifted to the throne of mercy. He might be persuaded to do so by the guilty party doing penance, by the intercession of the righteous or the souls of the dead, and sometimes also by other circumstances. The popular practical kabbalah produced many examples of actions designed to influence the attributes of *din* and *raḥamim*. Employed appropriately, numerical techniques could be used to perform manipulations of words and meanings, and this too could effect changes in the heavenly reality. Below is an example of one such manipulation, published in the anthology *Rafa'el hamalakh*:

Take 160 coins. Let the rich man take large silver ones, and the poor man smaller ones. But let there be 160 of them. The mystery of this number lies in the value of the words *ets* [tree], *tselem* [image], and *kesef* [silver, money]. For humans are known as 'trees of the field' [Deut. 20: 19], they were created 'in God's image' [Gen. 1: 27], but they can be bought with silver. But all money is known as silver, for a woman is bought for silver that is coinage of copper.

To begin with, the number of coins [should be] counted out in such a way as to form the following four groups. The first will number ten times 5, the second five times 10, the third six times 5, and the fourth five times 6 [these represent the numerical value of the letters which make up the Tetragrammaton] . . . All together, they give 160. Now mix the groups into one and take from it first 31 coins to make a separate group. And say out loud [the numbers] 1, 2, 3, 4, etc. until the thirty-first coin is reached. And then recite the verse: 'God's faithfulness never ceases' [Ps. 52: 3]. [Do this] with the intention of reinforcing the attribute of grace [*ḥesed*] comprised in the [divine] name El [the letters of this name add up to 31].

Next take coins from the large group up to the number 64, which is the sum

---

[50] According to T. H. Koydanover, at the hour of sickness 'a heavenly court is in session; the defence is justifying [the person's actions], the prosecutors are enumerating their wrongs and mistakes before the Holy One, may his name be blessed'; see *Kav hayashar*, 112.

of the word *din* [judgement]. But do not count this number out loud, only focus your thoughts on it, because it is the number of [harsh] judgement. Make of them one group, and after a short while take from it coins and count out 17, concentrating your thoughts on the great name Ahavah. And make from these 17 coins a separate group. Then take coins from the former group again, to the number of 21, thinking of the great name Ehyeh, and from them also make a separate group. Then take the remaining coins, to the number of 26, thinking of the great name Yahveh, and make of them a separate group . . . The number 64, meaning *din*, has thus been broken down into the three numbers of the three sacred names . . . which constitute the three attributes of mercy [*midot harahamim*] . . .

Now take up the coins from the fifth group and count them out until you reach 65. But before counting, focus your thoughts on the sacred name Adonai, which is 65. And it is composed of the letters of *din* [and] *a*. And the mystery of the full letter *a*, *alef*, lies in its combination [anagram] with the most supreme *pele* [miracle], in which [there is] but full mercy. Thus *a* sweetens the three letters of *din* in the name Adonai.[51]

Kabbalistic manipulations, however, required knowledge that was largely inaccessible to ordinary people, meaning that they did not occupy a prominent place in therapeutic practices that approached sickness as a manifestation of sin. The negative impact of sins against God and one's neighbours could be neutralized by performing a good deed or an appropriate *mitsvah*. According to the rabbinic tradition, three things had the power to save one from death: prayer, repentance, and alms (*tefilah*, *teshuvah*, and *tsedakah*).[52] The traditional Jewish community in eastern Europe developed this thought after its own fashion, interweaving it with beliefs of a different character. The ill, changing winds which followed the festivals of Pesach (in the spring) and Sukkot (in the autumn), and were so detrimental to those with lung diseases and to infants, were thought to be connected with the misdeeds that were often perpetrated in festive periods. As it was written in the book of Job (1: 5): 'When a round of feast days was over, Job would send word to them to sanctify themselves, and . . . make burnt offerings, one for each of them; for Job thought: "Perhaps my children have sinned and blasphemed God in their thoughts."' In order to lift the odium of sin from oneself and one's community, and thus to protect

[51] Rosenberg, *Rafa'el hamalakh*, 77–8.
[52] According to the Talmud, *RH* 16*b*, four things could bring salvation, the fourth being a change of name.

oneself from the effects of the weather, one should undertake a fast known
as *sheni ḥamishi vesheni*—as its name indicates, to be observed on the second
and fifth day of the week and on the second day of the subsequent week in
the month after these festivals (Iyar and Heshvan respectively). This custom, which had its source in a text from the Mishnah well known in the
early Middle Ages, was observed above all in Ashkenazi culture.[53] It is
worth noting, though, that at the end of the nineteenth century the significance of fasting diminished somewhat. In times of epidemics in particular,
medical professionals appealed to the populace not to forgo food so as not
to render their already compromised immune system any more susceptible
to infection. Notes exhorting people not to fast during outbreaks of cholera
are even featured in traditional medical vademecums.[54]

Acts of contrition, alms, and prayer tended to be linked to the peniten-
tial period around Rosh Hashanah and Yom Kippur. On occasion, however,
these pious means of warding off death might be enacted independently of
the festivals, and of each other. One situation in which the three acts would
be observed to the letter was where they were intended as a means of keeping a child alive. As mentioned above, the death of a child—something still
extremely widespread around 1900—was interpreted as a divine punishment for the sins of its parents, and as such the parents and other members
of the immediate family were expected to undertake propitiatory action.
Even before their child was born, both spouses were advised to perform
*tsedakah*, contemplate their sins, and say the 'Aneinu' prayer, customary for
fast days, every evening.[55] If at birth the child proved to be sickly, they
might designate the day of its birth or another day of the week of their
choice as a permanent fast day until the child reached halakhic adulthood—
13 in the case of a boy or 12 in the case of a girl. Another, related custom was
lighting candles in commemoration of the mishnaic sage Rabbi Meir Ba'al
Hanes (Meir the miracle worker) on that day. If one could not fast, there
was the alternative option of giving alms in the amount of eighteen coins,
which might be of particular significance to women who were pregnant
again or nursing the child. If these steps proved efficacious and the child did
survive, it was to be given candles and money to perform the almsgiving.
It would also be taught a prayer that was written out in the shape of the

[53] BT *Ta'an.* 15*b*; Lipiets, *Sefer matamim*, 131; Hirshovitsh, *Minhagei yeshurun*, 132–3.
[54] Those suffering from epilepsy were also advised against fasting; Rosenberg, *Rafa'el
hamalakh*, 51, 69; id., *Der malekh refoel*, 61.                    [55] Wilff, *Imrot shelomoh*, 98.

menorah, the candelabrum of the Temple in Jerusalem.[56] Alms for the soul of Rabbi Meir Ba'al Hanes would also be given in other difficult or perilous situations; the almsgiving would be accompanied by a prayer, the central feature of which would be the repetition several times of the words *elaha deme'ir aneni* (God of Meir, answer me). According to one talmudic tale, this short prayer had the miraculous power to call down divine aid.[57] Collections of Yiddish *tkhines* (supplications) also contained longer texts to be recited when placing alms in the Rabbi Meir tin. These included the overt plea for 'the granting of full recovery' to a sick child.[58]

The importance of charity in Jewish therapeutic practices is revealed in an analysis of them in the broader context. The custom of making votive offerings to the synagogue was widespread in Ashkenaz, as the numerous Torah scrolls, *parokhot*, Elijah's thrones, and similar furnishings and fittings testify,[59] but alms to the needy seem to have been far more highly regarded than donating ritual objects. Assuming that 'To do what is right and just [*tsedakah*] is more desired by the Lord than sacrifice' (Prov. 21: 3), one could expect to achieve more by helping a poor person than by making any other sort of offering to God. Alms were not always direct in character; indeed, the most highly valued act of charity was one that remained anonymous for both parties.[60] In this context, financing the repairs to or renovation of the *beit hamidrash*, the *mikveh*, or especially a poorhouse or homeless shelter might be interpreted as aid to the poor.

Alms featured in some way in almost all health-related practices, forming an element of a variety of rituals. A pregnant woman who wished to take precautions against miscarriage would drape her belly in seven cubits of material which had lain on the Torah ark of the synagogue for seven days, and after having been safely delivered of her baby, would give some of the fabric to the poor.[61] If an infant was ill, its mother would be advised to bake as many loaves of bread as would fit in its cradle, and give them to the poor.[62] In case of jaundice the advice was to place a variety of herbs in a

[56] *Ets ḥayim*, 99; Wilff, *Imrot shelomoh*, 110; Rosenberg, *Rafa'el hamalakh*, 33; Lilientalowa, *Dziecko żydowskie*, 70–1.

[57] BT *AZ* 18*a–b*; Rosenberg, *Rafa'el hamalakh*, 82; Lilientalowa, *Dziecko żydowskie*, 70.

[58] See *Mekor dimah*, 342–3.

[59] See e.g. An-sky, *The Yiddish Ethnographic Programme* (Yid.), 177; Rechtman, 'Some Customs and Their Folk Explanations' (Yid.), 250.

[60] Ganzfried, *Kitsur shulḥan arukh*, 34: 1–16.         [61] Lilientalowa, *Dziecko żydowskie*, 26.

[62] Elzet [Złotnik], 'Some Jewish Customs' (Heb.), 370.

bottle, place the bottle into the dough for a loaf of bread, and bake it. The bread was given away, and the contents of the bottle administered to the patient several times a day.[63] The anthology of women's prayers *A naye shas tkhine* recommended that almsgiving be accompanied by a protective formula against the evil eye, comprising eleven quotations from the Hebrew Bible, all beginning and ending with the letter *nun*.[64] According to the most popular Yiddish-language biblical anthology, the *Tsene urene*, which was intended as a resource for women, *tsedakah* during pregnancy was only effective when combined with the act of biting off a piece of an *etrog*, as a protective measure guarding a woman against death in childbirth.[65]

Measures involving *tsedakah* were also taken by patients on their deathbed. It was widely believed that even if almsgiving could not avert every type of death, it could certainly prevent *mise-meshune* (sudden or tragic death).[66] The family of an agonal patient would organize a collection in their town and donate the entire sum raised to the needy, as *pidyon hanefesh*. The value of the donation would depend on the wealth of the patient: wealthy families were expected to sacrifice larger amounts than others. Redemptive purchases were also practised. According to Lilientalowa's notes, the money collected from family members would on occasion be used to buy oranges, at that time considered a luxury. The fruit would be given to the patient, and in this way the sins of the family members would be redeemed.[67] The most dramatic step, as a last resort, was sacrificing all of the patient's worldly possessions: the house door would be opened wide, closets and drawers thrown open, and all who wished could come and take whatever they wanted. If the step had the intended effect, and the person was cured, people would return the items to their owner.[68]

To the traditional Jewish community, prayer could have a bearing on health primarily as a regular form of fulfilment of divine service. The sin of neglect, as mentioned above, affected not only the human soul but also the body. In the face of sickness, prayer took one of two basic forms, which corresponded to the two aspects of folk religiosity termed by Kazimierz

---

[63] Lew, 'Lecznictwo i przesądy', *Izraelita*, 48, p. 505.

[64] *A naye shas tkhine*, 154–5. See T. H. Koydanover, *Kav hayashar*, 95.

[65] J. Ashkenazi, *Tsene urene*, 13.

[66] Lipiets, *Sefer matamim*, 15. The term was the Yiddish equivalent of the Hebrew *mitah meshunah*, unusual death. In earlier sources it was sometimes a synonym for apoplexy. See Lilientalowa, *Obrzędy pogrzebowe*, fo. 117.          [67] Lilientalowa, *Choroby, lecznictwo*, fo. 49.

[68] Zelkovitsh, 'Death and Its Accompanying Moments' (Yid.), 164.

Moszyński the 'attitude of supplication' (*stosunek prośby*) and the 'attitude of injunction' (*stosunek nakazu*).[69] These seem broadly to have corresponded to the element of cult and the element of folk belief in religious life, or to the *loshn koydesh* (Hebrew) and the *mame-loshn* (Yiddish). Prayers in Hebrew and Aramaic, as well as their Yiddish translations, conformed strictly to the rigid structures bestowed on them by the rabbis. In effect, they did not venture beyond subordinacy and proclamations of the glory and might of the Creator, the Ruler of the World. If they did express a request, they often did so with caveats such as 'may Thy will be done' or 'He in His mercy will bring peace upon us'. Prayers composed in the vernacular were entirely different in tone, with the accent often shifting from supplication to negotiation, and even adjuration. In this respect the Jews seemed to emulate their Slavic neighbours, for whom sacrifices to their deities bore the characteristics of an exchange of goods. The first branch of traditional Judaism where prayers of this nature were recognized as legitimate was Polish hasidism. One of the leading proponents of the movement, Levi Isaac of Berdychev, who for a time also held rabbinic functions in Ryczywół, Pińsk, and Żelechów, was himself the author of a number of such popular prayers, which continue to be published in collections of sabbath hymns to this day.[70]

Rabbinic tradition maintained that prayer had the power to neutralize adverse turnings of the stars. The Talmud (*Yev.* 64*a*, *Suk.* 14*a*) contains a story which tells how Abraham, on sighting the planet Jupiter in the western reaches of the sky and interpreting this as a sign that he would never have children of his own, made supplication to God. The Creator first reassured him that the stars cannot affect the fate of the righteous, but then almost immediately moved Jupiter to the east of the sky, thus allowing the patriarch to father a son. According to the Zohar, similar interventions averting the influence of the stars in response to prayer were elicited by other biblical heroes, above all Hannah, the mother of Samuel, who also suffered from infertility.

Confession of sins was seen as an important way of attaining reconciliation with the Creator, and one traditionally practised in cases of mortal

[69] *Kultura ludowa Słowian*, 235–44.

[70] One of the best known is the hymn beginning: *Reboyne shel oylem, lomir makhn a bayt* (Lord of the world, let us make an exchange), in which the tsadik offers God an exchange of human sins for the divine blessings of 'children, health, and money'; *Zemirot leshabat kodesh veyom tov*, 163–4.

threat. The Talmud taught that anyone who fell ill or found themselves in mortal peril should confess as if they were a prisoner sentenced to death.[71] This confession took the form of the Vidui prayer. The author of the halakhic code *Ḥokhmat adam* cited a variant of this prayer which included the following words: 'I thank You Lord God . . . for healing me with Your hand and putting me to death by Your hand. If it be Your will, You will restore me to full health, for You are a merciful, healing God, and if I die, may my death be an atonement.'[72] Those visiting the patient were obligated to urge them to recite it, but there were conflicting opinions on the matter among the populace. The author of the book of customs *Ta'amei haminhagim* noted that women (whom he equated with ignoramuses) saw such entreaties as omens of imminent death, but he himself believed that they had real potential to contribute to prolonging life.[73]

It was important that the patient's confession be accompanied by authentic remorse. If they wept, this might be a good sign, suggesting the possibility of a rapid return to health.[74] The liturgy for Yom Kippur incorporated a public confession of sins, which included the prayer 'Al ḥet', accompanied by the beating of breasts. The Talmud averred that though the gates of prayer leading to heaven might sometimes be closed, the gates of tears never were (*Ber.* 32*b*). While at other festivals it was chiefly adult men who filled the synagogue, services on the Day of Atonement were attended by all, even small children. The faithful would beat their breasts and sob as they confessed their sins, listing them in a whisper so that Satan the accuser would not overhear them and exploit them at the trial before the heavenly tribunal. They would also entreat God to dismiss the words of the accuser and instead hear out the defence.[75] In popular understanding, the dying person's confession was an act of redemption not so much of the soul as of the body, racked by endless agonal torment. For the sufferer could not leave this world until they had confessed (*oprufn*, *opshrayen*) their sins and attempted to make good any wrongs they had done.[76] Interestingly, the same words were used when someone attempted to exhort a dying patient to return from 'the other side' by means of weeping or wailing, and the patient regained consciousness even after

[71] BT *Shab.* 32*a*.
[72] Danzig, *Ḥokhmat adam*, 217.   [73] Sperling, *Ta'amei haminhagim oyf ivri taytsh*, i. 107.
[74] Lilientalowa, 'Wierzenia, przesądy i praktyki', 106; Khayes, 'Death-Related Beliefs and Customs' (Yid.), 296.   [75] Lilientalowa, *Święta żydowskie*, ii. 104–5.
[76] Zelkovitsh, 'Death and Its Accompanying Moments' (Yid.), 153.

several days of agony. Nonetheless, popular wisdom left no doubt that a person in such a condition would not live long (certainly no longer than three days), or would be no more than a body without a soul. They would be said to be 'wandering as if called', in reference to their torpor. Although it was universally believed that this *oprufn* (summons) could not but have an effect on their body and cause them yet greater suffering, it had a huge redemptory role. A person who had been recalled to this life three times was to be given a new name; they were as if reborn, and all their sins from their 'previous life', as the preceding period would thenceforth be termed, were forgiven them.[77]

One interesting consequence of considering illness to be a punishment for sins committed by the sufferer's parents was the custom of selling children (*opkoyfn a kind*), which was widespread throughout the Jewish community but was also documented in the Slavic environment.[78] This took the form of an actual transaction, accompanied by the payment of a coin and the pronouncement of the appropriate formula. In one story by An-sky this coin was a five-kopeck piece, and the ritual had to be enacted in the presence of two witnesses.[79] *Opkoyfn a kind* was conducted by devout women: the coin would be wrapped in a sabbath serviette and held above the head of the 'merchandise', and the contract was considered concluded when both parties took hold of the edges of the serviette.[80] With the change of family membership came the change of the child's father's name.[81] According to one manuscript, although the child remained in the home of its original parents, it was thenceforth to be referred to not by its name but as 'that one'.[82] Rabbinic authorities accepted this custom, which represented not the sale of the child's physical body but the binding of its fate to the fate and merits of another family, preferably one in which the children thrived

[77] Weissenberg, 'Krankheit und Tod', 359; Khayes, 'Death-Related Beliefs and Customs' (Yid.), 296–7; Zelkovitsh, 'Death and Its Accompanying Moments' (Yid.), 165.

[78] Moszyński, *Kultura ludowa Słowian*, 276; Podbereski, 'Materyały do demonologii ludu Ukraińskiego', 73. Sick livestock would be 'sold' in the same way; see 'Omens and Remedies' (Yid.), 291.          [79] An-sky, 'Khane the Cook' (Yid.), 12.

[80] Rechtman, 'Some Customs and Their Folk Explanations' (Yid.), 250.

[81] Lilientalowa, *Dziecko żydowskie*, 74. In the *yizkor* book of Pruzhana there is a story of a woman who sold one of her sons for three *groszy* and he was the only one of her children to survive; see Fayvushinski, 'The Folklore of Pruzhana' (Yid.), 204.

[82] *Segulot urefuot*, JTS, MS 9862, 101. Among the Slavic surnames used by Jews in the regions of present-day Belarus and Ukraine there are some that testify to the popularity of this practice of 'selling' a child and treating it as that of another, or as a foundling, e.g. Naydus ('foundling'), Niemoy or Nimoy ('not mine').

and did not die—a sign of divine grace. This is also the spirit of the recommendations in *Sefer ḥasidim* and in many books of customs.[83] Once the child reached a 'safe' age—for instance when a boy started to study the Scriptures (5–6 years old) or reached barmitzvah age and ritual maturity (in both cases the Torah provided protection from demons)—he would be bought back by his parents, again in a highly ceremonial atmosphere and to the accompaniment of the necessary formulas. He would nonetheless continue to refer to his 'interim' mother as 'mother', and she would be invited to his wedding and other celebrations organized for him by his biological family.[84] If the child was not bought back, it was thought to have been inscribed in the heavenly registers as the child of its adoptive parents. If it was a boy he would say Kaddish for the souls of his adoptive parents but not for those of his biological parents.[85] This custom was primarily applied in relation to young children; according to at least some sources, however, adults could also 'sell' their own illness or sins and in this way free themselves from their negative consequences.[86]

[83] Judah Hehasid, *Sefer ḥasidim*, 160. See Wilff, *Imrot shelomoh*, 111; Rosenberg, *Rafa'el ha-malakh*, 18; Lipiets, *Sefer matamim*, 84. On occasion the child might be sold to a community institution, such as the *ḥevrah kadisha*; Zimmels, *Magicians, Theologians and Doctors*, 143–4.

[84] Rechtman, 'Some Customs and Their Folk Explanations' (Yid.), 250–1.

[85] Lilientalowa, *Dziecko żydowskie*, 75.

[86] Benet, Sheloshah sefarim niftah.im, 78a. See the description of the ritual sale of sins in Charap, 'Zum Volksglauben der Juden in Polen', 18–19.

CHAPTER TEN

# FESTIVALS AND RITUALS

CENTURIES of incessant struggles with the reverses of fate prompted people to undertake complex manoeuvres in an attempt to ensure well-being for themselves. These sometimes took ritualized form, becoming inextricably bound up with the theology and ethical norms prevailing in a given culture, and in time being incorporated into everyday prayers and more broadly defined divine service. The Ashkenazi community in eastern Europe was no different in this respect, though the character and cultural attributes of these relations were nonetheless unique. As in other traditional communities, the service of God was a significant element of day-to-day life, and it gained further importance around the time of annual festivals and family rituals. The lines between the quotidian and the festive, the ordinary and the sacred, were sharply drawn. They were expressed in the dress worn by members of the community, by the appearance of their surroundings, by the distinctive customs, the many interdictions surrounding feast days, and so on. Festivals were considered a time of 'divine favour', as expressed in this excerpt: 'As for me, may my prayer come to you, O Lord, at a favourable moment' (Ps. 69: 14). It was believed that things that could not be entreated from the Creator on an ordinary day became possible during the recital of the festival liturgy or at the festive table. One value that was given special prominence in the context of religious rituals was health. The area of everyday and festive observances was one of the most colourful manifestations of the cosmology of the traditional Jewish populace. The religiously motivated health-related practices of the Jews differed from those of their Christian neighbours chiefly in content, less so in form. Within both traditions, the annual cycle of such protective rites and rituals was closely linked to the liturgical calendar. This resulted in a host of deeply entrenched notions as to the link between health issues and observances and obligations regulated by halakhah and Jewish custom.

The spring festival of Pesach is preceded by the ritual of searching every nook and cranny of the home for ḥamets (food items containing leaven) and the subsequent incineration of the bread or cake crumbs found in the search. The strength of the association of this custom with the biblical story of the Israelites baking matzah before fleeing from Egypt often eclipsed its more practical aspect of cleaning, and devout tales ascribing hero status to famous rabbis and tsadikim emphasized above all the religious and moral aspect of the search for ḥamets. This does not mean, of course, that during Pesach—or indeed on any of the other festivals—Jews were indifferent to the issue of health. Likewise, European folklore knows a number of similar rites relating to spring cleaning, many of which incorporate warnings of consequences such as rotting, decaying, and sickness if they are not carried out. According to one hasidic story, the tsadik Mordkhele of Mikolaiv (now in southern Ukraine) was studying Torah on one of the semi-festive, 'intermediate' days of Pesach when somebody came to him to ask him to pray for a perilously sick man. 'He should have done the search for his ḥamets. Find the ḥamets and throw it away, and he will recover', the tsadik reportedly answered. And indeed, half a loaf of bread was found in the sick man's house.[1]

In many towns and villages in eastern Europe, an interesting folk rite was performed before Pesach: parkhe. Its name was a reference to the name Pharaoh (Heb. paroh), the Yiddish word for sickness, parkh or parekh, and to one of the Egyptian plagues ('It shall . . . cause an inflammation breaking out [pore'aḥ] in boils on man and beast'; Exod. 9: 9). The ritual was usually played out on Shabat Hagadol (the sabbath before Pesach), and involved young men roaming the streets of their town looking for fellow residents with skin diseases such as mange—though any bald or balding men would do just as well. Anyone who answered to the description would be regaled with the irreverent rhyme Halelu, halelu min hashamayim, kol haparkhes lemitsrayim (Glory, glory from heaven, all the scab-heads to Egypt), and presented with a train ticket accompanied by the recommendation that they pack their bags quickly because the train from Budzanów (or whatever their town was called) to Egypt would not be waiting long. This 'leper-hunt' would often take the form of a procession with drums and other instruments, and, carried at its head, a straw figure dressed for a journey (in

---

[1] Even, *From the World of Hasidic Leaders* (Yid.), 107–8. Devout women observed the custom of purifying in the fire the needles they were to use to sew up the goose-necks to be cooked for Pesach. Some even kashered the door handles. See Shoys, *The Book of Jewish Festivals* (Yid.), 34.

trousers, overcoat, etc.). In some places 'leper lists' would be displayed in public, in either alphabetical or hierarchical order, with a list of what the exiles would need for such a long journey: a pot of chicken broth, pickled gherkins, and a comb.

The Seder meal, when matzah and other traditional dishes would be on the table, had its own series of prophylactic and protective practices. The holy night of Pesach was known as *leil hashimurim*, the night of especial divine protection. There was a widespread belief that on this night demons were powerless to cause harm, and so a shorter version of the Shema prayer was said on retiring. Nonetheless, certain traditions connected with the Seder were interpreted specifically as prophylactic. The custom of opening wide the door to the house during the reading of the Haggadah passage beginning *Shefokh hamatekha al hagoyim* ('Pour out your fury on the nations', Ps. 79: 6), which has been explained as an expression of faith in divine providence, took on a protective aspect in the context of the even number of glasses of wine that every adult Jew should drink during the Seder. It is written in the Talmud: 'If one drinks in pairs, his blood is upon his head.' In order to avert this danger, one had to take a look outside the house between the second and third glasses.[2] Another belief documented in the sources was that reading out the song 'Ḥad gadya' from the Haggadah would protect Israel from jealous looks cast by the angels (and hence from the evil eye).[3] Other Seder customs included practices designed to ensure material well-being. The sources mention that anyone hoping to get married in the immediate term should eat a piece of roast meat,[4] while fulfilling the commandment of eating unleavened bread was said to guarantee success in finding a source of income for the whole year ahead.[5] In respect of health, the most important element of the Seder was the hiding of the pieces of *afikoman*. Kept safe, and sometimes even suitably preserved, these would serve over the ensuing months as protection from the dangers that might lie in wait for travellers, and could help with many problems, including mice.[6] They were one element of procedures used to protect children from the

[2] BT *Pes.* 110a; Hirshovitsh, *Minhagei yeshurun*, 128–9; Yeushsohn, *From Our Old Treasure* (Yid.), 429.

[3] Because the angels in the other world could not celebrate Pesach as the Jews on earth did; Ashkenazi, 'The Evil Eye' (Heb.), 109.

[4] Lilientalowa, 'Przesądy żydowskie', 640.          [5] Lifshits, *Segulot yisra'el*, 100b.

[6] Rosenberg, *Rafa'el hamalakh*, 25; Buchbinder, 'Jewish Omens' (Yid.), 250; Benet, *Sheloshah sefarim niftaḥim*, 76a. Some authorities maintained that hanging up the *afikoman* for the year

evil eye, and would be placed under the child's pillow along with a few grains of salt.[7] The *afikoman* was also particularly sought after as a charm for carrying a pregnancy to term,[8] and for ensuring an easy birth.[9] According to hasidic tradition, the tsadik of Dzików attached great importance to the numerical value of the word itself and connected it to the phrase 'the more they increased' (Exod. 1: 12).[10] Another form of protection from the potential danger of a difficult delivery was said to be a morsel of the *maror* eaten at the Seder, hung round the neck of the birthing woman.[11]

Of still greater importance for matters of health was the cycle of autumn festivals, which began with a long period of penance in the month of Elul. This led up to the festival of Rosh Hashanah (the Jewish new year), commemorating the work of creation, which fell on the first day of the seventh month, Tishrei. It was followed by the Day of Atonement, Yom Kippur, when the fate of the people was decided for the year to come. Elul, the month of repentance, was characterized by the blowing of the shofar (ram's horn). *Az men blozt, vert kalt* (When they blow, it starts to get cold), it was said, suggesting a link between this custom and the approaching autumn chill.[12] According to the Midrash, on hearing the sound of the shofar, the Creator would leave his throne of judgement, where he issued stern verdicts, and go to sit on the throne of forgiveness, which lent mercy to his verdict.[13] The month of Elul also marked the beginning of a period of frequent visits to family graves. People living near and far, even those in remote villages, would descend upon the towns and divide their time between visiting relatives and going to the cemetery. This was a busy season for stonemasons, for the local *shammosim*, whose task it was to show people to the right graves, and for those who recited the 'El male raḥamim' prayer for the souls of the dead. It was also the beginning of the 'high season' for beggars and professional mourners. Though Jews gave alms all year round, in Elul and the days leading up to Yom Kippur, when the

---

disgraced what was a divine gift, and anyone who did so would lose their source of income. It was better, they claimed, to carry the *afikoman* on one's person, to guard against the detrimental effects of desire. See *Ets ḥayim*, 118; *Passover Haggadah* (Heb.), 140.

[7] Lilientalowa, 'The Evil Eye' (Yid.), 257.        [8] Rosenberg, *Rafa'el hamalakh*, 61.

[9] Ibid. 63. It was nonetheless considered prudent when putting the *afikoman* into the labouring woman's mouth to remember to take it out again as soon as the baby was born, in order not to put the woman in mortal danger.        [10] Benet, *Sheloshah sefarim niftaḥim*, 76a.

[11] Wilff, *Imrot shelomoh*, 101; Lifshits, *Segulot yisra'el*, 69b.

[12] Einhorn, 'Folk Proverbs' (Heb.), 341.        [13] See *Vayikra rabah*, 29: 3.

atmosphere of penitence was all-pervading, the faithful were especially keen to give *tsedakah* as a form of spiritual expiation. One former resident of the town of Gliniany recalls: 'The weeping and wailing of the women carried all across the cemetery, and was so heart-wrenching that it could have moved a stone to tears. At the graveside the "Ma'aneh lashon" was recited in Yiddish translation, and anyone who could not read could pay a scholarly Jewish woman a few kreutzers to do it for them.'[14] In Orla the prayers would be read by an elderly woman known as a *zogerke* or *beterke*, using the *Ma'avar yabok* prayer book.[15] According to folklore, the souls of the dead awaited these annual visits impatiently. In the month of Elul and on the eve of Yom Kippur, as on the anniversary of their death and on the fast day 9 Av (the anniversary of the destruction of the Temple in Jerusalem), they would come back to earth to hear out their loved ones and take their pleas back with them directly before the throne of the Almighty. Since in the popular imagination the heavenly tribunal was highly bureaucratized, the verdict was imagined to be issued in writing. Throughout the festive period in the month of Tishrei, until the last days of Sukkot, the Jews would petition their deceased parents, relatives, and friends to intercede for them with God, that he might record them 'for a good year' and 'send down' *a gutn kvitl*—a receipt confirming this positive decision. They would also pray at the graves of righteous, holy men, especially hasidic leaders, whose intercessionary activity was the subject of many popular stories.

During the period of the Days of Awe, another widespread custom was that of measuring the cemetery and graves with string, which was later used to make wicks for candles. In Orla the length of a cemetery would usually be measured by two women: one holding the ball of string and slowly paying it out, and the other holding the end of the string to take the measurements.[16] In Ukraine there would sometimes be three of them, reciting *tkhines* and measuring the cemetery from the entrance, from right to left, while a single grave might be measured by one woman alone.[17] In Pruzhana the cemetery would be measured using cotton thread, to the accompaniment of the following rhyme: 'I have a mother Tseytele, it is for her soul that I [am making] this wick, the thread is wound round strong and long, long.' Next, the thread would be dipped into a bowl of wax and cut into lengths, from which

[14] 'Jewish Festivals in the Shtetl' (Yid.), 62.
[15] Khayes, 'Death-Related Beliefs and Customs' (Yid.), 312.
[16] Ibid. 295.      [17] Weissenberg, 'Das Feld- und das Kejwermessen', 39–41.

candles would be made.[18] According to the author of *Sefer matamim*, the fundamental significance of this custom of *kvorim mestn*, which was also practised in emergencies, lay not so much in measuring as in pacing the cemetery with prayer on one's lips, and hence in a symbolic cordoning off of the space occupied by death.[19] As well as string, pieces of canvas might also be used, and these would be given out to the poor at the culminating point of this operation. The measuring ritual was sometimes carried over into other borderline spaces, such as crossroads. A person who was seriously ill might also be measured, and the string used to make a wick for a candle. This candle would then either be taken to the synagogue or buried in the cemetery, wrapped in a shroud.[20]

There were a number of types of such candles. Long, thin ones, called *stotshik*, were used by those studying Torah and saying the midnight prayers. They would also be cut up to make Hanukkah candles, or candles given to boys to light their way home from *ḥeder*. Candles for Yom Kippur, which were known as *reyne neshome likht* (candles of a pure soul), were made with particular deceased loved ones in mind, and donated for use in the synagogue before the festival began. These were often very tall—according to one testimony from Orla they were the height of the person for whom the intercession of the dead was desired.[21] Yet others, called *lebedike likht* (living candles), were made for the living, for parents or children, and burned at home. If one of these candles fell over, or burned down too fast, this was taken as an ill omen.[22] One man from Horokhiv in Volhynia recalled that his grandmother would make large candles for the synagogue which had to last a whole day and night. The candle-end served his father during the Havdalah ceremony ending the sabbath, as a *segulah* guaranteeing a source of income. His grandmother also made smaller candles, which were burned at home for the souls of the living. On the morning of the day before Yom Kippur she would take a large piece of wax, soften it in water,

[18] Fayvushinski, 'The Folklore of Pruzhana' (Yid.), 202.     [19] Lipiets, *Sefer matamim*, 91.
[20] Lilientalowa, 'Wierzenia, przesądy i praktyki', 106. According to her, measuring the cemetery was intended as a substitute for measuring a patient. See also Hirshovitsh, *Minhagei yeshurun*, 205.
[21] Khayes, 'Death-Related Beliefs and Customs' (Yid.), 295; Weissenberg, 'Das Feld- und das Kejwermessen', 41. Olga Goldberg-Mulkiewicz reported that there were instances of candles being made so as to correspond in weight to that of the patient. See Goldberg-Mulkiewicz, 'Obrzędy żałobne i pogrzebowe Żydów polskich', 103.
[22] Buchbinder, 'Jewish Omens' (Yid.), 254; Elzet [Złotnik], 'Some Jewish Customs' (Heb.), 352; Zelkovitsh, 'Death and Its Accompanying Moments' (Yid.), 161.

knead it like dough, and 'lay out' the wicks into it, reciting a separate *tkhine* for each family member as she did so.[23] In the small town of Bursztyn in Galicia (now Burshtin, Ukraine) the services of the Jewish women who performed this ritual were expensive, and not everyone could afford to have a Yom Kippur candle made from fresh beeswax with the names of their relatives recited in the process. 'Only old Rokhele Hamer would make them for free, as a good deed, but even she would only do so for a select few'; she would also take care of impoverished women in childbirth.[24] In Bełz the local tsadik took it upon himself to sit with the women as they drew the wicks through the melted wax, and preach moralizing sermons to them as they worked. This would take place in the synagogue, and crowds of hasidim would gather outside. At other hasidic courts preaching such words tended to be the domain of the tsadik's wife.[25] The melted wax from a candle burned in the synagogue at Yom Kippur would be used in treatments for ailments such as earache.[26]

Artefacts connected with the festival of Sukkot, such as the *sukah* (booth), construction of which began on the evening after the end of the Day of Atonement, and the *lulav* bundle, were also of some importance in Jewish folk medicine. The Talmud grants exemption from the commandment to dwell in the *sukah* to those whom it would cause sadness, and to the sick and their carers.[27] A later interpretation of the religious law altered this perspective, shifting the emphasis to the requirement for the *sukah* to be free of cares and sickness. This thought was supported by the words of the psalm, 'He will shelter me in His pavilion on an evil day' (Ps. 27: 5). For this reason, some hasidic authorities, among them Solomon of Radomsko (the Tiferet Shelomoh) and Menahem Mendel of Vizhnitz (the Tsemah Tsadik), recommended fulfilling the *mitsvah* of erecting the *sukah* and living in it for seven days as a panacea for all manner of problems, including health issues,[28] as a way of ensuring healthy offspring,[29] and to ensure longevity.[30] Other rabbis embellished this conviction with greater detail, stressing the

---

[23] Varad, 'Every Jewish Festival with Its Own Atmosphere' (Yid.), 47–8. The practice of reciting *tkhines* while making the candles is mentioned as early as Sarah bat Tovim's eighteenth-century *Sheloshah she'arim*. See e.g. Zinberg, *A History of Jewish Literature* (Yid.), 290.

[24] Schwarz, 'Characters and Personalities' (Yid.), 263–4.

[25] Mekler, *Fun rebns hoyf*, 264; Unger, *Hasidism and the Jewish Festivals* (Yid.), 65.

[26] Segel, 'Materyały do etnografii Żydów', 327.                      [27] BT *Suk.* 25*b*–26*a*.

[28] Lifshits, *Segulot yisra'el*, 88*a*; Sperling, *Ta'amei haminhagim umekorei hadinim*, 346. See Rabinovitsh, *Tiferet shelomoh*, 60*a*.          [29] Lifshits, *Segulot yisra'el*, 12*a*.          [30] Ibid. 147*b*.

protective function of the *sukah* in times of plague.[31] The tsadik Naftali of Ropshitz averred that building a *sukah* was the only religious obligation that the devout Jew fulfilled with every part of his body.[32] Thus, if any body part were to be damaged by sin, fulfilment of this commandment could bring atonement, which was equivalent to healing.

Of immense and solemn significance for curative practices was the Four Species (Heb. *arba'ah minim*), a bundle composed of four types of plant: a date palm frond (*lulav*), three myrtle branches, and two willow branches, all bound up with palm rings, and an *etrog* (citron). According to one traditional interpretation, each component of the bundle corresponded to a part of the human body, the most important being the *etrog*, which was identified with the heart, the seat of spiritual life and morality. For this reason the Torah mandated the selection of a fresh, unblemished specimen, which in turn would have a beneficial effect on the bearer's ethical qualities.[33] Both the palm and the fruit were imported from the Mediterranean basin. The *etrog*, which spoiled far faster than the date palm branch, could not be kept until the next year, so people would try to procure a new one before every Sukkot. The peel of the old one would often be used in treating complaints, including loss of voice (laid on the lips, or placed under the tongue),[34] tinnitus (fried in oil infused with Mediterranean herbs),[35] rashes (made into preserves),[36] and nosebleeds (coarsely grated),[37] and prophylactically as a protection from snakes.[38] The linen cloth in which the *etrog* was kept was also used for various types of treatment; it might be incorporated into compresses for aching legs or painful knees,[39] or for curing erysipelas.[40] Inhaling the fragrance of the *etrog* was traditionally recommended to pregnant women, either so that their babies would smell sweet,[41] or to guarantee a

[31] Sperling, *Ta'amei haminhagim umekorei hadinim*, 598.

[32] Unger, *Hasidism and the Jewish Festivals* (Yid.), 128. The author of the *Kav hayashar*, however, stated that whoever fulfilled the *mitsvah* of erecting a shelter properly diminished the power of Lilith; see T. H. Koydanover, *Kav hayashar*, 237.

[33] Sperling, *Ta'amei haminhagim umekorei hadinim*, 346–7.

[34] Halpern, *Mifalot elokim*, 14*a*; Rosenberg, *Rafa'el hamalakh*, 22; *Segulot urefuot*, JTS, MS 9862, 20. Aside from the *etrog*, other remedies recommended for loss of voice were a willow branch and the *afikoman*; see Rubinstein, *Zikhron ya'akov yosef*, 32*a*, 34*a*.

[35] Rosenberg, *Rafa'el hamalakh*, 10; id., *Der malekh refoel*, 6–7. On the subject of *etrog* peel oil for tinnitus see Lilientalowa, *Choroby, lecznictwo*, fo. 51.

[36] Rosenberg, *Rafa'el hamalakh*, 74; Lilientalowa, *Dziecko żydowskie*, 69.

[37] Halpern, *Mifalot elokim*, 14*b*; *Segulot urefuot*, JTS, MS 9862, 20.

[38] Rubinstein, *Zikhron ya'akov yosef*, 89*b*.          [39] Rosenberg, *Rafa'el hamalakh*, 88.

[40] *Segulot urefuot*, JTS, MS 9862, 113.          [41] Wilff, *Imrot shelomoh*, 56.

boy.[42] A woman struggling with a difficult birth (or hoping to avoid one) would be told to bite off the top of the *etrog* (Heb. *pitam*), which, according to the author of *Rafa'el hamalakh*, was particularly efficacious on Hoshana Rabah after prayer.[43] An equally effective use of the fruit was to boil it up and serve it to a pregnant or birthing woman in the form of a preserve on Tu Bishvat (15 Shevat).[44]

The other elements of the Four Species might also be used in treatments of various types, especially if they had been left for some time after Sukkot. Preserving the *lulav* bundle in its entirety was believed to offer protection from major misfortune. Sometimes it would be hung up, its components still bound together, above the front door after prayers on Hoshana Rabah, and left there until Passover, when it would be burned along with the *hamets*, and the remains cast into the fire as the matzah was being baked.[45] Finely ground pieces of the Four Species mixed with mother's milk and baked were thought to bring good luck.[46] Rings made from the *lulav* were used to guard against cholera,[47] rheumatism, and the evil eye.[48] The willow branches might be brewed like tea and served as an infusion with sugar to a married couple who could not have children.[49] The same remedy was also said to be effective protection from fever.[50] The myrtle branches were burned on Saturday evenings during Havdalah, and the aroma not only added to the solemn mood of the end of the sabbath, but also offered protection from the forces of evil.[51] On occasion the *lulav* would also be used in a smudging ritual to provide protection from the evil eye.[52]

Human life as understood by traditional Jewish society was divided into successive stages, each of which was marked by important ritual events. With these events came a change in status, and this engendered the loss or

---

[42] Fayvushinski, 'The Folklore of Pruzhana' (Yid.), 203.

[43] Lilientalowa, *Coitus, ciąża, poród*, fo. 2, no. 11; ead., *Święta żydowskie*, i. 88; ead., *Dziecko żydowskie*, 20; Rosenberg, *Rafa'el hamalakh*, 62; Lifshits, *Berit avot*, 3a; Bastomski, *At the Source: Jewish Proverbs* (Yid.), 109.

[44] Sperling, *Ta'amei haminhagim oyf ivri taytsh*, i. 86. See 'In the Quarter of the Kabbalists' (Heb.), 333.     [45] Sperling, *Ta'amei haminhagim oyf ivri taytsh*, i. 85–6.

[46] Rosenberg, *Der malekh refoel*, 38.

[47] Segel, 'Wierzenia i lecznictwo', 54; Lew, 'O lecznictwie i przesądach', *Izraelita*, 35, p. 296; Kotik, *My Memoirs* (Yid.), 315.

[48] Lilientalowa, *Święta żydowskie*, i. 74; ead., 'Additions: The "Evil Eye"' (Yid.), 434.

[49] Rosenberg, *Rafa'el hamalakh*, 29.

[50] Lew, 'Lecznictwo i przesądy', *Izraelita*, 50, p. 530.

[51] Lilientalowa, *Święta żydowskie*, i. 88.     [52] Lilientalowa, *Dziecko żydowskie*, 51.

gain of particular attributes, rights, and obligations. Without these rituals the change in status could not ensue, which affected the person's position and often led to their exclusion from a given social group. For boys, these rites of passage were circumcision on the eighth day of life, barmitzvah on reaching the age of 13, marriage, and death. In the case of women, the only two events of major significance were the last two in that list. These were occasions that engaged not only the individuals and members of their immediate family, but often the entire local community. Each of the rites signalling the advent of a new phase of life was likewise of significance for health-related practices. On the one hand the folk imagination considered the change in status to be a moment when the person concerned was vulnerable to mortal danger, attack by the forces of evil, or other hazards. On the other, this caesura presented an opportunity to perform actions which in other circumstances would have been ineffective, since in that brief moment of existence in the liminal zone between old and new, the individual gained access to powers and attributes that were out of reach to other people. Just as it is impossible to understand Jewish medical beliefs without reference to their relation to the liturgical calendar, so it is important to remember that family celebrations and other ceremonies ordained by the Torah or by custom incorporated elements that spoke to the folk imagination in the context of health. Membership of the community began with birth and ended after death, with burial in the ground, or when memory of the person in question faded. Throughout their life, every community member participated in rites of passage as either the main character or a bit-part actor, and each rite had a bearing on various aspects of their happiness and prosperity.

The birth of a boy was a much-desired event in the culture of east European Jews, and augured blessings. Nonetheless, it also brought a host of potential dangers; these were far more common for boys than for girls. From the age of 13, men were bound by the commandments of the Torah, and it was the man who said Kaddish for his parents after their death. Men also held ritual and public functions, could include in their prayers pleas for salvation, and might even be admitted before the face of God to present them in person. For all these reasons, Satan was thought to use every available means to hinder the descendants of Abraham in their fulfilment of the Law. His wrath was mainly focused, however, on the covenantal act, following which the child would be forever bound by the obligations of the

Torah.[53] From the very first moments of his life, a baby boy was an enemy of the forces of evil, and he was in the greatest danger over the seven days preceding the circumcision ceremony. This sign of the covenant brought him under the protection of the God of Israel, and rendered him considerably safer. Prior to that moment, however, he could be safeguarded only by the performance of various prophylactic practices.[54]

During the birth itself, news of the labour should not be allowed to reach the ears of women outside the mother's immediate circles, as it was believed that their sympathetic sighs of *oy vey* would increase her pain.[55] After the birth, care was taken that outsiders should not have access to the baby, and even the name that was to be given during the upcoming ceremony would be a closely guarded secret. The infant and its mother would lie in a closed room hung with drapes; both the curtains and the walls would be festooned with *kimpet-brivelekh* (confinement letters) or *shir-hamaylesn* (psalms). These bore the words of Psalm 121, including the excerpt reading 'The Lord will guard you from all harm' (Ps. 121: 7), as well as a whole series of other symbolic texts and signs. The standard elements of this popular amulet included the exhortations to 'tear Satan apart' and not to tolerate sorceresses (Exod. 22: 17); the names of the patriarchs and matriarchs of Israel; and the Hebrew phrases *adam veḥavah penimah* (Adam and Eve in the middle—sometimes inscribed within a geometrical figure) and *lilit vekol kat deileih ḥuts* (Lilith and all the hosts of her servants outside). It might also include the initials of the words of Psalm 91: 10: 'no harm will befall you, no disease will touch your tent'.[56] Such amulets might be beautifully decorated, made by the *sofer* with great care, though they could just as well be printed or reproduced using other techniques. There were also very simple ones written in a cursive hand, but they all repeated the standard form.[57] The same *shir-hamaylesn* were sometimes sewn into the red cap and pillow that would accompany the boy during the circumcision ceremony.[58] The curtain concealing the new mother and her infant,

---

[53] Lipiets, *Sefer matamim*, 47.

[54] The primacy of male offspring in Jewish culture is addressed by authors including Lilientalowa, *Dziecko żydowskie*, 22–4. Practices designed to protect boys, such as tying red strings or amulets to the baby's body or to its cradle, were also used for girls, but the solicitousness of the traditional community was far greater when it was a boy's health that was at stake.

[55] Lilientalowa, *Coitus, ciąża, poród*, fo. 1, no. 7.

[56] Weissenberg, 'Das neugeborene Kind', 85.

[57] Ibid. 86.                              [58] Ben-Ezra, 'Customs' (Yid.), 174.

the threshold, and the door frame would be studded with needles, and a locked padlock would be hung on the door.[59] In addition, a person conversant with conjuration and lifting charms would draw a circle on the wall using a piece of charcoal, and write in it the phrase *adam vehavah huts lilit* (Adam and Eve without Lilith).[60] Any openings in the chimney flue would be kept blocked, and often a broom and an axe—implements used in anti-demonic rituals—would be inserted into them.[61] The woman would not be left alone; she would be tended to by other women in her family, hired midwives, or *vartorins* (nurses).[62] A fire was kept burning at all times if possible, and sacred texts would be studied in another room in the house.

The most dangerous days in the period between the birth and the circumcision ceremony were thought to be the third,[63] the fifth,[64] and above all the seventh, because this was the day when the candle or oil lamp in the woman's room was changed.[65] On the eve of the circumcision the protective measures were stepped up. Young boys with their *heder* teacher or his assitant (*bahelfer*) were invited into the main room of the house to recite anti-demonic prayers. 'Shouting "Good evening, *mazl tov!*", they start to repeat after their *bahelfer* the Keriyat Shema, the "Shir hama'alot", and finally the "Shehakol" and the "Bore minei mezonot" [blessings]', one former resident of the village of Bóbrka recalled.[66] In another version of this custom, the *heder* boys would come to the new mother's home every evening, and every evening they would add to the evening prayer the names of the guardian angels Michael, Gabriel, Uriel, and Raphael, and recite the 'Viyhi no'am' and the 'Hamalakh hago'el' prayers (Gen. 48: 16).[67] They would also speak aloud the cursed names of Lilith which she herself revealed to the prophet Elijah, and which, according to legend, had the power to render her harmless.[68] In exchange for this favour, the

[59] Lilientalowa, *Dziecko żydowskie*, 31–2.

[60] Lifshits, *Berit avot*, 5b; Pulner, 'Obryadi i povirya', 106; Zoller, 'Lilith' (Yid.), 125. Similar methods were adopted to guard against plague; Segel, 'Wierzenia i lecznictwo', 54.

[61] Segel, 'Wierzenia i lecznictwo', 58; id., 'Materyały do etnografii Żydów', 319; Lew, 'O lecznictwie i przesądach', *Izraelita*, 38, p. 363; Lilientalowa, 'Dziecko żydowskie', 146; Shlaferman, 'The Folklore, Customs, and Stories of Kazimierz' (Yid.), 172.

[62] See Rivkind, 'Notes on Words' (Yid.), 12; Shoys, 'A Jewish Child is Born' (Yid.), 59; Axenfeld, *The Kerchief* (Yid.), 23–4.     [63] Moszyński, *Kultura ludowa Słowian*, 276.

[64] Lew, 'O lecznictwie i przesądach', *Izraelita*, 40, p. 382.

[65] Segel, 'Materyały do etnografii Żydów', 319.

[66] Kh. S., 'Childhood Years in Boyberke' (Yid.), 176.

[67] Lilientalowa, *Dziecko żydowskie*, 32; Fayvushinski, 'The Folklore of Pruzhana' (Yid.), 105.

[68] Benczer, 'Jüdische Volksmedizin', 120–1. On occasion these names (Abitu, Abizu, Ikforu,

children would be given honey cakes or other delicacies (in Pruzhana and Horodets these might be peas and broad beans, with the exception of the seventh day,[69] while in Szydłowiec the treat was honey bagels shaped like links in a chain[70]), and on occasion even a little sweet cherry brandy. The eve of the circumcision was known by the name *vakhnakht*, or night of vigil.[71] The *mohel* would come to the house to examine the baby and place the circumcision knife at the head of his cradle. In this way, if the ceremony was to fall on the sabbath he would not have to break the rule prohibiting the carrying of objects between the private and public spheres. Moreover, the knife was a tool held to be an effective form of protection, and so it was often brought even earlier.[72] In some cases, other objects with the power to ward off evil would be placed under the child's pillow along with the knife (a *talit*, a prayer book, or a bulb of garlic).[73]

The examination of the child was taken seriously, for a sick baby should not be circumcised until he has regained his strength. The *Kitsur shulḥan arukh* held that the *mohel* and the midwife were responsible for watching for any indications of illness. In more serious cases it was also imperative to wait seven full days from the child's recovery and only perform the ritual on the eighth. In the most serious instances, and where previous children from the same marriage had died in infancy (perhaps as a result of the procedure), the circumcision was to be postponed for a longer period.[74] The *mohel* would examine the boy using methods typical for traditional medicine. He would check to see that his skin and eyes were not yellowish, and look at his nails, palms, and feet. He would insert his finger into the child's mouth to check that it was cool and moist, and that the child reacted by sucking. One cause of infant death was thought to be blisters on the palate which prevented sucking, and this belief corresponded with the Slavic perception of oral thrush. If the child exhibited no natural sucking reflex, the

Shatruna, etc.) would be written on amulets, in the belief that knowledge of them enabled one to counter the actions of the maleficent demoness. See Buchbinder, 'Jewish Omens' (Yid.), 256–7; Folmer, 'A Jewish Childbirth Amulet for a Girl', 53–4.

[69] An-sky, *The Yiddish Ethnographic Programme* (Yid.), 31; N.C., 'Places of Learning in Pruzhana' (Yid.), 105. The Yiddish word for broad bean, *bob*, was explained as an acronym for the words *barukh atah bevo'akha*, 'Blessed shall you be in your comings' (Deut. 28: 6), i.e. 'Welcome'; Kastrinski, 'Two Grandmas' (Yid.), 184.

[70] Rosenzweig-Blander, 'Lifestyle, Customs, Remedies' (Yid.), 154.

[71] Marcus, *The Jewish Life Cycle*, 47.    [72] Ibid. 77.    [73] Segel, 'Wierzenia i lecznictwo', 58.

[74] Ganzfried, *Kitsur shulḥan arukh*, 163: 5. See BT *Shab.* 134*a*.

standard procedure was to take a piece of thin linen, wrap it around one's finger, and massage the inside of its cheeks to burst the blisters.[75] A manual for hasidic *mohalim* published in Kraków in the late nineteenth century, describing these methods, explained what symptoms to look out for to distinguish between minor ailments (for example a rash appearing because of excess 'bad blood') and potentially dangerous ones (such as pox).[76] This classification was largely based on the views of Maimonides and on information in the halakhic codes. A yellow skin tone was thought to indicate insufficient blood, and redness to suggest that the blood had not circulated to the limbs, but remained between the skin and the muscles.[77] It was the *mohel*'s responsibility to assess the child's condition after the circumcision procedure. If a warm bath was deemed necessary—something which on the sabbath represented a contravention of the religious laws—it would be prepared as if for a sick person.[78] Circumcision in itself mandated a few days' reconvalescence for the child because it often led to a brief deterioration in his health. Unlike Christian baptism, circumcision was not unanimously regarded as a life-saving measure, and sources indicate that this was often a bone of contention between the populace and more enlightened rabbis.[79] What is more, in the late nineteenth century, awareness of the dangers inherent in certain diseases spread rapidly. Manuals for *mohalim* warned that men suffering from venereal diseases should not take on this role owing to the danger of infecting the child when sucking off the blood (*metsitsah*). They also included information on alternative ways of conducting the *metsitsah* procedure and on contemporary methods of hygiene for disinfecting the instruments and the *mohel*'s hands.[80]

Being asked to play an important role during a child's circumcision as *kvater* or *kvaterin* (the person who brought the infant into the room at the beginning of the ceremony, godfather/godmother) was much vaunted as a cure for infertility for both men and women,[81] though such a cure was not

---

[75] Benet, *Sheloshah sefarim niftahim*, 74b; Lifshits, *Segulot yisra'el*, 2b. Cf. Moszyński, *Kultura ludowa Słowian*, 195–7.                    [76] J. Levin, *Ḥotam kodesh*, 25b–26b.

[77] *Shulḥan arukh*, 'Yoreh de'ah', 263; J. Levin, *Ḥotam kodesh*, 27a–b.

[78] J. Levin, *Ḥotam kodesh*, 39a.            [79] See Petrovsky-Shtern, *The Golden Age Shtetl*, 230–3.

[80] J. Levin, *Ḥotam kodesh*, 62a–b. *Metsitsah* (suction to clean the wound) is the third step of the circumcision rite, which was traditionally performed orally (*bepeh*). Since the nineteenth-century controversy on the hygienic consequences of this operation, *metsitsah bepeh* has been conducted only by the most strictly Orthodox groups.

[81] An-sky, *The Yiddish Ethnographic Programme* (Yid.), 36, 177. Participation in the circumcision ceremony as the *kvater* (Ger. *Gevatter*) was proposed in the ethical literature as the first

guaranteed. The woman acting as the *kvaterin* would sometimes also bathe the infant. If she did, she would drop a few coins into the water as a kind of payment for the nurse. Otherwise she might pay the midwife to perform this duty.[82] Among Sephardi Jews the custom of infertile women swallowing the foreskin of the circumcised infant was deeply rooted. In Ashkenazi culture it was not so common, though a number of sources indicate that it was known around 1700. The author of *Rafa'el hamalakh*, though disapproving of it, nonetheless confirmed that advice of this nature had reached eastern Europe via popular health-related literature.[83] In many cases the severed foreskin was employed in other ways, however. According to some sources, a man trying for a child should take the foreskin from the *mohel* as soon as he cut it off, place it on the ring finger of his left hand for half an hour or so, and then after the ceremony burn it to ash. He should then drink this ash in a good wine on the day of his wife's ritual bath, some of it in the morning, some in the afternoon, and the rest in the evening.[84] Another recommended remedy, both for infertility and for the problem of the deaths of several of one's children in infancy, was to examine the *mohel*'s knife.[85] Women in difficult labour were advised to drink from the cup over which the blessing had been said during a circumcision ceremony.[86] At the same time, pregnant women were strongly warned against accepting the role of *kvaterin*, and also against participating in any other practices said to be effective as aids to conception.[87]

The issue of stopping the bleeding after the circumcision recurs in Jewish folk medicine testimonies very frequently. Because it was at the intersection of religious ritual and traditional treatment practices, it should come as no surprise that Jewish authors devoted considerable space to it,

step in atoning for the sin of masturbation; *Ets ḥayim*, 72. In pious etymology the term *kvater* was traced back to the Hebrew word *ketoret* (incense). See Gelbard, *Otsar ta'amei haminhagim*, 414.

[82]  Rivkind, *Jewish Money in Life, Culture, and Folklore* (Yid.), 40–1. See Weissenberg, 'Das neugeborene Kind', 87.

[83]  Rosenberg, *Rafa'el hamalakh*, 6; Patai, *On Jewish Folklore*, 406. See Agnon, *The Bridal Canopy*, 208.

[84]  *Segulot urefuot*, JTS, MS 9862, 27. According to another custom, the foreskin would be placed into the sand-filled chest in which the Yom Kippur candles were burned, and then burned itself; Lilientalowa, 'Dziecko żydowskie', 148; Ben-Ezra, 'Customs' (Yid.), 174.

[85]  Wilff, *Imrot shelomoh*, 97; J. Ashkenazi, *Tsene urene fun harav hekhasid*, 2.

[86]  Elzet [Złotnik], 'Some Jewish Customs' (Heb.), 363.

[87]  Lilientalowa, *Dziecko żydowskie*, 34. Lilientalowa also mentions the custom of women who were trying to conceive shaking the baby before passing him to the *kvaterin*.

both in healthcare manuals and in autonomous publications addressing various matters connected with the sign of the covenant. Generally speaking, most of the methods used were relatively common in staunching bleeding of all types. They tended to be natural in character, and included *moylmel* (lit. the *mohel*'s flour), made from finely ground charcoal, the shell of an egg from which a chicken had hatched, crushed rowan berries, powdered frog, and horse manure. Dressings were made using a mixture of vinegar and vodka, 'Galician bluestone' (copper[II] sulphate), iron drops, and rose ointment.[88] Many of these and other, somewhat more refined, remedies—the latter bearing de rigueur German or Latin names—were preferably to be bought from the pharmacy. Moreover, warm compresses, of pig's blood, for instance, would be applied to the infant's belly.[89] Methods involving magic were also widely used in addition to and in combination with natural remedies. The *mohel* and the *sandek* (the man holding the baby during the circumcision ceremony) were expected to be God-fearing, and to ritually purify themselves of their sins before the ceremony, expressing true repentance, otherwise their actions might present a direct threat to the child's health.[90] The family would often be prepared to go to great lengths to have a rabbi or hasidic rebbe perform the ceremony, in order that their piety might influence the child's future, even to the extent of saving him from death.[91]

The sign of the covenant could not, however, provide full protection from evil. Premature and sickly babies would have to undergo a host of protective procedures, among them having curses removed and wearing *baytelekh* (pouches containing protective items), as well as canvas cloths made from the offcuts of a funeral shroud. Practice of certain religious rituals to be performed by all boys might in such cases likewise be perceived as a form of prophylaxis. As early as the eighteenth week of life, baby boys would be dressed in an ornamental yarmulke.[92] Similarly, from their earliest years—as soon as they could distinguish between good and bad—they would be trained to wear *tsitsit* (ritual fringes, tied to the vest-like

---

[88] Rosenberg, *Rafa'el hamalakh*, 24; Lifshits, *Berit avot*, 95*b*–6*b*; Segel, 'Materyały do etnografii Żydów', 326; Lilientalowa, *Dziecko żydowskie*, 36; U. Weinreich, 'Beliefs: Remedies for Warts' (Yid.), 63. Samuel Weissenberg noted that in the early twentieth century, the use of dressings in place of *moylmel* became increasingly widespread ('Das neugeborene Kind', 87).

[89] *Segulot vekameyot*, JTS, MS 10082, 8*a*; Wilff, *Imrot shelomoh*, 103; Lifshits, *Berit avot*, 96*b*.

[90] Wilff, *Imrot shelomoh*, 103.          [91] Schwarzbaum, 'The Efficacy of Prayer', 283.

[92] Lew, 'O lecznictwie i przesądach', *Izraelita*, 40, p. 382.

undergarment called *talit katan*), which was treated by society at large not only as fulfilment of a commandment (Num. 15: 37–41; Deut 22: 12) but also as a protective measure. Stories of unfortunates who had fallen into the clutches of evil because they had left the house without their *tsitsit* were staples of the folk legend repertoire. It was considered exceedingly feckless to take any sort of journey, or even to venture into Christian streets, or anywhere near churches or non-Jewish cemeteries, without it.[93] 'The *tsitsit* is to the body what the mezuzah is to the home', according to the author of the vademecum *Rafa'el hamalakh*,[94] and a prudent man would be said to 'believe in God and the *tsitsit*'.[95] Wearing it conscientiously was a great *segulah*: through the protection it provided from sin, it was a guarantee of having healthy children.[96] According to numerous sources, placing the *talit katan* beneath one's head induced good sleep,[97] gazing on the *tsitsit* was said to ease aching eyes[98] and generally succour the sick,[99] knotting the strands was a way of avoiding fever,[100] and biting off the threads (rather than cutting them off) brought relief from toothache.[101]

Most of the recommendations listed above were applicable only to men, though in some cases women might also benefit from the protective properties of the *tsitsit* despite not wearing one. Making the thread from which the fringes were to be plaited, for instance, was considered one form of pious activity that a woman should undertake in order to avoid a difficult birth.[102] And in fact the woman did have an item of clothing that served a similar purpose to the *talit katan*: the apron. Wearing an apron was not a halakhic requirement, but a custom related to the virtue of modesty and Ashkenazi norms of conduct. Many ethnographic anthologies state that a woman who went out without it (sometimes also without a garter) would be laying herself open to attack by dybbuks and demons. This was of particular significance in the case of a pregnant woman, who, furthermore, should not carry anything in her apron (*trogn* means both to carry and to be pregnant), because in so doing she might bring difficulties on herself during the birth.[103]

[93] Lifshits, *Segulot yisra'el*, 22a.                [94] Rosenberg, *Rafa'el hamalakh*, 81.
[95] I. Bernstein, *Jewish Proverbs and Sayings* (Yid.), 49.
[96] Rosenberg, *Rafa'el hamalakh*, 17.                [97] Segel, 'Wierzenia i lecznictwo', 49.
[98] Ibid. 74.                [99] Sperling, *Ta'amei haminhagim oyf ivri taytsh*, ii. 51.
[100] Segel, 'Wierzenia i lecznictwo', 60. A similar method, but on a scarf, is mentioned in Tarlau, 'Volksmedizinisches aus dem jüdischen Russland', 144.
[101] *Segulot urefuot*, JTS, MS 9862, 80.                [102] Lifshits, *Berit avot*, 5a.
[103] An-sky, *The Yiddish Ethnographic Programme* (Yid.), 21–2. It was forbidden to carry meat

Entrance into adulthood for Jewish boys came on reaching the age of 13, and constituted a significant rite of passage. The boy, who was referred to as a 'son of the commandment' (*bar mitsvah*), would be called up to read the Torah in the synagogue; there would also be a celebratory meal, and he would be given presents, one of which was a set of *tefilin*. In the case of women, adulthood was a function of biology. According to religious law a girl ceased to be a child on reaching the age of 12, but no equivalent celebration to the barmitzvah was held to mark the occasion. She became a woman with menarche. Confirmation of this fact was limited to a slap in the face from her mother, sometimes even without any explanation. Folk wisdom explained it as a way of ensuring that she retained colour in her cheeks, or as a warning against the enigmatic 'evil deed'. Sometimes this slap was said to ensure regularity of the monthly cycle, to which end other steps were also taken, for instance red ribbons were worn. It is important to stress that adulthood in Judaism means obligation in the commandments, and this applies to both women and men in accordance with the roles they perform within the family and society.[104]

The first event that irrevocably changed the status of both boys and girls was marriage.[105] Marriage was one of the most significant institutions of the traditional Jewish community. Around the time of a wedding, interest in omens and ways to ensure eternal good fortune for the new couple increased greatly. Even the choice of the day on which the ceremony was to take place was important. Like some of the communities around them, the Jews considered Tuesday to be the most auspicious day of the week. It was on this, the third day of Creation, that God had twice pronounced his work 'good'.[106] According to some sources, however, anyone wishing to marry a widow should choose Thursday as a safer day.[107] There was also a general belief that some matches should be avoided altogether, for one's own good and that of any future children. Marriage to a woman who had already buried two (or, according to other versions, three) husbands was considered risky, for instance; likewise to a virgin who had survived two (or three)

in one's apron, for instance, as this was said to cause infantile eczema; see Lilientalowa, 'Wierzenia, przesądy i praktyki', 161.

[104] Fels, 'Zabobony lekarskie u Żydów', 4; Elzet [Złotnik], 'Some Jewish Customs' (Heb.), 369. Szychowska-Boebel, *Lecznictwo ludowe na Kujawach*, 69.

[105] See e.g. 'Marriage'; Sperber, 'Marriage', 354–5.

[106] Y. Bergman, *Jewish Folklore* (Heb.), 33.          [107] Wilff, *Imrot shelomoh*, 13.

fiancés.[108] It was inadvisable to take a wife from a family of epileptics or lepers, as this increased the risk of incidence of the disease in one's own offspring. Marriage of a father and his son to two sisters (or a woman and her daughter to two brothers) was also thought foolhardy, as was wedding the sister of one's previous wife if there were sons from the previous union, and likewise contracting several marriages with any one family.[109] There was also pressure on the potential bride, who was warned that her behaviour could have a bearing on the qualities of her future husband. If an unmarried girl sang at table or was immodest, she could expect a madman for her betrothed, and if she sat at the corner of the table she would have to wait seven years to find a match.[110]

As the greatest blessing for a married couple was children, many customs revolved around the fertility of the future bride and groom. On the sabbath before the wedding, when the young man was led to the synagogue and called up (*ufrufn*) to read a passage of the Torah, the women would shower him with nuts and almonds from the women's gallery. According to the *Sefer matamim*, the nuts were a form of propitiatory offering for the youth's sins, while the almonds were directly connected with fertility.[111] During the *badekns* ceremony just before the wedding when the young man covered the face of his bride with her veil, those present recited the words spoken to the biblical Rebecca: 'O sister! May you grow into thousands of myriads' (Gen. 24: 60). The couple would again be showered with rice, nuts, and grains of wheat directly after the vows were sealed, while they were still standing beneath the *hupah* (wedding canopy), to the sound of shouts of the biblical commandment 'be fruitful and multiply' (Gen. 1: 28). The ceremony itself was held in the evening, in the open air, under the stars, which were the subject of God's promise to Abraham that he would have numerous offspring (Gen. 15: 5).

[108] Wilff, *Imrot shelomoh*, 4. Such a woman was dubbed a *katlanes* (murderess). The Talmud advised against such marriages in view of the woman's inauspicious constellation (BT *Yev.* 64*b*). The mortality of a man's wives was explained in less colourful language, but it was likewise considered a problem. For this reason, a fourth wife returning from her wedding ceremony was advised to enter the house not through the door but through the window; Lilientalowa, 'Wierzenia, przesądy i praktyki', 170.

[109] On the one hand this was justified by citing the belief that like couples tended to be unlucky, while on the other there was an awareness of the danger of diseases caused by incestuous unions. See Wilff, *Imrot shelomoh*, 12–13; *Segulot urefuot*, JTS, MS 9862, 97; Bastomski, *At the Source: Jewish Proverbs* (Yid.), 108. Cf. 'Tsava'at rabi yehudah heḥasid', 10.

[110] Grunwald, 'Aus unseren Sammlungen. II', 8.

[111] Lipiets, *Sefer matamim*, 33. See Prilutski and Lehman, 'Jewish Proverbs' (Yid.), 27.

In the transition period between one state and the next, the betrothed were vulnerable to attack by the forces of evil. In order to prevent this, numerous protective measures would be undertaken. Before the wedding the couple would go to the cemetery to ask their dead parents or any other deceased relatives for forgiveness for sins they might have committed, and to invite them to the forthcoming ceremony.[112] During the week preceding the wedding (at the latest from the day of the *ufrufn*), neither would be left alone, owing to the perceived threat of demonic activity. On the day of the ceremony the betrothed had to fast and make confession of their sins in the form also used on Yom Kippur ('Al ḥet'). Both would be dressed in white, and the groom would wear a *kitl*, the robe in which he would eventually be buried. Beneath the *ḥupah* the bride would circle her husband seven times, so giving him protection from demons.[113] After the 'consecration' of the bride and the recital of the traditional seven blessings, the ceremony was concluded with the consumption of wine from a glass that was then smashed. This echoed the smashing of the plates at the drawing up of the prenuptial contract that preceded the marriage; both actions were variously interpreted—as commemoration of the destruction of the Temple, as a gesture testifying to the irreversible character of the obligations being undertaken, or as an act of banishment of all forces of evil. The bride's veil covering her face during the *badekns* ceremony might also be seen as protection from curses. Nonetheless, if a cat ran under the *ḥupah* and between the couple, it was considered a bad omen, and a sign that neither would live the year out.[114]

Some of the artefacts connected with the wedding ceremony were treated as magical and used in the treatment of various complaints. The betrothed couple also enjoyed a status that in the folk imagination had connotations of magical potential, and material elements of the ritual were available for the benefit of all. Eating the leftovers from the married couple's first meal or using the ritual bath after the bride's immersion ahead of her wedding night were both claimed to cure women of infertility.[115] An epileptic, a child suffering from cramps, and the dying might all expect to experience relief when a *ḥupah* or a bridal dress was laid on them;

---

[112] Lilientalowa, 'Wierzenia, przesądy i praktyki', 111; Weissenberg, 'Eine jüdische Hochzeit in Südrussland', 61.                                          [113] Sperber, 'Marriage', 354–5.

[114] Zelkovitsh, 'Death and Its Accompanying Moments' (Yid.), 159.

[115] Segel, 'Wierzenia i lecznictwo', 57.

a similar effect might be achieved with a *talit*.[116] *Vasermun*, the infantile sickness I have discussed earlier, was treated using a glass of water into which a wedding ring and a few grains of millet had been placed.[117] The ring was a popular cure for a stye if rubbed over the affected eye.[118] During a hasidic wedding there would be queues to hand the groom, like in other circumstances the tsadik, *kvitlekh* in the hope of being given help.[119] The groom, in turn, would hand out *shirayim*, also in the manner of a tsadik; the Sanzer hasidim claimed that on his wedding day the groom was blessed with a unique sanctity which far exceeded that of any 'ordinary' holy man.[120] The special status of the groom was also indicated by his exemption from reciting the Shema prayer on his wedding night and every successive night before the next sabbath until the marriage was consummated (*Ber.* 16a). In some east European shtetls care was also taken that those who led the couple to the *ḥupah* were not childless, though the survey conducted by An-sky suggests that taking on this role might equally have served as a *segulah* for fertility.[121]

The last major events in a person's life were death and burial. There were a number of types of death, according to the ethical literature, awaiting people of varying degrees of spiritual elevation. A just and virtuous person would die a *mise binshike*, an easy death in their sleep, through a heavenly kiss. 'He was a righteous man' was the phrase used in towns including Brest to refer to someone who had not suffered on their deathbed.[122] A misdoer would suffer a *mise meshune*, a sudden, unnatural death, associated with convulsions and suffering. The vast majority of people died slowly, because the heavenly scales on which their sins and good deeds were weighed could not establish unequivocally whether or not they deserved to die yet.[123] The Jewish community employed a dedicated phraseology to speak about dying. The agonal state began at the point when the dying person began to choke, to 'struggle with death', which was accompanied

[116] Lilientalowa, 'Wierzenia, przesądy i praktyki', 107, 172; ead., 'Dziecko żydowskie', 152. Covering the patient with a *kitl* had a similar effect; Khayes, 'Death-Related Beliefs and Customs' (Yid.), 297.

[117] Khotsh, *Segulot urefuot*, 8; David ben Aryeh Leib, *Sod hashem*, 33; Lilientalowa, 'Dziecko żydowskie', 149; Grunwald, 'Aus Hausapotheke und Hexenküche II', 145.

[118] Lilientalowa, 'Wierzenia, przesądy i praktyki', 174; Ben-Ezra, 'Customs' (Yid.), 176.

[119] Unger, *Pshiskhe and Kotsk* (Yid.), 72.      [120] Meisels, *Vihyitem li segulah*, i. 136.

[121] An-sky, *The Yiddish Ethnographic Programme* (Yid.), 146; Elzet [Złotnik], 'Some Jewish Customs' (Heb.), 359.      [122] Khayes, 'Death-Related Beliefs and Customs' (Yid.), 297.

[123] Zelkovitsh, 'Death and Its Accompanying Moments' (Yid.), 166.

by the 'appropriate music' or 'dead melody' (*toyter nign*)—the heavy breathing of the dying.[124] They would be said to be in a state of *hinerp(f)let*, a transition between here (*her*) and there (*hin*). The term *hinerplet* encompassed not only the death agony, but any loss of consciousness. Folk etymology translated the word as either *hin-her-flet* (that way, this way, flight) or *hiner-bet* (hen's bed; probably in connection with warnings against putting a hen's feather pillow under the dying person's head). Max Weinreich, however, traces its provenance to the Middle High German *hin-brit* (ecstasy).[125]

A patient in an agonal state was given solicitous care. Their bed should not be made of iron (perhaps so that they would not be wakened by its creaking),[126] but the key to the synagogue should be placed under their pillow; this was said to ease their suffering.[127] It was thought vital that they be left in peace; the bedclothes should not be straightened, the light should be extinguished, and they should not be repeatedly disturbed; if the house had only one room, they should be turned to face the wall.[128] Soiled bedlinen would be removed in the belief that it could prolong the death agony.[129] The pillow, if filled with chicken feathers, would likewise be removed; this latter custom was justified by the conviction that chicken feathers added to the dying person's suffering because they absorbed moisture, which was thought to increase discomfort and prolong the state of *hinerplet*.[130] Chairs were to be placed around the bed to prevent any part of the patient's body from hanging off. A limp limb might be an indication of imminent death, and it also rendered the dying person vulnerable to attack by the demons that lay in wait around the bed but could not actually

[124]  Ibid. 163–4. See *Yevrieiskaya narodnaya piesni*, 32.

[125]  M. Weinreich, *Geschichte der jiddischen Sprachforschung*, 192; Veynig, 'Doctors and Medicine in Jewish Sayings' (Yid.), 21.

[126]  Rechtman, 'Some Customs and Their Folk Explanations' (Yid.), 253.

[127]  Segel, 'Wierzenia i lecznictwo', 53.

[128]  If the patient turned to face the wall of their own accord, this might indicate imminent death, or if they died in that position it might be a sign that they had died angry, ashamed, or unreconciled with the living; Lilientalowa, 'Wierzenia, przesądy i praktyki', 107; Khayes, 'Death-Related Beliefs and Customs' (Yid.), 298–9.

[129]  Zelkovitsh, 'Death and Its Accompanying Moments' (Yid.), 166.

[130]  Sperling, *Ta'amei haminhagim oyf ivri taytsh*, ii. 4; An-sky, *The Yiddish Ethnographic Programme* (Yid.), 199; Weissenberg, 'Krankheit und Tod', 359–60; Segel, 'Wierzenia i lecznictwo', 53; Lilientalowa, 'Wierzenia, przesądy i praktyki', 107; Fayvushinski, 'The Folklore of Pruzhana' (Yid.), 200; Khayes, 'Death-Related Beliefs and Customs' (Yid.), 297, 313. Cf. Szukiewicz, 'Wierzenia i praktyki ludowe', 444.

get to it.[131] All those whose weeping, other behaviour, or even sight might prolong the death agony should leave the room. It was believed that a person who was very attached to their loved ones would not want to part from them, and would cling to this world even if it caused them pain. The sight of a weeping mother or child could cause extra suffering.[132] At the same time, every effort was made not to leave the dying person alone, and members of the family or funeral fraternity would keep vigil. Candles were lit to keep demons away.[133] Anyone keeping vigil at a deathbed alone might also be vulnerable to attack by demons, hence the belief that the more people surrounded the patient, the easier it would be for their soul to leave their body; indeed, a death that went unnoticed by other household members was considered a dishonour.[134] Sometimes it was also said that there should not be any unclean objects or people (such as non-Jews) in the room, as the patient might be unwilling to depart life in their presence.[135] Furthermore, since in Jewish culture all *mitsvot* performed by a woman were credited to her husband, if it was she who was dying, in order not to cause her additional pain he should assure her that he was ceding them to her (in order to help her gain entry to paradise).[136]

A seriously ill patient would not be addressed by name, as this might enable the angel of death to identify the person for whom he had been sent.[137] The widespread custom of changing a patient's name was justified in a similar way. The rabbis saw the genesis of this tradition in the biblical story of the renaming of Sarai to Sarah simultaneously with the divine promise of offspring.[138] This story gave rise to a number of different interpretations. According to one of the *midrashim*, Abram complained to God that the stars would not let him have children. The Creator answered that

---

[131] If an arm or a leg did slide out of the bed, however, it was not to be moved; Sperling, *Ta'amei haminhagim oyf ivri taytsh*, i. 108; Danzig, *Ḥokhmat adam*, 218.

[132] Lilientalowa, 'Wierzenia, przesądy i praktyki', 107; ead., *Dziecko żydowskie*, 72. See 'Tsava'at rabi yehudah heḥasid', 6, 8.

[133] Sperling, *Ta'amei haminhagim oyf ivri taytsh*, i. 108. See Aaron Berakhyah of Modena, *Ma'avar yabok*, 178.       [134] Khayes, 'Death-Related Beliefs and Customs' (Yid.), 298.

[135] Zelkovitsh, 'Death and Its Accompanying Moments' (Yid.), 167.       [136] Ibid. 167.

[137] Rechtman, 'Some Customs and Their Folk Explanations' (Yid.), 253. If a seriously ill patient suddenly began calling out to other, previously deceased, people by name, it was a sign that death was imminent; Zelkovitsh, 'Death and Its Accompanying Moments' (Yid.), 164. The tsadik Yehiel Mikhl of Złoczów believed that the patient's name should be used, but together with the word *refuah* (healing), which would bring light and vitality to them; Idel, *Hasidism: Between Ecstasy and Magic*, 78.       [138] BT *RH* 16b. Cf. Gen. 17: 15–16.

while Abram would not have children, Abraham would.[139] Contrary to widely held conceptions, however, changing the patient's name was not an exclusively Jewish custom, and is also encountered in Slavic folklore.[140] In Ashkenazi practice it tended to be implemented primarily in respect of infants, probably in view of their high mortality rate. If parents feared for their child's life—whether due to illness or past experience of the premature deaths of previous children—they would add or change its name to a 'trembling name' (*tsiterdiker nomen*). These new names suggested adulthood, and hence survival of the danger period, such as Alter, Alte, Zeyde, or Bobe,[141] or longevity and vitality, such as Hayim or Hayah;[142] animal names (Ze'ev Volf, Dov Ber, Tsevi Hirsh, etc.);[143] names indicating trust in divine providence, such as Ben-Tsiyon,[144] Joseph (the biblical Joseph was said to have been immune to the evil eye),[145] or Nathan;[146] or names incorporating God's holy names Yah and El (for example Shemaryah or Raphael).[147] Some rabbinic authorities recommended that the new name should not include any letters from the previous name.[148] If there had been previous infant deaths in the family, slightly different measures were taken. On the advice of the Vilna Gaon, a boy would be given as a second name the name of his deceased brother.[149] On occasion the name chosen (sometimes by the tsadik) might be the first name heard during the sabbath Torah reading in the synagogue.[150] In other cases the logic behind the choice of name was to garner divine grace for the child through a symbolic link between the name and a given festive period. For instance, if the child was born around the festival of Purim, it might be named Mordkhe, and if around the fast day of 9 Av, Menahem might be chosen (Heb. comforter; this was also a name for the month of Av).[151]

[139] *Bemidbar rabah* 2: 12. See also Schwarzbaum, 'Fate Tricked by Change of Name', in id., Studies, 285.                                    [140] See Libera, *Medycyna ludowa*, 57–8.

[141] Sperling, *Ta'amei haminhagim oyf ivri taytsh*, i. 99; Rosenberg, *Rafa'el hamalakh*, 18; Lipiets, *Sefer matamim*, 47–8; Lilientalowa, *Dziecko żydowskie*, 74.

[142] Lilientalowa, *Dziecko żydowskie*, 71.                    [143] Rosenberg, *Rafa'el hamalakh*, 18.

[144] Sperling, *Ta'amei haminhagim oyf ivri taytsh*, i. 102; Rosenberg, *Rafa'el hamalakh*, 18; Wilff, *Imrot shelomoh*, 111; Benet, *Sheloshah sefarim niftahim*, 74*b*; J. Ashkenazi, *Tsene urene fun harav hekhasid*, 2.                    [145] Landau, 'Zur Geschichte der jüdischen Vornamen', 8.

[146] Yunis, 'The Old Homeland' (Yid.), 73.

[147] Rosenberg, *Rafa'el hamalakh*, 18; Benet, *Sheloshah sefarim niftahim*, 74*b*. See Yunis, 'The Old Homeland' (Yid.), 85.                    [148] Zimmels, *Magicians, Theologians and Doctors*, 143.

[149] Wilff, *Imrot shelomoh*, 111; J. Ashkenazi, *Tsene urene fun harav hekhasid*, 2; *Segulot urefuot*, JTS, MS 9862, 25.

[150] Herzog and Zborowski, *Life Is with People*, 322.                    [151] Wilff, *Imrot shelomoh*, 108.

In a number of earlier Jewish sources we find suggestions that ill fate, and hence even death, might be evaded by moving to live elsewhere. In the practices of the Ashkenazim such advice, which was to be found in sources including the Talmud (*RH* 16*b*), the *Sefer ḥasidim*, and the Zohar, went largely unheeded, or at least the extent of its impact was negligible in comparison with the importance attached to changing a name. Granted, Ignatz Bernstein noted in his famous collection the saying *Meshane mokem, meshane mazl—amol tsum gutn, amol tsum shli-mazl* (You change your place, you change your luck—sometimes for better, sometimes for worse),[152] but the overt fatalism of this statement seems only to confirm the thesis that it was rarely taken literally in matters of health. Chaim Schwarzbaum cites only one source from eastern Europe, a remark noted in the hasidic anthology *Zikaron tov* about the tsadik of Niesuchojeże (Neskhizh), who, in addition to changing a patient's name, also recommended that they be moved to another room or another house.[153] And Henryk Lew advised that a mother whose previous children had died could avoid the death of a subsequent infant by nursing it not at home, but in someone else's home.[154] Any other examples in the literature tend to link moving house to a change in one's fate in the categories of success and prosperity rather than improved health.

Death was pronounced using tried and tested methods known from early medicine. A feather or a mirror would be placed under the patient's nose or by their mouth to check whether or not they were still breathing. A candle might be held close to their eyes to watch for a pupillary response to the light. The deceased would be pricked with a pin under the fingernail to elicit a reflex reaction. Blood would be let to check blood pressure,[155] and the pulse would be taken; wisdom had it that *Vi lang es varft zikh an oder, tor men nit farlirn di hofnung* (As long as an artery is pulsating, one must not lose hope).[156] If the eyes of the deceased remained open after death, this was taken to be a sign of nostalgia for the world of the living. It was nonetheless considered risky, because of the danger of the evil eye, and so apologies would be made to the deceased and their eyes (and mouth) would be closed. Leaving them open by an oversight could be an omen of the

---

152 I. Bernstein, *Jewish Proverbs and Sayings* (Yid.), 157.
153 Schwarzbaum, 'Change of Place Frustrates Fate', 290.
154 Lew, 'O lecznictwie i przesądach', *Izraelita*, 40, p. 381.
155 Zelkovitsh, 'Death and Its Accompanying Moments' (Yid.), 168.
156 Y. Tsherniak, 'Linguistic Folklore in Yiddish' (Heb.), 96.

imminent death of another member of their family.[157] As soon as death was announced, all the windows in the room would be opened in order to allow the soul to leave freely, and a glass of water and a rag would be left on the windowsill so that it could make its ablutions.[158] Sometimes small children would be taken out of the room; if they fell asleep they could easily be suffocated by the spirit of the deceased.[159]

The brief period available for access to the deceased was used for curative purposes. This was the moment in which to ask them for forgiveness and for intercession for the living. The family and neighbours of the deceased, and others who had had disputes with them in their lifetime, would come to them with requests.[160] Mourners ('lamenters') would come to the house, too. They needed no invitation; they would come of their own volition when they heard of the death, and would accompany the body, wailing, during the funeral cortège and at the cemetery. For this 'service', which was believed to awaken in the deceased the realization of the need to intercede for the living before the heavenly throne, they would demand payment.[161] Pleas lodged with a deceased person might include 'instructions'. During one cholera epidemic, a certain hasidic rebbe had supplications to God drawn up and signed by the entire body of the local rabbinic court, and he placed the document in the hands of a recently deceased man, whispering his request for intercession into the ear of the corpse as he did so.[162] The same belief inspired the inscription of the names of family members on the boards of the coffin holding the earthly remains of a tsadik from Sochaczew.[163]

Caution was to be exercised in the waiting period preceding the removal of the body from the house. It was thought dangerous to kiss the deceased farewell, especially for a small child.[164] Contact with the corpse might cause fright, a state of shock that could result in lasting trauma. It might also bring on or aggravate symptoms of epilepsy, and even have a

---

[157] An-sky, *The Yiddish Ethnographic Programme* (Yid.), 204; Lilientalowa, 'Wierzenia, przesądy i praktyki', 107; Khayes, 'Death-Related Beliefs and Customs' (Yid.), 299–300.

[158] Lilientalowa, 'Wierzenia, przesądy i praktyki', 107; Ch., 'Materiały do etnografii Żydów polskich', 438; Khayes, 'Death-Related Beliefs and Customs' (Yid.), 308.

[159] Khayes, 'Death-Related Beliefs and Customs' (Yid.), 305.

[160] Ibid. 301.                                                               [161] Ibid. 312.

[162] Veynig, 'Medicaments and Remedies among the Jews' (Yid.), 26.

[163] Wolrat, 'The Rabbi's Funeral' (Yid.), 95.

[164] Zelkovitsh, 'Death and Its Accompanying Moments' (Yid.), 177. Cf. 'Tsava'at rabi yehudah heḥasid', 6.

detrimental effect on one's memory.[165] In order to protect oneself from
adverse consequences, while saying one's farewells it was considered prudent to hold the deceased by their big toe or little finger. Rather than looking at their face, which should be covered (so as not to embarrass the
deceased and not to copy Slavic customs), one should look at their feet
(in Bereźno the custom was specifically to look at their toenails).[166] If a
child was overcome with fright, its hand would be placed on the corpse's
hand, or after the body was taken from the room, the child would be led
across the straw on which the body had lain. An adult in the same situation
would be advised to glance three times at their nails and up at the sky.[167]

Sometimes the body would be used in more instrumental ways. Even
early talmudic texts contain testimonies to the custom of leading a child by
the hand around a corpse as a foreign practice.[168] Ashkenazi sources offer
many examples of performance of similar rituals across eastern Europe.
Anyone suffering from epilepsy was advised to go up to the deceased, take
them by the hand, and make the following request: 'Take from me the
weakness of epilepsy, I beg of you. It can do you no harm, and you will be
doing me a favour.' Then, with the hand of the deceased, they should trace
around their own body three times, after which they should apologize for
the affront, and go home.[169] It was likewise believed that rubbing aching
teeth with the dead person's finger would bring relief.[170] Similar methods
were used to treat disabilities, above all in children.[171] A corpse's hand
might be rubbed over the affected area of the patient's body as treatment
for goitre, mange sores on children's heads, mats in the hair, erysipelas

[165] Rosenberg, *Rafa'el hamalakh*, 69; id., *Der malekh refoel*, 61; Lew, 'O lecznictwie i przesądach', *Izraelita*, 46, p. 446.

[166] Segel, 'Materyały do etnografii Żydów', 32; Bastomski, *At the Source: Jewish Proverbs*
(Yid.), 109; Khayes, 'Death-Related Beliefs and Customs' (Yid.), 307; Herzog and Zborowski,
*Life Is with People*, 36. In some shtetls (e.g. Szydłowiec), in spite of warnings that the sight of a
dead person's face was 'hard to forget', looking at it was considered a way of combating fright in
general; Zelkovitsh, 'Death and Its Accompanying Moments' (Yid.), 177.

[167] Lilientalowa, 'Wierzenia, przesądy i praktyki', 108. Walking across straw used for this
purpose (sometimes three times) after returning from a funeral was universally recommended
as a way of eliminating fear of the dead; Lilientalowa, *Obrzędy pogrzebowe*, 57, 209.

[168] Tosefta *Shab.* 7: 1.

[169] Rosenberg, *Rafa'el hamalakh*, 67; *Segulot urefuot*, JTS, MS 9862, 85. The source cited by
Rosenberg, a responsum of the Bratislava rabbi Moses Schreiber (Hatam Sofer, 1762–1839),
specifies that it should be the body of a non-Jew. Rosenberg himself makes no mention of this,
however. See Schreiber, *Ḥatam sofer*, 137b.     [170] Lew, 'Z ludoznawstwa', *Izraelita*, 22, p. 239.

[171] Elzet [Złotnik], 'Some Jewish Customs' (Heb.), 370; Frimer, 'A Podolian's Observations
on the Language in *Genarter Velt*' (Yid.), 46.

rashes, warts, large moles (nevi), hunchback (kyphosis), necrotic bone, swelling caused by splenomegaly, any kind of paralysis, blindness, and even curses, which might present in the form of any of the above-mentioned complaints. This practice was called *opshtraykhn* or *arumshtraykhn*.[172] Usually the hand was passed over the affected area three times, to the accompaniment of an incantation (such as 'Let all evil depart from my child'), followed by an apology to the deceased. Care was taken to ensure that the patient was the same sex as the deceased, and ideally younger. In the folk imagination, blood bonds also brought better therapeutic effect, and as such, a child might request help from a recently deceased parent or other relative.[173] On occasion a devout individual might give their consent to the performance of such rituals using their body after their death. This occurred in the case of a woman who lived in a rural settlement near Krynki (in north-eastern Poland); as a child she was cured of ulcers by having her body contours traced with the hand of a deceased religious Jew.[174]

The Jewish sources yield many more examples of use of dead bodies as a remedy for various problems. Touching a corpse was said to bring relief to people suffering from sweaty palms (palmar hyperhidrosis),[175] while turning the corpse face down was thought to be a way of avoiding an outbreak of fire in the household.[176] At the same time, pregnant women were warned against having any form of contact with the dead. As fascination (staring at certain objects or people as if powerless to look away) was potentially hazardous not only to them but also to their unborn children, gazing on a pale, yellowish body would inevitably, it was believed, bring on neonatal jaundice.[177] Moreover, the death of a close relative might suggest that they had made an unwilling sacrifice for the life of the child to be born.

[172] The same expression was used to denote the custom of pouring a raw egg over a bundle of birch rods in order to discover the source of the evil eye or fright. See Mark, 'The Language of the Comedy *Di genarte velt*' (Yid.), 75; Weissenberg, 'Krankheit und Tod', 359; id., 'Kinderfreud', 316.

[173] An-sky, *The Yiddish Ethnographic Programme* (Yid.), 205; Lilientalowa, 'Wierzenia, przesądy i praktyki', 111; ead., *Dziecko żydowskie*, 64; Zelkovitsh, 'Death and Its Accompanying Moments' (Yid.), 173; Khayes, 'Death-Related Beliefs and Customs' (Yid.), 306–7; Fayvushinski, 'The Folklore of Pruzhana' (Yid.), 202; Frimer, 'A Podolian's Observations on the Language in *Genarter Velt*' (Yid.), 46.

[174] Kositsa, *Reminiscences of a Woman from Białystok* (Yid.), 60–1.

[175] Lilientalowa, 'Wierzenia, przesądy i praktyki', 111.

[176] Zelkovitsh, 'Death and Its Accompanying Moments' (Yid.), 173.

[177] Lilientalowa, 'Wierzenia, przesądy i praktyki', 108; Khayes, 'Death-Related Beliefs and Customs' (Yid.), 305. Cf. Libera, *Medycyna ludowa*, 85.

The pregnant woman should thus not provoke the revenge of the deceased, and after the birth should see to it that her child was named after them.[178]

One object that had considerable therapeutic power by virtue of its connection with death was the shroud. The halakhah is fairly explicit in its prohibition of using either that item or any other piece of clothing or body part of the deceased for any purpose other than burial.[179] Nonetheless, folk practice departed sharply from these rules, as illustrated by the following laconic saying: *Krankayt brekht a din* (Illness breaks the law).[180] Anyone who had their shroud made at an early age, it was believed, could expect to enjoy a long life.[181] Scraps of the shroud were used as amulets for protection from conscription, for instance, or might be rubbed on the eyes in case of problems with vision. Such scraps, soaked in wax from the candle burned in the synagogue on Yom Kippur, were used to treat earache, and were generally thought to bring good fortune to the house.[182] Sewing a snippet of a shroud into a baby's swaddling clothes or children's clothes, or wearing a piece of it in a *baytele*, was said to offer protection from enchantments.[183] Scraps from the shroud in which a near-centenarian rabbi had been wrapped were also considered a *segulah* for a long life.[184] Offcuts from the shroud were used by women to make coarse shirts and yarmulkes for children. If a family was cursed with a high mortality rate among the children, or a couple had had a long-awaited child, the child would be dressed in such clothes for protection from enchantments and other misfortunes. It would have to wear them for several years (in Pruzhana and Horodets until the age of 8 or 10). These shirts resembled shrouds (as a sign that their wearer no longer needed one), and care was taken to ensure that they were free from fibre mixes prohibited by the halakhah.[185]

---

[178] Zelkovitsh, 'Death and Its Accompanying Moments' (Yid.), 169. This did not contradict the principle that a child should not be named after anyone who had died prematurely.

[179] *Shulḥan arukh*, 'Yoreh de'ah', 349; Danzig, *Ḥokhmat adam*, 228–9.

[180] G. Bernstein, 'Expressions and Proverbs' (Yid.), 53.

[181] An-sky, *The Yiddish Ethnographic Programme* (Yid.), 210. See Kuper, *The Jews of My Nostalgia* (Yid.), 227–8.

[182] Zelkovitsh, 'Death and Its Accompanying Moments' (Yid.), 172. Cf. Biegeleisen, *Lecznictwo ludu polskiego*, 157.

[183] Segel, 'Materyały do etnografii Żydów', 319; Lilientalowa, 'Dziecko żydowskie', 156; ead., *Dziecko żydowskie*, 49; Khayes, 'Death-Related Beliefs and Customs' (Yid.), 303.

[184] Kastrinski, 'Two Grandmas' (Yid.), 183.

[185] Khayes, 'Death-Related Beliefs and Customs' (Yid.), 307; Veynig, 'Medicaments and Remedies among the Jews' (Yid.), 29; Ben-Ezra, 'Customs' (Yid.), 175; Fayvushinski, 'The Folklore of Pruzhana' (Yid.), 204; Herzog and Zborowski, *Life Is with People*, 322.

The water that had been used to wash the deceased constituted a threat to human health. It could cause complaints such as pustules to anyone who stepped in it, and so it was poured out 'in a place where nobody goes' or 'over the fence'.[186] Nonetheless, it was sometimes drunk as medicine for alcohol addiction or other diseases.[187] If a close relative of the deceased happened to be suffering acute labour pains, she too would be given some of this water as a *segulah*.[188] The curative power of water obtained in this way was directly related to the ethical qualities of the person it had been used to wash in the ritual ablution. In Pruzhana, when a rabbi of great local esteem died, people 'fought' over the water used to wash his body, which was 'reused' to wash external complaints such as wounds, ulcers, or the feet of a child too weak to walk unaided.[189]

Quite aside from the practices of measuring and visiting graves before certain festivals, there were several other instances in which the cemetery figured prominently in the curative practices of the Jews. Grass from the graves of ancestors or pious leaders would be gathered and placed under the head of someone seriously ill (in places including Bielsk Podlaski). Sometimes it might also be accompanied by a scarf that had been laid on it; this was said to give the patient dreams of the deceased offering them a piece of fruit, and thereafter lead to their recovery.[190] The infertile might be helped by a piece of wood from a cemetery where a tsadik or righteous man was buried.[191] In some cases dust might be gathered from the grave of a person who had been important to a birthing woman or to her wider community, and given to her to drink in water.[192] Early nineteenth-century (and even slightly earlier) Ashkenazi manuscripts contain instructions on many other ways to use dust from graves as a charm for protection from the evil eye,[193] and descriptions of the cemetery as a place where anything used in

---

[186] The straw and feathers on which the deceased had lain were also thrown away; Fayvushinski, 'The Folklore of Pruzhana' (Yid.), 203; Khayes, 'Death-Related Beliefs and Customs' (Yid.), 302.

[187] Lilientalowa, 'Wierzenia, przesądy i praktyki', 112; Biegeleisen, *Lecznictwo ludu polskiego*, 331.                          [188] Zelkovitsh, 'Death and Its Accompanying Moments' (Yid.), 174.

[189] Fayvushinski, 'The Folklore of Pruzhana' (Yid.), 201.

[190] Fels, 'Zabobony lekarskie u Żydów', 2; Segel, 'Wierzenia i lecznictwo', 54; Khayes, 'Death-Related Beliefs and Customs' (Yid.), 296.                          [191] Wilff, *Imrot shelomoh*, 97.

[192] Segel [Schiffer], 'Alltagglauben', 273; Elzet [Złotnik], 'Some Jewish Customs' (Heb.), 366; Pulner, 'Obryadi i povirya', 106. Cf. Lilientalowa, *Obrzędy pogrzebowe*, fo. 253.

[193] e.g it was burned and worn inside the clothing as protection from charms; *Segulot urefuot*, Bibliotheca Rosenthaliana, HS. ROS. 444, 7a.

therapeutic practices would be thrown or poured away.[194] If there was a difficult, life-threatening birth at hand, prayers at the cemetery took the form of desolate laments known as *raysn kvorim* (tearing up graves), sometimes accompanied by the sound of the shofar. On other occasions, attempts would be made to reach the Creator directly, rather than via the intercession of the dead. To this end women would go to the synagogue to *raysn di shul*, or tear up the shul; they would open up the holy ark, in which the Torah scrolls were housed, and pour out their bitterness and woe before it.

The Jewish cemetery played an important role in times of cholera. In some cities and towns a non-Jew would be employed to guard the cemetery gate and refuse entry to funeral cortèges on the grounds that there was 'no more space'.[195] Legend had it that the new cemetery in Burshtin was founded as a *segulah* against cholera—the epidemic abated when the first dead were buried in it.[196] The graves of righteous men and deceased relatives were places where people went to pray for the plague to pass. The custom of organizing 'black weddings' for cripples or poor couples lent the cemetery considerable significance. Another ritual that took place there was the ceremonial burial of *sheymes*, fragments of Hebrew books and any scraps of paper bearing the name of God. The logic behind this was that such sacred script should not be left to rot on rubbish heaps but should be honoured by being laid to rest in the company of pious individuals. Further rabbinic justification for this custom—aside from the fact that it prevented an act of contempt against the Creator—was that it distracted people's thoughts from the misery of the plague. Jewish ethnographers, however, saw it as a form of substitute burial whose function was to save humans from death.[197] Similarly, items onto which all the misfortunes caused by the epidemic had been symbolically transferred would also be buried in the cemetery.

[194] *Segulot vekameyot*, JTS, MS 10082, 3a.
[195] Veynig, 'Medicaments and Remedies among the Jews' (Yid.), 29.
[196] Schwarz, 'Characters and Personalities' (Yid.), 268.
[197] Lipiets, *Sefer matamim heḥadash*, 62; Veynig, 'Medicaments and Remedies among the Jews' (Yid.), 30.

# PART IV

# UNCLEAN FORCES

CHAPTER ELEVEN

# DISEASES AS
# DEMONIC BEINGS

PREMODERN CULTURES saw diseases either as autonomous entities whose existence was closely bound up with that of humans or as entirely separate beings that could take possession of the human body and manifest themselves in the form of various symptoms (pain, stabbing sensations, swelling, redness, etc.). Some of these 'lived' in the body of their host as congenital to it, even vital for its proper functioning. Others were seen as harmful intruders. Naturally, the Jewish culture of eastern Europe was no exception to this rule. One conjuration recorded in the collection *Sefer laḥashim usegulot* employs the model of the prophet Elijah's dialogue with a demon, with the role of the malevolent Lilith taken in this particular example by a stabbing pain (*a shtekh*). The prophet commands it: 'Go up the mountain where three bears stand, one as green as grass, the second as yellow as wax, and the third as bitter as bile. Stab them! And do not touch the human X, son/daughter of Y, but be his/her healing.'[1] And among the Ruthenian conjurations for sprains used by the Jewish population of the region there is one which adjures the sprain not to be a 'vile spirit', not to break bones, not to plague the living, and so on.[2] Legends offering explanations for the aetiology of diseases often lent them human form and character; they roamed the world, settled down, and often suffered hunger and cold together with their hosts. A folk tale from Siemiatycze tells of a louse and a fever that were seeking a new home. They came across a peasant in a field, and decided to throw in their lot with him. However, while the peasant's ragged clothes proved the perfect home for the louse, his overworked body did not suit the fever at all. So it fled, and went to inhabit a squire

[1] Goldberg and Eisenberg, *Sefer laḥashim usegulot*, 9a; Heller, *Medicaments and Remedies* (Heb.), 64.
[2] Maggid, 'Inoyazichniye zagavori', 588–9. Cf. Wereńko, 'Przyczynek do lecznictwa ludowego', 200.

instead; from that time on, peasants have had fleas, and squires have been susceptible to fevers.[3]

This anthropomorphization of physical misfortunes had a variety of consequences for therapeutic practices. While infants were defenceless in the face of both physical attack and illness, many ailments were seen as insufficiently potent to strike down a person who had grown more robust with age. For this reason, older children were not separated from younger siblings afflicted by croup, in the belief that they were not at risk.[4] The demonic character of diseases invading the human body occasioned the use of remedies designed to confuse, frighten away, disgust, bribe, or starve the anthropomorphized complaint. In Dawidgródek (now David-Garadok, Belarus), for instance, the first remedy that was applied if a Jew fell sick was a strict diet and fasting.[5] The advice for treatment of fever was to douse the sufferer in water from a watering can when they were least expecting it; in addition to bringing their body temperature down, this was said to frighten the illness away.[6] One form of protection from various types of affliction that 'did the rounds' was to hang out a warning on the door such as 'Fever, whooping cough, and measles have already been here.'[7] Diseases that were imagined as unclean beings would be treated with a vast arsenal of magical remedies, including popular apotropaics. Some complaints were even perceived as allies; their presence in the body was accepted because it was believed to provide protection from worse misfortunes, or tolerated because it was thought that any attempt to remove them might prove fatal.

The most commonplace demonic affliction among east European Jews was *Plica polonica*, or 'Polish plait' (Pol. *kołtun*, Yid. *kolten*), whose name reflects the fact that it had for centuries been considered endemic to the population of the Polish Commonwealth and was not documented any-

---

[3] Y. Tsherniak, 'Linguistic Folklore and Narrative Style' (Heb.), 31. This story was known to the Christian world in various versions from at least the eighth century; see Brückner, *Literatura religijna w Polsce średniowiecznej*, 104.

[4] Lilientalowa, *Dziecko żydowskie*, 69. Likewise, in a situation where more than one person in a given household was suffering from the same illness, it was believed that the death of one would bring about the recovery of the others; see ead., *Obrzędy pogrzebowe*, fo. 303.

[5] Neumann, 'Our Town' (Yid.), 423.

[6] Lilientalowa, 'Kult wody', 12; Segel, 'Materyały do etnografii Żydów', 325. Cf. Haur, *Ekonomika lekarska*, 12.

[7] Segel, 'Materyały do etnografii Żydów', 321. Sometimes a sign would be displayed claiming that the patient was not at home; see e.g. Lew, 'Lecznictwo i przesądy', *Izraelita*, 48, p. 505, and 50, p. 530.

where else. In Ashkenazi culture it was treated as one more indication of the peculiarity of the Polish environment, as exemplified by Tuvyah Hakohen's statement in his encyclopaedic work *Ma'aseh tuvyah* that it was 'a dangerous disease affecting the people of this land'. Among the many remedies for *Plica polonica* which he listed, he included one given to his father in the mid-seventeenth century by an elderly Christian peasant woman.[8] In terms of the character and significance of *plica*, the Jewish community shared the vast majority of Slavic convictions, and to some extent these beliefs concurred with the stance of modern medical literature regarding the condition. It was known in Slavic folk culture as the external manifestation of a complaint called *gościec* (now termed rheumatoid arthritis; the word is related to *gość*, guest), or 'internal *plica*', and was believed to be a creature planted in the human body (hence 'guest' in the bones) which found its way out in the characteristic tangled, matted mass of hair, and in certain instances could cause rheumatic pain. The first practitioners of biomedicine identified this as two distinct ailments. The 'monstrous suffering of the hair' was a symptom of *plica*, while the 'racking in the limbs' was an indication of rheumatoid arthritis.[9] This interpretation was also documented in the specialist literature in Hebrew.[10] The presence of both these Slavic terms in Jewish folk medicine is most clearly visible, however, in Hebrew and Yiddish magic formulas; here, *kołtun* and *gościec* are not merely medical terms but the names of demonic creatures. One nineteenth-century manuscript contains the following text for lifting a curse:

In the name of the God of Israel, the Almighty, who cures all sickness in His people Israel, casts out all illnesses and all pains, and sufferings, and all unclean forces that exist in the world, and all evil spirits and demons in the world, so also in Your great mercy order the angels of mercy to protect X, son/daughter of Y, from the unclean forces known as *kolten*, that is: plaits, and all the nine types of impurity, that is *gościec*.[11]

Another manuscript reflects the belief that the ailment, which was evidence of the work of demons, might sometimes be the consequence of a

---

[8] Hakohen, *Ma'aseh tuvyah*, 97a–99b.
[9] Majer and Skobel, *Uwagi nad niektóremi wyrazami lekarskiemi*, 13.
[10] The mid-nineteenth-century edition of *Refuot ha'am* (the Hebrew translation of *Avis au peuple sur sa santé* by Samuel August Tissot) contains a mention of *ke'ev ha'evarim hanikra gostits* (pain in the limbs known as *gostits* [*gościec*]), which expresses the same conviction; see Lefin, *Folk Medicine* (Heb.), 84a.      [11] *Segulot urefuot*, Bibliotheca Rosenthaliana, HS. ROS. 444, 6b.

curse. The author of the conjuration would appeal to the illness, defined as a 'tangle of hair called *kołtuny*' and dwelling in 'a man or a woman, in the house, in the field, in the wood, in the wilderness . . . in the belly . . . in the head of a non-Jewish woman, in the belly button . . . in the knees, hands, legs, bones'.[12] At the same time, the formation of *plica* might be a deliberate attempt on the part of the disease to seek help. Rabbinic responsa of the earlier centuries contain indications that some medical practitioners actually recommended to Jewish women the cultivation of a *plica* by sprinkling their head with ashes as a type of cure.[13] This method was used into the twentieth century to combat sicknesses perceived to have been caused by provoking the *gościec*, believed to roam the body, causing a plethora of ailments. Released from inside the body in visible form as the *plica*, it could take a milder course. Testimonies gathered by scholars including Lilientalowa demonstrate that the folk imagination attributed to the *plica* the ability to draw out headaches and erysipelas.[14] However, it might demand the fulfilment of certain whims, using its host as a mouthpiece. For this reason, Lilientalowa noted, a child with a *plica* should not be refused anything, otherwise the *plica* would not stop short of 'twisting its limbs'.

Cutting off the daglock—the external symptom of the sickness—or throwing it away was thus out of the question, as this would have negative consequences. At best it might cause blindness or other permanent damage to the host's health.[15] The Poznań rabbi Akiva Eger described the case of a married woman who cut off her *plica* and soon afterwards lost her mind;[16] the consequences of imprudent treatment might even include death. Methods of removing the matted, felted hair were thus contingent upon a host of conditions that had to be observed for the patient's safety. The treatment procedure would be carried out only at a particular time of day, preferably before sunrise (and thus presumably also after sunset).[17] Rather than being cut off, the *plica* had to be burned at its base and allowed to fall off, and the

---

[12] *Segulot vekameyot*, JTS, MS 10082, 2*b*.

[13] Zimmels, *Magicians, Theologians and Doctors*, 99. Children were forbidden to put sieves on their heads for fear that they might develop 'mange'. But in the early twentieth century the reasons for cultivating afflictions of this nature might be entirely prosaic, e.g. the desire to evade military service; see Buchbinder, 'Jewish Omens' (Yid.), 258; Shabad, 'On Favus (Ringworm)' (Yid.), 159–60.    [14] Lilientalowa, *Dziecko żydowskie*, 62, 68.

[15] Ibid.; Lew, 'O lecznictwie i przesądach', *Izraelita*, 40, p. 382.

[16] Zimmels, *Magicians, Theologians and Doctors*, 99.

[17] Lilientalowa, 'Kult ciał niebieskich', 12.

process was to be staggered by burning one hair at a time.[18] If the patient was a small child, the unwanted *plica* could also be bitten off by its mother.[19] If it was vital to act at once, the patient should stand immersed in water up to their neck; the water formed a symbolic barrier against evil. It was also recommended that the cleansed head be massaged with spikenard. In order to prevent the affliction from returning, the severed *plica* would be wrapped in fabric (a stocking or a blanket) and put away in an inaccessible place (under the threshold, in the corner, or stuffed into a crack). Sometimes it might be left out on the road with a ransom of eighteen groszy in the hope that it would find itself another host.[20]

As mentioned above, in the popular conception the human body was the natural seat of all manner of beings, without which it could not exist. These were normally dormant, but in certain adverse conditions they would awake and make their presence painfully felt in some way. One example of such a creature was the *hartsvorem* (heart worm). Conjurations for expelling parasites from a sick person's body included caveats stipulating that they did not apply to this particular worm.[21] Worms were considered demonic and were associated with snakes, and hence with unclean forces. Moreover, they were to be found in dark, uninhabitable, putrid-smelling nooks and crannies, which was also where demons were believed to lurk. Jewish sources contain examples of magic incantations to drive out worms of different colours (usually white, black, or red),[22] conjurations in Yiddish borrowed from the language of the Christian environment, biblical quotes, and so on. The sources add little to our knowledge about the heart worm, though they do document the use, in the colloquial register, of the expression *grizhet/nogt vi a vorem in hartsn* (gnaws/wears one down like a worm in the heart), which was used metaphorically to refer to something that caused mental discomfort. There is also a clear connection here with the phrase 'to drown the worm', known from both Polish and Jewish literature and

[18] Lilientalowa, *Dziecko żydowskie*, 62.          [19] Weissenberg, 'Kinderfreud', 316.

[20] Rosenberg, *Rafa'el hamalakh*, 96; Lilientalowa, 'Wierzenia, przesądy i praktyki', 173.

[21] *Segulot urefuot*, Bibliotheca Rosenthaliana, HS. ROS. 444, 7a; *Segulot vekameyot*, JTS, MS 10082, 9b; Goldberg and Eisenberg, *Sefer laḥashim usegulot*, 9b; Benet, *Sheloshah sefarim niftaḥim*, 75a; Rubinstein, *Zikhron ya'akov yosef*, 69a; *Sefer hatsadik r. yosef zundl misalant*, 66.

[22] *Segulot urefuot*, Bibliotheca Rosenthaliana, HS. ROS. 444, 7b; Goldberg and Eisenberg, *Sefer laḥashim usegulot*, 9b; Khotsh, *Segulot urefuot*, 8–9. Cf. Biegeleisen, *Lecznictwo ludu polskiego*, 5. Certain other illnesses were also, like worms, imagined as entities of various colours. In one source we find a much-altered Slavic incantation for cataracts, in which the affliction was referred to as white, or various shades of grey. See Heller, *Medicaments and Remedies* (Heb.), 20.

meaning to seek solace in alcohol.[23] The conviction of the existence of a creature of this nature, which lived in the human heart and was an intrinsic element of life, was shared by the folklore of other central and east European nations. Provoked by its human host's actions, it might make its presence felt in various ways—by causing general fatigue, nausea, stomach problems, and the like.[24] Yiddish also had the term *hartsgeshpan*, which described a slightly different complaint: pain in the region of the heart and stomach, which in German-language sources was identified with asthma. In the colloquial language of the Ashkenazi Jews it became synonymous with divine decree, as reflected in sayings such as: *S'iz nit keyn man, s'iz hartsgeshpan* (It's not a man, it's *hartsgeshpan*).[25]

In the late nineteenth century, according to Lilientalowa's notes, the womb was imagined as a frog, or more generally as a creature with several arms—a description also found in non-Jewish sources. In pregnant women it was thought to hold the foetus in place with these arms, and if for any reason it let it go too soon, a miscarriage would ensue.[26] Other sources seem to corroborate this belief, even if they do not make direct reference to it. In one anthology compiled by Benjamin W. Segel, there is a mention of a miscarriage prevention method used in pregnancy: if the woman felt that the foetus in her uterus was dropping, she—or rather her uterus—should undergo a smudging procedure using rectified spirit and buckwheat. This was probably conceived as a way of mollifying or calming the creature functioning in the woman's body independently of her will.[27] The suggestion that smudging 'down there' with pepper or mustard was appropriate for a woman in labour was probably based on the conviction that this would induce contractions and thus ease the child's delivery.[28]

[23] e.g. *Hot men zikh tsezetst un genumen tsiyen fun fleshl, fartrinken dem vorem, vos hot eybik genogt* ('They sat down and began to take slugs from the bottle to drown the worm that was always gnawing at them'); Berlinski, *The First Generation* (Yid.), 27; *Er hot nokh opgetretn in a shenk, fartrunken dem vorem vos totshet in im biz veytik* ('And then he stepped into a tavern to drown the worm that was gnawing him to the quick'); Knapheys, *A Boy from Warsaw* (Yid.), 89.
[24] Cf. Grimm, *Deutsche Mythologie*, 1112; Biegeleisen, *Lecznictwo ludu polskiego*, 7–8.
[25] Halpern, *Mifalot elokim*, 25a, 29a, 44a; Goldberg and Eisenberg, *Sefer laḥashim usegulot*, 17a. See Landau, 'Sprichwörter und Redensarten', 342; Kosover, 'Jewish Sayings and Their Origins' (Yid.), 202–3. Cf. Grimm and Grimm, *Deutsches Wörterbuch*, ii. 1246.
[26] Lilientalowa, 'Wierzenia, przesądy i praktyki', 160–1. Cf. Moszyński, *Kultura ludowa Słowian*, 184. The Latvians, Lithuanians, and Kashubians also imagined the uterus as a frog, and similar beliefs were also found in the German lands; Moszyński, *Kultura ludowa Słowian*, 213. [27] Segel, 'Materyały do etnografii Żydów', 325.
[28] Plaut, *Likutei ḥever ben ḥayim*, 7a; Rosenberg, *Rafa'el hamalakh*, 63; J. Ashkenazi, *Tsene*

Jews shared the ancient belief in the 'wandering womb'. After the birth of a child, the uterus was thought to be restless, trying to find the baby, and its movements were what induced the afterpains. However, it became particularly restless in women who were unable to conceive for long periods, or who generally avoided sexual relations.[29] This latter conviction should be viewed in the context of beliefs surrounding hysteria (Gr. *hystera*, uterus), a certain mood that affected women and bore the hallmarks of a disease of the soul.[30] The leading proponents of ancient medicine advised that a 'wandering womb' had to be taken care of, otherwise it could cause physical and psychological problems. It could be calmed by marriage, or, more accurately, by regular sexual relations. According to Hippocrates, 'if the woman does not have intercourse with her husband, and her belly is emptier [than it should be] . . . the womb displaces itself. For the womb is not wet on its own, because the woman has not had sexual intercourse, and there is an open space, because the belly is emptier, so it turns on itself, and is drier and lighter than normal.'[31] While the traditional Jewish community did not openly articulate this conviction, collections of folklore contain hints showing that it was a deeply rooted belief. The popular kabbalistic pamphlet *Mifalot elokim* included advice on subjects such as headaches in women caused by amenorrhoea. This problem was one of a broad catalogue of issues attributed to a 'wandering womb' by ancient medicine.[32] Folk songs often portrayed young girls tragically in love as hysterical maidens suffering anguish caused by longing. The most common symptoms of this condition, aside from emotional instability, were general weakness, exhaustion, and headaches. A girl who did not find consolation would inevitably meet a sad end, and certain death:

> Mame der kop tut mir vey,
> Shik nokh a dokter, oder tsvey,

*urene fun harav hekhasid*, 3; Lilientalowa, *Coitus, ciąża, poród*, fo. 10, no. 44. The vademecum *Imrot shelomoh* also contains advice on smudging with olibanum (frankincense); see Wilff, *Imrot shelomoh*, 101.

[29] Lilientalowa, 'Wierzenia, przesądy i praktyki', 160–1.
[30] See e.g. Buczkowski, *Społeczne tworzenie ciała*, 153–4; King, 'Once Upon a Text', 205–46.
[31] Whiteley, *Hippocrates' 'Diseases of Women'*, 4.
[32] Halpern, *Mifalot elokim*, 43*b*. Robert Burton, citing authorities including Hippocrates, attributed women's melancholic states to the 'wandering womb'. This caused menstrual blood, which was contaminated and a danger to their health, to have difficulty leaving the body, and the vapours it gave off gave rise to problems including headaches; see Burton, *The Anatomy of Melancholy*, 274–5.

S'kumt oyf mir an ek,
Mayn gelibter iz avek.[33]

Mamma, my head aches; help me, do!
Send for a doctor, or two,
I am dying, certainly,
My beloved has left me.

Hysteria was only one of the indications of a wandering womb. As in
the case of *gościec*, an equally significant symptom of its various movements within the woman's body were the ailments affecting the parts which
it visited. The remedial actions taken in such cases often included magic
incantations intended to persuade the uterus to return to its rightful place.
The oldest Hebrew conjurations used in these instances date back to the
period when the influence of Hellenic culture was at its height. The *Sefer
harazim* included a prescription for this problem that was copied from
a Greek original.[34] Another medieval source contains a Judaeo-German
incantation which begins with the words *Ber muter lig dikh* (Womb, be
still!) and entreats the uterus 'by nine generations and by nine pure Torah
scrolls, and by nine angels'.[35] There is also a formula in Yiddish, dating
from as recently as the early twentieth century, which was used by a quack
healer to charm the '*heyb muter* in the woman', so that the uterus would
return to the rightful region of the body. The healer was supposed to recite
the formula with their right hand on the patient's navel.[36] While most of
the sources analysed for this study stress the feminine aspect of this problem, it was in fact potentially a universal issue, because according to folk
conceptions, men also had a uterus.[37]

The primary issues associated with a 'wandering womb' were abdominal pains and gripe. This is the interpretation proffered by scholars of
German folklore, such as Jacob Grimm, who identified the gnawing *Hach-*

[33] Rozental, 'Folk Songs' (Heb.), 348. A slightly different variant of this song is listed in the
collection *Yevrieiskaya narodnaya piesni*, 158. One way to assuage uterus pain was to perform a
smudging procedure by burning hairs taken from the woman's husband, perhaps as a substitute
for sexual intercourse; see Rosenberg, *Rafa'el hamalakh*, 12; *Segulot urefuot*, JTS, MS 9862, 73.

[34] Bohak, *Ancient Jewish Magic*, 237.

[35] Perles, 'Die Berner Handschrift des kleinen Aruch', 28; Trachtenberg, *Jewish Magic and
Superstition*, 200–1. See Khotsh, *Segulot urefuot*, 11; David ben Aryeh Leib, *Sod hashem*, 34.

[36] *Segulot urefuot*, JTS, MS 9862, 42–4. See a similar conjuration, also referring to a woman
and recited with the hand on her navel, in Goldberg and Eisenberg, *Sefer lahashim usegulot*, 2a.

[37] Lilientalowa, 'Wierzenia, przesądy i praktyki', 161.

*mutter* or *Bärmutter* as gripe.[38] The same term figures in a similar meaning in *Refuot ha'am*.[39] One of the stories attributed to the tsadik Mordecai ('Motl') Twersky of Chernobyl, in turn, cites the case of a man who came down with *heyb muter*, which the author interpreted as 'belly fever'.[40] In such cases, the 'wandering womb' was treated with large doses of natural remedies. In *Emunat shemuel*, a collection of responsa compiled by rabbi Aaron Samuel Koydanover (1614–76), there is a discussion of consent for treatment of this complaint during Passover with compresses made from barley or oats, which were otherwise forbidden during the festival as *hamets* (products which may ferment and become leavened).[41] A number of other herbal remedies and methods to counteract this ailment, which was 'particularly widespread in women', were also listed in the pamphlet *Mifalot elokim*, including smudging, compresses, and the use of purgatives.[42]

In the folk understanding, it was in the nature of some diseases to 'attack' whole populations. In the nineteenth century, when the peoples of eastern Europe were repeatedly decimated by cholera, this plague was personified in demonic form. In Lublin, for instance, it was thought to be a tall, shrivelled, scabrous woman who, on arriving in the city, had announced her presence to one of the Jewish community officials. When the same official saw her leaving, the epidemic abated.[43] In Kraków the Jews accused a recently arrived man of having brought the disease, and plied him with gifts to persuade him to leave the area.[44] Mystical methods were ubiquitously employed to combat plague, the most widespread being symbolic isolation. 'At such times people would wear rings made from the *lulav*, and four

[38] Grimm, *Deutsche Mythologie*, 1111.
[39] Lefin, *Folk Medicine* (Heb.), 84b.     [40] Bodek, *Mifalot hatsadikim*, 22–3.
[41] A. S. Koydanover, *Emunat shemu'el*, 26a. The word *febra* (fever or ague) was sometimes used to denote a head cold and chill (*febris catarrhalis*), while various stomach complaints, producing symptoms such as diarrhoea, might be called intestinal chills; see Barukh of Shklov, *Derekh yesharah*, 9a. Oat or barley compresses and baths were used for a range of abdominal problems, including enlarged spleen (Schneersohn, *Sefer refuot*, 14; Rosenberg, *Rafa'el hamalakh*, 15), kidney stones (Rosenberg, *Der malekh refoel*, 60), and intestinal chills (Rosenberg, *Rafa'el hamalakh*, 87; Lew, 'Lecznictwo i przesądy', *Izraelita*, 47, p. 493).
[42] Halpern, *Mifalot elokim*, 7a–b. The recipes for concoctions to combat a wandering womb, recorded in the pamphlet *Sha'ar efrayim*, 23b, date from around the same period.
[43] Levin, *From the Good Old Days* (Yid.), 122–3.
[44] Kopff, *Wspomnienia z ostatnich lat Rzeczypospolitej Krakowskiej*, 138. 'Bad air' (miasma), which was often seen as the cause of disease, could also take the form of a pig. According to folklore, the killing of one such pig with the silver rod of the tsadik of Przeworsk brought an end to the spread of the disease; see Nagelberg, 'Das Ipisch bei galizischen Juden', 286.

young girls would be harnessed to a horse collar and would plough up a
strip of land on the outskirts of the town, on the side from which the cholera
had come', recalled Yehezkel Kotik, who was originally from Kamenets
(now Belarus). The custom of ploughing up a symbolic demarcation line to
protect a settlement is also known from Slavic sources.[45] Another response
to the threat of plague was the practice of reciting, at the four corners of the
town, passages from the Bible relating to the incense offering. This was
accompanied by solemn processions with Torah scrolls and the celebration
of black weddings in cemeteries. In private homes many preventative measures might be taken: a locked padlock might be hung on the door and the
walls would be daubed with charcoal (creating a symbolic wall of fire),[46] an
onion and a bulb of garlic would be hung in the window,[47] or a notice displayed on the door frame that the disease should pass over the house.[48]

   In this context it is worth taking a moment to discuss amulets for
protection from cholera. The *Rafa'el hamalakh* contains several interesting descriptions of objects of this type. They were to be written on kosher
parchment, after a ritual bath, and in observance of the rules for writing
sacred texts. They were usually hung up in the house, or worn on the forehead or around the neck of the sufferer, though on occasion they might be
swallowed at the first sign of symptoms, as in the case of an amulet from
Jerusalem attributed to Rabbi Akiva Eger.[49] In order to work as intended,
many amulets had to be used in conjunction with other items. A diagram
created by the tsadik Mordecai of Trisk depicted a kind of kabbalistic
incense burner for the symbolic burning of fragrant spices to the accompaniment of recitation of angelic names and appropriately selected biblical

---

[45] Kotik, *My Memoirs* (Yid.), 315.
[46] Segel, 'Wierzenia i lecznictwo', 54. The daubing of the walls of the room with charcoal
was intended to protect the birthing woman from the forces of evil; see Lifshits, *Berit avot*, 5*b*;
Pulner, 'Obryadi i povirya', 106.                      [47] Rosenberg, *Rafa'el hamalakh*, 52.
[48] Weissenberg proffers a copy of the handwritten statement: 'Khaya-Reyzl, daughter of
Leah, is not at home.' See Weissenberg, 'Krankheit und Tod', 357.
[49] Rosenberg, *Rafa'el hamalakh*, 50; Veynig, 'Medicaments and Remedies among the Jews'
(Yid.), 29; Lilientalowa, *Choroby, lecznictwo*, fo. 357. This is echoed in the collection of advice to
be followed during epidemics entitled *Shemirot usegulot nifla'ot*, 22. This 'imbibing' of the
sacred names should be performed using only kosher wine, from a ritually purified vessel; see
Rosenberg, *Rafa'el hamalakh*, 112. R. Akiva Eger of Poznań is mentioned in the context of one
more widely disseminated method for combating cholera: during an epidemic in 1831 he is said
to have recommended swallowing nine mustard seeds every morning on an empty stomach; see
e.g. Rosenberg, *Rafa'el hamalakh*, 52; Lew, 'Lecznictwo i przesądy', *Izraelita*, 47, p. 494; Segel,
'Materyały do etnografii Żydów', 325.

quotes.[50] In other cases the efficacy of the amulet depended on the con-current use of herbs, also believed to offer protection from demons. The recipe compiled by the kabbalist Hayim Vital (1542–1620), a student of Isaac Luria, required the image of an open hand to be drawn on parchment together with a number of combinations of letters and names. Then leaves of the common rue, gathered on the fourth day of the week at a full moon and before sunrise, with the intention, expressed vocally, that they were being gathered for X, son/daughter of Y, should be shredded using a gold coin, wrapped in the parchment, and hung around the neck.[51] Rue leaves were also recommended for wearing with another parchment amulet, which comprised some of the 'canonical' protective texts generally accep-ted by rabbis and kabbalists (such as the words of Ps. 106: 30 interspersed with the letters of the name of God, and the phrase *Shadai kera satan*, 'May the Almighty tear Satan apart').[52]

Of particular note is an amulet that is mentioned not only in the context of epidemics, but also as a deterrent against demons and the evil eye. This was the *baytele* (bag) mentioned earlier: a leather or linen drawstring pouch filled with certain protective objects and hung around the neck of the person at risk (usually a child). According to the translators and editors of the Yiddish edition of Yehudah Yudl Rosenberg's *Rafa'el hamalakh*, that book contained the most efficacious (and rabbinically approved) version of the amulet for convulsions, which came from the tsadik Israel of Kozie-nice (Koznits). 'This *segulah* is indeed known [also] to other holy men [*gute yidn*], but in terms of helping, it does little, usually no good at all', the editors complained, citing inaccuracies arising from the oral convention as the reason for this, and averring that 'if performed less than precisely, the *segulah* will not work'.[53] The authentic amulet, as recommended by the tsa-dik, comprised a chamois leather glove filled with hyssop from the Land of Israel, gastroliths taken from the stomachs of cockerels (or of hens for women), needles, deadly nightshade (the 'devil's herb'), mercury, and com-mon rue (as the main ingredient). It also contained nutshells fused together with tar and bound up, which were to be filled with three almonds, some peppercorns and salt crystals, and a live spider. Almost all of these ingredi-ents were included for their specific apotropaic effects.[54] The glove should

---

[50]  Rosenberg, *Rafa'el hamalakh*, 57.
[51]  Ibid. 53.                      [52]  Ibid. 54.                      [53]  Rosenberg, *Segulot urefuot*, 26.
[54]  Some of these ingredients were to be purchased from a pharmacy; see Sosnowik, 'Mater-ial on Jewish Folk Medicine in Belarus' (Yid.), 165.

be tied up with a red cord—a widespread form of protection from enchantments—and as the amulet was being placed about the patient's neck, to hang just below the heart, the following words in Yiddish were to be spoken: 'This is a *segulah* of the Magid of Koznits, son of Perl, a righteous man of blessed memory, that epilepsy might have no power here.'[55]

The reservations of the translators of Rabbi Rosenberg's work regarding other, supposedly less effective variants of the amulet should themselves be treated with reserve. First of all, it can be assumed that an objective study of the effectiveness of the item would bring similar results. Secondly —and this seems even more important—such *baytelekh* were employed extremely widely, and were in fact more commonly disseminated by mothers, grandmothers, and next-door neighbours than by tsadikim or other holy men. For vomiting, and also for teething, a small sachet would be filled with walnut shells holding almonds, pepper, salt, and a live lizard.[56] For fright the sachet would be filled with rue, belladonna, and pigeon droppings.[57] Lilientalowa cites an example of a sachet, intended as protection from spells, which contained pepper, salt, a spider, pins, crayfish eyes, earth from beneath the threshold, a piece of material from a shroud, and a goose-feather quill filled with lead.[58] And there are many more examples. Evidence of the immense popularity of these *baytelekh* as protective measures against epidemics is the fact that they continued to be used en masse by successive generations of Jewish émigrés in America. In periods of epidemics whole classes of children would wear sachets of this type around their neck to ward off the polio or influenza that was threatening them.

These *baytelekh* were the most elaborate form of repellent worn by

---

[55] Ibid.; Rosenberg, *Rafa'el hamalakh*, 69. The same amulet is discussed briefly by Lilientalowa, who cites as her source 'the book of the angel Raphael'; *Dziecko żydowskie*, 60.

[56] Rosenberg, *Rafa'el hamalakh*, 44. Lilientalowa's version makes mention of a heart-shaped sachet containing stolen salt, pepper, and allspice for teething pain (*Dziecko żydowskie*, 46), and for teething convulsions a sachet holding amber received from a 'good Jew' (a holy man, perhaps a tsadik), the child's nail clippings, three locks of its hair (cut from three sides of its head), mercury, a spider, salt, and earth from a cemetery (*Dziecko żydowskie*, 59).

[57] Rosenberg, *Rafa'el hamalakh*, 79.

[58] The sources also mention earth from the cemetery, hair from a dog's tail, a cock's or hen's comb (depending on the gender of the 'patient'), coal, and soot from the stove; see e.g. Plaut, *Likutei hever ben hayim*, 8b; Weissenberg, 'Südrussische Amulette', 369; Lilientalowa, *Dziecko żydowskie*, 49; ead., 'The Evil Eye' (Yid.), 256–7; Fayvushinski, 'The Folklore of Pruzhana' (Yid.), 203. Weissenberg also notes the custom of the sufferer carrying earth from the Land of Israel under their arm; see Weissenberg, 'Palästina in Brauch und Glauben der heutigen Juden', 261.

those at risk from various types of threat; the protective agents were not always placed in a bag. Sometimes mothers would simply wrap a clove of garlic, a piece of amber, or some salt in a handkerchief, or sew it into their child's clothing (especially in the nine days leading up to the fast of Tishah Be'av, when Torah study—and hence the protection this afforded—was curtailed). Items carried in the pockets could be just as effective.[59] Peony root, known since antiquity as a remedy for convulsions, and recommended by Galen to be worn in a little leather bag around the neck, was often used by the Jews in slightly different forms. It might be placed under the sufferer's pillow[60] or sewn into their clothing.[61] Folk aetiology, which linked epilepsy to spells, attributed to this natural remedy the power to repel the evil eye. There was even a Hebrew amulet, cited in full by Lilientalowa,[62] which mentioned the wearing or carrying of peony seeds, and many different texts, both printed and in the form of manuscripts, testify to the consumption by epileptics of *Radix paeoniae*; analogies with this custom may also be found in sources for the ethnography of the Slavs.[63]

When protective and preventative measures failed, however, the preferred course of action taken by folk medicine tended to be the forcible eviction of the ailment from the body it occupied. One method of expelling demonic forms—independently of naturalistic interpretations—was to induce sneezing in the sufferer.[64] A mid-nineteenth-century manuscript from the library of the Leszno *ḥevrah kadisha* contains the advice that sneezing caused by placing an appropriate substance under the nose can put a

[59] Sosnowik, 'Material on Jewish Folk Medicine in Belarus' (Yid.), 164; Lilientalowa, 'The Evil Eye' (Yid.), 257; salt was sometimes sewn into the pillow used during the ritual of *pidyon haben*, the redeeming of the firstborn (to guard against spells); Lilientalowa, 'Additions: The "Evil Eye"' (Yid.), 433.

[60] Halpern, *Toledot adam*, 10. An example of a technique to prevent children from dying from epilepsy, which involved inserting selected items into the mother's pillow (e.g. a piece of whetstone and trimmings from horses' hooves) before childbirth, is to be found in the collection of Goldberg and Eisenberg, *Sefer laḥashim usegulot*, 19b.

[61] Berger, *Imrei yisra'el*, 7b. On the subject of the links between the moon and the peony, and on the use of peonies in the ancient world, see Stol, *Epilepsy in Babylonia*, 125–6.

[62] Lilientalowa, 'Dziecko żydowskie', 147; Spinner, 'Zur Volkkunde galizischer Juden', 95–6.

[63] *Segulot urefuot*, Bibliotheca Rosenthaliana, HS. ROS. 444, 8b; Eliasberg, *Marpe le'am*, Pt I, 127; Berger, *Imrei yisra'el*, 6b. Cf. Talko-Hryncewicz, *Zarys lecznictwa ludowego*, 121.

[64] Authorities in humoral pathology stressed that sneezing cleared and strengthened the brain; see Andrzej of Kobylin, *Gadki o składności członków człowieczych*, 23. Popular Jewish opinion also held sneezing to be healthy because it 'tore apart' headaches; see Lilientalowa, *Choroby, lecznictwo*, fo. 122.

patient back on their feet.[65] This provides the context for the traditional wishes of health, which verged on a ritual, requiring the patient to say the words: 'I await your deliverance, O Lord!' (Gen. 49: 18), to which those standing around were to respond: *Tsu gezunt!* or *Asuse!* (Aram. *Asuta*, Your health!).[66] When the one sneezing was a child, the person responsible for performing the ritual was its mother. In this case, the wish would be: *Tsu gezunt, tsum lebn, tsum vaksn, tsum kveln* (Your health, your life, your growth, your joy),[67] or: *Shtark zolstu zayn, gezunt zolstu zayn, vaksn zolstu* (May you be strong, be healthy, and grow),[68] though this popularly took rhyming form, for example,

> *Asuse!*
> Frum un alt
> Hundert yor alt
> Raykh un zelik
> Nisht shlemielik![69]
>
> *Asuse!*
> Devout and old
> A hundred years old
> Rich and happy
> Not a clot!

If a sick child sneezed, this might indicate that they would soon recover; if the youngest child at the sabbath table sneezed, this was taken as evidence of the presence of the prophet Elijah, and as a good omen for the new week.[70] These beliefs in no way contradicted the conviction that the human soul departs the body through the nose, and that sneezing in even the symbolic presence of a dead person (for example while reminiscing about them) presaged one's own death. Belching could also help to rid the body of disease. The standard reaction to a baby burping was to say:

---

[65] Goldstein, *Halikhot olam*, 52. Goldstein is referring to *roytel zaft*, perhaps meaning *Rautensaft* (rue juice); see Buck, *Medicinischer Volksglauben*, 39.

[66] Lipiets, *Sefer matamim*, 75; Buchbinder, 'Jewish Omens' (Yid.), 256. According to tradition, it was only with the intercession of the patriarch Jacob (or Isaac) that people stopped dying from sneezing, an action which blew the soul out of the body; see Lilientalowa, 'Przesądy żydowskie', 281; ead., *Dziecko żydowskie*, 67; Gilad, 'Wise Words' (Heb.), 144.

[67] 'Aus unseren Sammlungen. II', 7.                    [68] Weissenberg, 'Kinderfreud', 316.

[69] Grunwald, 'Aus unseren Sammlungen. Teil I', 35.

[70] Lew, 'O lecznictwie i przesądach', *Izraelita*, 40, p. 383, and 42 (1897), p. 407. Another good prognosticator in children was sweating from the soles of the feet, which, like sneezing, was also significant according to humoral pathology; see Weissenberg, 'Kinderfreud', 316.

*A greps aroys, a gezunt arayn* (Burp out, health in).[71] Similar words were said if a child coughed,[72] and if it was having trouble clearing its throat or was choking on something, it might be helped with a slap, by blowing in its mouth, or with other similar actions.[73]

One category of methods used, while not for all illnesses, nonetheless fairly extensively, was 'shaking', beating, or even 'chopping' an illness or complaint out of the body. A recommended technique in the case of infantile convulsions was to hold the child by its head and knock its feet several times against the door frame—presumably the threshold.[74] And one of the standard treatments for a cold was whipping with a bundle of twigs in a steam bath, for which humoral pathology also found justification.[75] 'Chopping' was used above all in the case of an illness called *ripkukhn* (early German medicine knew the term *Rieb-Kuchen*, which could denote a sense of 'hardness in the side'[76]). Jewish sources tended to translate it as abdominal flatulence or enlarged spleen (or more rarely liver), a symptom of the 'English disease' (rickets).[77] For this reason one of the remedies used to treat it was the fresh spleen of a pig or a cow, which was applied as a compress to the swollen site, or used for 'pulling through' (the recommended way of doing this was to cut the meat into a 'ring' and 'pull' the patient's body through it from head to foot three times). The cut of meat was then hung up over the mantelpiece to dry out along with the disease.[78] The most popular method of combating *ripkukhn*, however, was to lay the sick child on the threshold, place a washing paddle, plank, or kneading trough on top of the child, and strike this piece of wood repeatedly with a meat cleaver (or washing paddle). The operation, which was to be repeated over a period of three days, was to be accompanied by the following dialogue, conducted over the threshold: 'What are you chopping?' '*Ripkukhn.*' 'What are you chopping it with?' 'An axe.' 'So chop better!', or: 'What are you hacking?'

---

[71] 'Aus unseren Sammlungen. II', 7. Cf. Lilientalowa, *Dziecko żydowskie*, 67.

[72] Lilientalowa, *Dziecko żydowskie*, 61.

[73] Ibid. 67.                                    [74] Segel, 'Wierzenia i lecznictwo', 56.

[75] Shlaferman, 'The Folklore, Customs, and Stories of Kazimierz' (Yid.), 172.

[76] Crato, *Johannis Cratonis . . . ausserlesene Artzney-Künste*, 199. See Grimm and Grimm, *Deutsches Wörterbuch*, v. 2500.

[77] Halpern, *Mifalot elokim*, 44a; Khotsh, *Segulot urefuot*; Lilientalowa, *Dziecko żydowskie*, 65; Rosenberg, *Segulot urefuot*, 23; Alfabet, 'Materials for the Study of Idiom' (Yid.), 70; Opatoshu, 'From My Lexicon' (Yid.), 119.

[78] Lilientalowa, *Dziecko żydowskie*, 64; Rosenberg, *Rafa'el hamalakh*, 37; id., *Segulot urefuot*, 23.

'*Kra*!' 'Hack it to smithereens!'[79] It is worth noting that the Slavic residents of Belarus used similar methods to treat an illness they called *bryzie* (biting), which has been translated as hernia caused by a sickness 'biting into the body'.[80]

In the popular consciousness, since diseases entered the body from outside, there had to be a way of extracting them again and removing them from the immediate environment. In the above-mentioned example of *ripkukhn*, another method used by the Jews was to draw it out onto the surface of the body in the form of ulceration. These ulcers would be induced using the tried and tested method of smearing the body with mustard and honey or wrapping it in a piece of cloth smeared with those substances. For better effect the child patient should be placed in a hot stove three times.[81] These compresses, and even specially prepared mustard plasters, were also used in the case of puncture wounds, vomiting, and suffocation.[82] Indeed, they were widely used in herbalism, and were also prescribed, sometimes in processed form (as an essential oil, or blended with rectified spirit) by biomedical practitioners. If simply drawing out the disease did not help, however, sometimes attempts to expel it beyond the limits of the place of residence were undertaken. The hope in such cases was that these steps would render it impossible for the complaint to return via the same route. A child with diphtheria, for instance, should be taken out of the town via the first toll gate, and brought back in via the third (or taken out to a crossroads).[83] In case of a fever, the patient should run out of the house, through the streets, and into a field, pick up a stone, throw it, and then run away again without looking back.[84]

[79] Alfabet, 'Materials for the Study of Idiom' (Yid.), 63; Lilientalowa, *Dziecko żydowskie*, 65. Some sources do not mention this dialogue, and speak only of striking a pot (e.g. one for making cholent) with a meat cleaver eighteen times in three cycles before sundown; Lew, 'O lecznictwie i przesądach', *Izraelita*, 42 (1897), p. 407. Other measures taken to treat *ripkukhn* include that described in a recipe from Szkłów (Shklov), which required ten units of Epsom salts and fifteen drams of semolina to be boiled up in water and drunk morning (on an empty stomach) and evening until the symptoms subsided; *Sefer hatsadik r. yosef zundl misalant*, 67.

[80] Wereńko, 'Przyczynek do lecznictwa ludowego', 151; Moszyński, *Kultura ludowa Słowian*, 201.

[81] Lilientalowa, *Dziecko żydowskie*, 64; Rosenberg, *Rafa'el hamalakh*, 37; id., *Segulot urefuot*, 23. Cf. Libera, *Medycyna ludowa*, 34.

[82] Sperling, *Ta'amei haminhagim oyf ivri taytsh*, ii. 106, 108; Rosenberg, *Der malekh refoel*, 32, 49. [83] Fels, 'Zabobony lekarskie u Żydów', 4.

[84] Lew, 'Lecznictwo i przesądy', *Izraelita*, 50, p. 530. Cf. Udziela, *Medycyna i przesądy lecznicze*, 184.

In this period, procedures performed using various types of 'props' were hugely popular. Many curative rituals involved hiding certain objects belonging to the patient—usually hair, or finger- or toenails—in a hollow tree (for instance an aspen or an almond tree) or in a crevice in a wall. The idea was that the sickness should follow the hidden objects, which were in some rather vague way perceived as at once part of the body and growths, offshoots, or secretions from it. Hiding them or symbolically shutting them away somewhere was seen as a chance to rid oneself of the ailment too. A ritual of this nature might be enacted on the threshold: a hole would be drilled in the door frame (on the right) and afterwards stopped up with an aspen peg. In other cases a location at a certain distance from human habitation might be preferred: in a field or under a tree, for instance. If the patient was strong enough, the act would be performed in their presence at the place where the objects were to be hidden. If not, the hair and nails would be pressed into a piece of soft wax, which a person close to the patient would take to the selected site. As they were being placed into the hole, a formula would be recited, such as 'Take what is yours, and take this child's cough'—though often longer formulas taken from the vernacular of the environment might also be used. Those present would then leave the site of the ritual as quickly as possible and without looking back.[85] A very similar method for removing an enchantment involved placing nail clippings into a blown-out eggshell, which would then be rolled to a milestone—a place that represented both a real and a symbolic border—at a distance from the affected person's home.[86]

Other objects used in rituals of this nature included things that could absorb the ailment by being pressed to the affected site (an apple, a potato, or a cabbage stalk, all of which were used in the case of warts). For various eruptions on the skin, string or other types of thread (a horse hair, or a thin piece of wire) might be used, either to tie around the wart or for magical numerology practices involving tying as many knots in the thread as there were growths. Animals might also be used as media. A black cockerel would be swung around the head of an epileptic three times (to absorb the illness), and would then be ripped apart above the patient as a sign of the destruction of the illness. After the performance of the ritual, the objects used

---

[85] Berger, *Imrei yisra'el*, 7*b*; Goldberg and Eisenberg, *Sefer laḥashim usegulot*, 7*a*; Plaut, *Likutei ḥever ben ḥayim*, 8*a*; Rosenberg, *Rafa'el hamalakh*, 45, 67; Sperling, *Ta'amei haminhagim umekorei hadinim*, 579.       [86] *Segulot urefuot*, Bibliotheca Rosenthaliana, HS. ROS. 444, 6*b*.

would usually be buried in the ground, thrown onto the rubbish heap, or buried in manure, in the hope that they would rot, and with them the disease.[87] In larger towns they might also be dropped into storm drains, with the words: 'Just as I don't know where [the object] will end up, so I don't know where my [name of sickness] will end up.'[88] Other recommended courses of action seem to have functioned on a similar basis, often with the addition of elements of kabbalah (names, Bible quotes). As a cure for fever, a number of sources advocated cutting up an apple into three or four pieces, or selecting nine large almonds, writing an appropriate label on each one (Yid. *opshraybn kadokhes*), and then eating them one after the other.[89] In many cases, rituals of this type would be enacted by a well, river, or stream. Standing with their back to the water, the person performing the action would throw the given object over their shoulder and then hurry away as quickly as possible.

Sometimes it was believed that an effective way of ridding oneself of an illness was to pass it on to someone else. This was usually achieved by 'planting'. Jewish sources document a plethora of ways of 'planting' objects via which the ailment could be transmitted in places frequented by others (at crossroads or forks in the road, or on the marketplace). Hasidic leaders including Tsevi Elimelekh of Dynów and Menahem Mendel of Rymanów even managed to find religious justification for this custom, citing the following verse from the book of Numbers (5: 2): 'Instruct the Israelites to remove from camp anyone with an eruption or a discharge.'[90] These practices led to tensions between the Jews and the Christian population, which recognized them for what they were on the basis of their own mythology.[91] The peasants in the Rymanów region were convinced that Jewish bakers added to their leaven water that had been used for the ritual washing of the dead; that they put nail clippings and even entire digits in their dough for

[87] *Segulot urefuot*, JTS, MS 9862, 48; Segel, 'Materyały do etnografii Żydów', 32; Lew, 'O lecznictwie i przesądach', *Izraelita*, 41, p. 394; Lilientalowa, 'Wierzenia, przesądy i praktyki', 173; ead., *Dziecko żydowskie*, 64.

[88] U. Weinreich, 'Beliefs: Remedies for Warts' (Yid.), 63.

[89] Rosenberg, *Rafa'el hamalakh*, 84–5; Plaut, *Likutei hever ben hayim*, 9a; Segel [Schiffer], 'Alltagglauben', 273. See Mark (ed.), *Great Dictionary of the Yiddish Language* (Yid.), iv. 1971. The connection between fever and water is emphasized by the recommendation to label four apples with the names of the four rivers which issued from the biblical Garden of Eden: the Gihon, the Pishon, the Tigris, and the Euphrates, and then eating them as treatment for the disease; Isaac ben Eliezer, *Refuah vehayim miyrushalayim*, 34.

[90] Kanarvogel, *Ta'amei mitsvot*, 18b (194).     [91] Biegeleisen, *Lecznictwo ludu polskiego*, 9–10.

bread rolls; and that the roads were littered with the clothes of cholera victims—not only rags but also items in good condition, so that someone
would be tempted and take them.[92] Many of these beliefs were reflected in
Jewish sources—and they are numerous, so it is worth making mention of
a few of the more typical examples. One cast-iron guarantee for ridding
oneself of a cold or fever was said to be smearing one's nasal discharge (or
spitting) on one's neighbour's door handle (ideally three times); another
was simply to discard a used handkerchief in a highly frequented place.[93]
A recommended course of action for epilepsy was to hang up a shirt belonging to the sufferer at a crossroads, stick a needle into it, and tie a coin
to it.[94] In Orla, the method for ridding oneself of a boil or abscess was to
rub the affected site with a pretty ribbon or other eye-catching trifle that
someone might be tempted to pick up, and then drop the contaminated
item in the street. In Bereza Kartuska the same principle was suggested for
flushing cockroaches out of one's house: one should catch twelve speci-
mens, put them in a bag and tie it up, and then throw them into a peasant's
cart without its owner noticing. This was said to make the vermin move to
his house.[95]

Other examples of treatment methods included 'revulsion' or 'spoiling'
(*paslen a krankn*, lit. rendering the patient unpalatable). Some complaints,
above all those caused by curses or spells, could be relieved by rendering
the sufferer's body unattractive to malevolent external forces. One of the
most typical strategies was washing a sick child[96]—and for prudence' sake
its siblings also—in its mother's urine.[97] Another commonplace practice
was to lay the child on the ground and urinate on it in such a way as to
shower its face and mouth. As menstruating women were one category of

[92] Potocka, *Mój pamiętnik*, 167–9.

[93] Fels, 'Zabobony lekarskie u Żydów', 5; Lew, 'O lecznictwie i przesądach', *Izraelita*, 49, p. 475; Segel, 'Wierzenia i lecznictwo', 55. Even simply talking to someone about having a cold could elicit one in that person: Lilientalowa, *Choroby, lecznictwo*, fo. 5.

[94] Lilientalowa, 'Wierzenia, przesądy i praktyki', 163.

[95] Khayes, 'Death-Related Beliefs and Customs' (Yid.), 326. For a similar method for removing cockroaches, see 'Omens and Remedies' (Yid.), 286.

[96] In Horodets this method was mainly used for 'cuts, punctures, swelling, and earache', while dog urine was also used for warts; Ben-Ezra, 'Customs' (Yid.), 176. See also U. Wein-reich, 'Beliefs: Remedies for Warts' (Yid.), 62.

[97] Landau, 'Notes and Comments on *Yidishe Filologye*' (Yid.), 330–1. This is the most common translation for the phrase *paslen a kind* in Yiddish dictionaries; see Alexander Harkavy, *Yiddish–English–Hebrew Dictionary* (Yid.), 374: 'to rub the face of a child with urine (thus removing the effects of an evil eye)'.

those who disseminated enchantments, they could not do this.[98] Erysipelas, which, according to Lilientalowa, was considered particularly responsive to 'degrading' strategies, should be smeared with faeces—ideally those of the patient themselves, or fresh horse droppings.[99] This method was known to Polish early modern medicine, which recommended compresses from cow dung mixed with vinegar,[100] to be used for a range of skin complaints. The faeces of an infant not yet introduced to solids were recommended for smearing on an anal fistula ('an abscess from which pus has flowed for many days').[101] Boils and mange could be treated with dog faeces (sometimes mixed with honey and egg), while for pimples pigeon droppings were preferred.[102] The term *paslen* was also used to refer to smashing a clay vessel over a child lying on the ground or in a cradle covered with a kneading trough, an action that sometimes accompanied the procedures described above.[103] According to some sources, convulsions were a sign that a *gilgul* —the errant soul of a sinner—was in the process of taking over the sick person's body. Smashing a pot or plate over the child's face was a way of preventing this.[104]

[98]  Segel, 'Wierzenia i lecznictwo', 60; Lilientalowa, *Dziecko żydowskie*, 58.

[99]  *Segulot urefuot*, JTS, MS 9862, 11; Lilientalowa, *Dziecko żydowskie*, 68.

[100]  Haur, *Ekonomika lekarska*, 127.                    [101]  Rosenberg, *Rafa'el hamalakh*, 59.

[102]  For treatment of boils, see *Segulot urefuot*, Bibliotheca Rosenthaliana, HS. ROS. 444, 10*b*. The same ingredients—dog's faeces mixed with honey—were also used to treat throat ulcers; Lilientalowa, *Dziecko żydowskie*, 63. For mange, the faeces were to be applied in the form of an ointment made using quicklime, privet, and 'bluestone' (*Blaustein*, copper(II) sulfate, or vitriol of copper); *Segulot vekameyot*, JTS, MS 10082, 8*b*. For the treatment of pimples, see Rosenberg, *Rafa'el hamalakh*, 66; *Segulot urefuot*, JTS, MS 9862, 108.

[103]  Schiffer, 'Alltagglauben', 170; Friedländer, 'Volksmedizin', 33; Sosnowik, 'Material on Jewish Folk Medicine in Belarus' (Yid.), 164. A similar *segulah* for a child who had fainted apparently involved covering their face with the inverted vessel and tapping the base with a stick; Meler, *Besorot tovot*, 50.

[104]  Akalovich, 'Zamietki o yevrieiskoy narodnoy demonologii', 139; Friedländer, 'Volksmedizin', 33.

# CHAPTER TWELVE

# DEMONS AND WITCHES

P EOPLE BELIEVED that an illness or other health issue could be the work of supernatural beings such as demons, devils, or witches. Unlike the diseases discussed above, these creatures were thought to do their mischief not by directly entering the victim's body, but usually by using magic. One conjuration for curing the childhood condition known in Yiddish as *tsemenik* (cradle cap), for instance, expressed the conviction that its power came from Lilith and her maleficent demons.[1] Folk demonology was not a systematized science, however, and the distinctions between spells, demons, and creatures of the other world (the angel of death or the devil) were somewhat poorly defined. One and the same text might be used in incantations offering protection from the evil eye, or on seeing a 'no-gooder' (Yid. *nisht-guter*) or a witch.[2] This makes it all the easier to understand the reason for the lengthy list of dangers enumerated in a single breath in popular incantations, such as: 'O God, cure X son/daughter of Y if s/he has worms in his/her belly, if s/he has the fright or anxiety, or is under a spell, or has any other weakness anywhere up to the top of his/her head, that s/he may be completely cured.'[3] It is also important to remember that any illness, even one not obviously associated with demons, rendered the victim vulnerable to threats from such quarters. Thus fear of talking about the patient's health may have been due to a preference for passing over ailments in silence, in the hope that this would avert any greater danger. One consequence of the belief in the particular susceptibility of the sick to attacks by unclean forces was the custom of holding night vigils in patients' homes and ensuring regular visits to them during the day by members of the *bikur ḥolim* fraternity.[4]

---

[1] Goldberg and Eisenberg, *Sefer laḥashim usegulot*, 5b–6a. According to the lexicon of Polish dialects *Słownik gwar polskich*, the term *ciemienica* might denote either *ciemieniucha* (cradle cap) or *ciemiennik* (a disease of the tongue). See Karłowicz, *Słownik gwar polskich*, i. 229.

[2] See e.g. Linetski, *The Hasidic Boy* (Yid.), 30; Lilientalowa, *Dziecko żydowskie*, 56; Lilientalowa, 'The Evil Eye' (Yid.), 268.

[3] *Segulot urefuot*, Bibliotheca Rosenthaliana, HS. ROS. 444, 7b–8a.    [4] See p. 62 above.

In the popular imagination humans were constantly surrounded by demons and the like, though not all of these creatures drew satisfaction from making mischief. Ghosts and demons were thought to inhabit specific places, or to be in the habit of behaving in particular ways, and, left in peace, they would not interfere in human affairs. Their natural habitats were woodlands, marshlands, and open fields. Anyone facing the prospect of spending the night in a field ought to wear a bulb of garlic around their neck for safety.[5] More specifically, the seat of all *shedim* was the ground. All evil beings were born or lived under the ground, and hoarded their treasures there jealously. Caves and potholes of all types were considered dangerous places—gateways to the underworld, as it were. Thus anyone who had a dream about digging in the earth was destined to die imminently.[6] In the folk consciousness, any interference in a sphere perceived to be the domain of unclean forces was bound to render the meddler vulnerable to a more or less violent reaction on the part of those forces.

The practical ramifications of this belief were visible in superstitions surrounding matters such as building and moving into a house. If someone was building a house on a plot that had never previously been built on, they should not move in immediately, but instead wait a year. If the house was already built, the moving-in process should incorporate a series of preventative measures. Recommendations of this type, to be found in the Jewish ethical literature, indicate that their intention was not so much to destroy the demonic beings as to propitiate them. Lilientalowa considered the act of burying a coin or organizing a feast at this point in the process to be a vestige of the ancient practice of making sacrifices to the earth and its demonic inhabitants.[7] Other sources, too, advised preparing a hearty meal for devout scholars or paupers, or sacrificing a cockerel and a hen for the latter group. The 'consecration' of the house (*khanukes-bayis*) was accompanied by Torah discourses, the singing of the psalm for the dedication of the Temple (Ps. 30), and the 'Sheheḥeyanu' thanksgiving blessing.[8] Pious

---

[5] Grunwald, 'Aus unseren Sammlungen. Teil I', 98; Lilientalowa, 'Przesądy żydowskie', 643; Segel, 'Materyały do etnografii Żydów', 323.

[6] This may be the reason for the certain popularity among Jews of curses such as 'May the ground swallow you up!'; Lilientalowa, *Ziemia w wierzeniach żydowskich*, fo. 5r.

[7] *Ziemia w wierzeniach żydowskich*, fo. 4r. The same reasoning may have been behind the warning not to step on the threshold when entering the new house; see *Śmiecie*, fo. 31, no. 205.

[8] Rosenberg, *Rafa'el hamalakh*, 15–16. The consecration involved holding a cockerel and hen while reciting phrases from the book of Ezekiel (the opening words of Ezek. 45: 18 and the closing words of Ezek. 45: 20): 'You shall cleanse the Sanctuary . . . to purge the Temple', taking

authors added the caveat that a place where the entire Torah had not been read should not be inhabited at all.[9] Since circumstances did not always permit waiting a year from the construction of the house until moving in, the new residents were advised to ask a *sofer* to write suitable amulets on kosher parchment and place them above the front door and the windows. Another option was to take a bundle of new thread and press it into the cracks around the windows and doors, repeating on each occasion: 'I am hereby putting in place an iron barrier for protection from evil spirits and all evil diseases, as it is written: "When you build a new house, you shall make a parapet for your roof, so that you do not bring bloodguilt on your house if anyone should fall from it" [Deut. 22: 8].'[10] These actions were performed in addition to fulfilling the requirement to mount a mezuzah on the door frame.

It was not only new buildings, however, but also old ones, and in particular those that had stood empty for long periods of time, that were believed to be inhabited by demons. Entering a ruined house at night was considered as dangerous as disturbing the peace of the dead. There was also a whole host of rules to be observed when moving into old houses. Windows and chimney flues should never be walled up entirely (a small crack should always be left), or new ones knocked through in solid walls. Aside from the practical issues, the reason for this was the danger of disturbing the peace of the resident demons, who would be prepared to defend their domain in a manner that presented a risk to human life and health. On moving in, the first thing to do was to bring a gift of bread and salt (and according to other sources also a candle and some sugar).[11] One former resident of the town of Pińczów remembered that a local hasid (a carpenter by trade) had taken this course of action on his rebbe's advice before moving into a house that had previously been inhabited by consumptives.[12] And one folk tale told of a healer who took a salted challah every Friday to the *lets* (jester, clown) that inhabited his attic. If he failed to do so, the demon

the fowl to the *shoḥet* and monitoring the slaughter, and giving the meat to the poor; see Rechtman, 'Some Customs and Their Folk Explanations' (Yid.), 261.

[9] Segel, 'Wierzenia i lecznictwo', 50.      [10] Rosenberg, *Rafa'el hamalakh*, 16–17.
[11] Buchbinder, 'Jewish Omens' (Yid.), 258; Segel, 'Wierzenia i lecznictwo', 60; Bastomski, *At the Source: Jewish Proverbs* (Yid.), 104; Ben-Ezra, 'Customs' (Yid.), 175. Cf. 'Tsava'at rabi yehudah heḥasid', 8–9. Hasidic tradition cites the tsadik Meir of Przemyślany, who recommends that among the first items to be taken into a new house should be a candle, honey, bread, and coffee; Meisels, *Vihyitem li segulah*, 88, 90.
[12] Himmelblau, 'Medical Aid in Pińczów' (Yid.), 216–17.

would wreak havoc in his home, and even blackmail the man and kidnap his children.[13]

Currying favour with such capricious creatures as demons took considerable effort. Moving house, for example, involved taking a series of preventative measures: on moving out it was prudent to leave at least one item behind, such as nails in the wall or the mezuzah, otherwise it would not be possible to go back for three (or in some versions seven) years. And if it did prove necessary to move back into the original house, before going back one should first leave a cockerel and a hen in it for a day and a night, then live in it for a week with them, and finally slaughter them and give the meat to four paupers.[14] Cobwebs should always be swept out of a house in which one was planning to live, because they were a seat of husks of sin. Moreover, as the saying went, cobwebs appeared in places where there were cares and worries.[15] The utmost caution was also recommended in the immediate vicinity of one's house. Men who went out to empty chamber pots at night should clutch the knots of their *tsitsit* tightly, and first warn the demons by repeating the words: *Hit zikh!* (Watch out!) three times.[16] If they did not, they could expect to go blind[17] or be possessed by a dybbuk.[18] This latter warning is indication that people harboured fears not only of demons but also of errant souls. According to traditional belief, at night the souls of the dead would return to their old home and linger outside the windows, sometimes weeping and wailing. Sinners were said to be unable to find peace after death, and to scavenge on rubbish heaps under cover of night, looking for their discarded (rather than burned, as was the custom) fingernails.[19]

Left alone and undisturbed, demons lived peaceably among humans as

---

[13] Brod, 'Judendeutsche Sagen und Schnurren', 344.

[14] T. H. Koydanover, *Kav hayashar*, 73; Sperling, *Ta'amei haminhagim oyf ivri taytsh*, ii. 11; Rosenberg, *Rafa'el hamalakh*, 15–17; Buchbinder, 'Jewish Omens' (Yid.), 258; Lilientalowa, 'Przesądy żydowskie', 642–3.

[15] Sperling, *Ta'amei haminhagim oyf ivri taytsh*, ii. 43; Segel, 'Wierzenia i lecznictwo', 50; 'Omens and Remedies' (Yid.), 294.     [16] Bastomski, *At the Source: Jewish Proverbs* (Yid.), 102.

[17] Segel, 'Materyały do etnografii Żydów', 322.

[18] Grunwald, 'Aus unseren Sammlungen. Teil I', 70. Women were popularly believed to be at risk of infertility for such imprudent behaviour; Goldberg and Eisenberg, *Sefer laḥashim usegulot*, 10a.

[19] 'Aus unseren Sammlungen. II', 9; Khayes, 'Death-Related Beliefs and Customs' (Yid.), 308. In the Bukovina region it was considered especially dangerous to be out alone at night on Wednesdays and Sundays. The presence of the souls of the dead was thought to be signalled at such times by wailing, and there was no shortage of those who claimed to have heard it; see Kaindl, 'Die Juden in der Bukowina', 159.

just another element of the local landscape. Jewish folklore is full of tales of benevolent guardian spirits akin to the Slavic *domovoi* (the ancestral protective spirit or deity of a house).[20] One typical example was the *lantukh*, a creature with a long tongue and chicken feet, known for its mischievous tricks. It would sit in the synagogue and do penance for its sins on Yom Kippur, but it was also fond of copulating with women.

Places considered holy and which were reserved for the enactment of rites and rituals, such as the synagogue, the *beit midrash*, or the *mikveh*, were by no means out of bounds to incorporeal beings. The *lantukh* itself would sit about in synagogues and flick its tongue at those who came in for morning prayers. In this context, one very interesting story is that of a Jew who suffered from a chronic infection on his foot. One day he was told in a dream by a holy man (probably the prophet Elijah) that the affliction had entered his body when, alone in the *mikveh*, he had been bitten on the foot by a devil (*makhshit*). In Opatów there were said to be demons on the steps of the *beit midrash* that tore the caps from the heads of the hasidim who frequented it. It took the tsadik Abraham Joshua Heshel to put a stop to the mischief by having a cast-iron bar made that bore his name, and which he put up in the attic of the building.[21]

One of the best-known spirits considered at least partly domesticated was the *shretele* (also known as *lapitut*), a sprite which lived in the chimney, under the bed, or under a cover. If left in peace, for a prearranged fee it would help out, deliver work that had been commissioned and completed, and even mind the children.[22] Having a demon of this type was associated with financial prosperity and general well-being. Thus if a woman pouring melted fat into a pot did not say aloud that the vessel was almost full, with the help of the house sprite she would be able to continue pouring fat into it *ad infinitum*.[23] If the sprite had drunk vodka from a bottle it was believed that humans would be able to drink from it without the level in the bottle going down.[24] The blue flame that sometimes appeared on the stove shelf would shower with riches anyone who threw a slipper at it—on condition

[20] See Moszyński, *Kultura ludowa Słowian*, 604–712.
[21] *Atarat tsadikim*, 26; Pintshevski, 'Opatów and the Rise of Hasidism' (Yid.), 58.
[22] Akalovich, 'Zamietki o yevrieiskoy narodnoy demonologii', 151–3. See 'Tales and Traditions' (Yid.), 167–73; Agnon, *The Bridal Canopy*, 48.
[23] Loewe, 'Jüdische Volkserzählungen aus Polen', 62.
[24] Silverman-Weinreich (ed.), *Yiddish Folktales*, 343.

that they told no one about it.[25] According to another story there were demons who, at the request of the rebbe, would protect the Jewish community from the local squire's insatiable greed.[26] Even crickets had supernatural attributes; a cricket in the house meant good fortune and money, and if it also sang loudly, the householders could expect good health to boot. But all this would evaporate if the cricket was called up to form part of a *minyan* (*Griln, kumt tsum minyen in bes-medresh arayn!*; Crickets, come to the synagogue [to pray] in the *minyan*). Good luck was also bound to evaporate if one allowed a child to climb out through the window to relieve itself in the yard (because going out via the window was considered highly improper).[27]

According to legend, almost every type of demon could be persuaded to help humans, and whether or not one was successful in this mission depended chiefly on one's cunning. In one story, an unclean creature living in a well helped a Jew amass a great fortune, in exchange for which the man agreed to remove from the same well the body of his malicious wife, whom he had drowned.[28] According to another tale, the malevolent *kapeliushniki* (known in other variants as *shretelekh*), which had a bad name for milking cows at night and worrying grey horses, would become the slaves of anyone who managed to steal (or burn) their caps.[29] There were certain circumstances which were believed to make exploitation of these demons much easier. They were subject to similar laws of nature as humans, and were also bound by the laws of the Torah. They could be ordered before a tsadik or religious court in cases where a sinful person had died childless and his home was being haunted by his demonic 'children', and the demons would sometimes invoke biblical inheritance precedents. Negotiations with them were conducted in a manner typical of Jewish commercial custom. The talmudic legacy (*Ḥul.* 105*b*) includes the story of a pack of demons brought to trial for destroying a barrel of wine. The hasidic literature is full of tales of the dead, errant souls, and dybbuks being brought before religious courts, interrogated, and judged fairly. Similar motifs abound in contemporary

---

[25] Lilientalowa noted that covering the flame with an apron would mean that one would have to dig deep for the treasure. Throwing a shoe at it ensured that the precious find would be on the surface; *Śmiecie*, fo. 30, no. 199. On returning home, one should never call out to one's child by name, because it may just have found a treasure, and both the child and the treasure would then disappear; Buchbinder, 'Jewish Omens' (Yid.), 251.

[26] 'Aus unseren Sammlungen. II', 23–5.          [27] 'Omens and Remedies' (Yid.), 278.

[28] Silverman-Weinreich (ed.), *Yiddish Folktales*, 83–4.

[29] Ibid. 344; Buchbinder, 'Jewish Omens' (Yid.), 250–1.

Jewish fiction. One novel by Alter Kacyzne contains a scene in which a trader is haggling with a demon, both of them using talmudic terminology, and the trader's clinching argument is the principle *ta'ut goy mutar* ('It is permitted to financially benefit from the business error of a non-Jew', *BK* 113b).[30] When a deal with a demon proved disadvantageous, however, the formal aspects of the pact and its documents, recorded in heaven, would be questioned; the date of the verdict and the name of the living person would be contested, and even attempts made to destroy the relevant documents and so to thwart Satan or the angel of death.[31]

Nonetheless, the dominant trope in folk tales is of demons harming or causing damage to humans, and even bringing death on them. Unclean forces often operated in disguise, luring their victims to apparently safe places, such as taverns on lonely roads or devout homes in distant villages. They would often take the form of animals, both wild and domesticated. One well-known story tells of a trader or carter who, on his way through a wood (or marsh) found a sheep (or calf, or goose). He put it in his cart, though it seemed strangely heavy, and returned home, pleased with his unexpected find. All of a sudden, however, the animal jumped up, burst out laughing, and took to its heels. According to the tale, this proved that the incident was a prank played on the man by unclean forces.[32] Demons were less likely to take on the form of respected Jews, though such cases are to be found in the ethical literature.[33] They were far more likely to be disguised as strangers, in particular beguiling women and mysterious 'Germans' (*daytshl*)—Europeanized apostate Jews.[34] Tricked or forced into entering a

[30] Kacyzne, *Shtarke un shvakhe*, 262.

[31] Schwarzbaum, 'Charity Thwarts Fate', in id, *Studies*, 278–80). In one of his humor-esques, An-sky recounted a discussion which the popular wit Motke Habad of Vilna conducted with the angel of death. When the 'knife was at his throat', the wily Jew saved himself by claim-ing the false identity of Alter, son of Hayim Katz. The heavenly missive was not to be deceived, however, and even permitted himself the sarcastic remark: 'Aha! My favourite Jewish tricks, here we go again! Assumed names! Counterfeit papers!', to which Motke, not missing a beat, retorted: 'Come here and prove that they're counterfeit!' An-sky, 'A Letter from the Other World' (Yid.), 101–2.

[32] See e.g. Loewe, 'Jüdische Volkserzählungen aus Polen', 61–2; M. Weinreich, 'Lantukh: The History of a Jewish Demon' (Yid.), 219–20; Yunis, 'The Old Homeland' (Yid.), 77–8.

[33] See e.g. the story of the *mohel* lured by a demon disguised as a devout rural Jew (T. H. Koydanover, *Kav hayashar*, 76–9), or the tale of the woman who wanted to get up for the *selihot* morning prayers but worried that the synagogue assistant would forget to knock for her (Loewe, 'Jüdische Volkserzählungen aus Polen', 62–3).

[34] Akalovich, 'Zamietki o yevrieiskoy narodnoy demonologii', 153. See Unger, *The Hasidic World* (Yid.), 159.

seemingly safe building, Jews should take care not to eat or drink anything offered by the host, and not to accept any gifts. If they passed the test, everything around them would fall away and return to its real form.[35]

Among the demons that tried to take advantage of humans were wraiths and ghosts, often referred to by their Slavic names.[36] These were said to be able to take various forms, even those of a deceased husband or wife, in order to visit a particular man or woman and be intimate with them. In this respect they were similar to the she-demon Lilith, and, as in the case of nocturnal emissions, after a visit from them a ritual bath in the *mikveh* was mandatory.[37] The belief in such creatures feeding on human vitality (represented by sexual potency) complemented the strict morality of the traditional community, serving as a warning to sinners and an explanation of mysterious, unknown phenomena for the pious. Carnal relations with such spirits produced sickly offspring that tended to die shortly after birth.[38] According to Lilientalowa's sources, it was most often unmarried men who fell victim to wraiths, who would suffocate them and suck their blood through their nipples. The prophylactic steps that could be taken to gain protection from these demons included 'squeezing milk' out of a baby's breast while bathing it, and placing one's shoes by the bed 'facing backwards'.[39] One folk tale told of a Jewish tailor who was sewing clothes for some peasants on Christmas Eve, when he suddenly felt an overwhelming fatigue. He knew that it was a wraith trying to send him to sleep to suck milk from his breast, so he resisted, which sent the wraith into a rage, and she tangled and knotted his thread. When the tailor cut through one of the

[35] See e.g. Silverman-Weinreich (ed.), *Yiddish Folktales*, 356.

[36] Opatoshu, *From My Lexicon* (Yid.), 91. The apparition would often take the form of a person called Mara Marovitch or Moritz Marovitch. In the collection compiled by Goldberg and Eisenberg (*Sefer laḥashim usegulot*, 4b–5a), the editors included two conjurations that had been used on a wraith accused of letting loose on a human evil beings by these names.

[37] Lilientalowa, 'Wierzenia, przesądy i praktyki', 154.

[38] Dik, *Old Jewish Sayings* (Yid.), 35–6. In another version, known from the book of Zohar, they produced children who suffered from epilepsy; see e.g. Berger, *Imrei yisra'el*, 5a; T. H. Koydanover, *Kav hayashar*, 51. A woman could also harm her child and give birth to a blind baby if she thought about a man other than her husband, as happened to the woman in this song: *Di mame hot gehat a makhshove zore, / Iz deroys gevorn a blinde tsore* ('Mama had an inappropriate thought / and a blind unfortunate was what became of it'); Taglicht, 'Lieder aus Slovakei', 61.

[39] Lilientalowa, 'Dziecko żydowskie', 145; ead., 'Wierzenia, przesądy i praktyki', 150. Cf. Moszyński, *Kultura ludowa Słowian*, 188–9. Shoes were also turned to point away from the bed in times of plague.

knots, the next morning a dead witch was found outside his house, and the attacks of the wraith ceased.[40]

Witches and warlocks also used deception. The Hebrew term *mekhashe-fah* is a biblical concept, first mentioned in the book of Exodus, in words that are often used in amulets: 'You shall not tolerate a sorceress' (Exod. 22: 17). It was usually women who were suspected of practising black magic, and as explanation for this fact, tradition cites the story that grew up around the biblical phrase: 'The divine beings saw how beautiful the daughters of men were and took wives from among those that pleased them' (Gen. 6: 2). According to one *midrash* much cited in the ethical literature, the angels Samyaza (Aza) and Aza'el not only took human lovers, but also taught them manipulations using the ineffable name of God.[41] The Creator's choice of the exclusively feminine word *mekhashefah* was seen as evidence of women's innate tendency towards uncleanness, one indication of which was menstruation. During a woman's period, tradition had it, 1,450 types of demons gathered on her fingernails. According to the *Kav hayashar*, sorceresses not only demonstrated characteristics typical of menstruating women, but also preferred to stall their actions until their own monthly period.[42] Folk culture also knew of male sorcerers. According to the ethical literature, however, they deserved to be put to death for a different reason: because they drew their powers from sexual relations with animals.[43]

The image of witches gathering by night on bare mountains to commune with devils and at their urging making mischief among their communities was not alien to Jewish culture.[44] One resident of Felsztyn recalls: 'We believed in magic, in witches, lame old *goy* women who could steal the milk from a cow, and even from a nursing mother'.[45] Among the reasons cited for hiding nail and hair clippings and not throwing away worn-out clothes was the fear that they might be misused by those who practised black magic. In order to blind someone, for instance, a witch needed a hair of her victim, which she would thread through the eye of

---

[40] Silverman-Weinreich (ed.), *Yiddish Folktales*, 360.

[41] J. Ashkenazi, *Tsene urene*, 25; Lew, 'O lecznictwie i przesądach', *Izraelita*, 36, p. 306. See Graves and Patai, *Hebrew Myths*, 104–6. This motif first appeared in the apocryphal book of Enoch.

[42] Even stepping on a menstruating woman's nail clippings, with or without shoes on, was enough to unleash harm; T. H. Koydanover, *Kav hayashar*, 49–50.

[43] Zaler, *Yalkut yitshak*, 62.           [44] Piątkowska, 'Ludoznawstwo żydowskie', 809.

[45] Kling, 'The Unwritten Book of My Mama's Remedies' (Yid.), 561.

a frog and then set the creature free. However, it was not hard to render a witch harmless; all that was required was to draw a single drop of her blood, with a needle for instance.[46]

Among the most dangerous sorcerers and sorceresses in the Jewish folk imagination were Catholic and Orthodox priests, and squires and their wives. One of their signature attributes was the skill of shape-shifting, in particular metamorphosing into animals. In this form they were said to creep into Jewish streets and homes to harm the lonely, the weak, and children. For this reason it was ill advised to let a cat into the house after dark,[47] and there was a whole list of other preventative actions to be taken at the mere sight of a Christian clergyman (making the fig sign, throwing a pin at them, reciting an incantation, etc.).[48] In a story recorded by Leo Wiener, the son of an impoverished Jewish entrepreneur even finds his way into the service of the pope, who proves uniquely skilled in taking various animal forms (horse, elephant, or lion) at will.[49] Jewish children were also warned about itinerant beggars, who were said to beat their victims with sticks, catch them and bundle them into huge bags, and even throw them down wells. These were mysterious figures who punished children for disobedience to their parents. According to reminiscences gathered from the Mazovia region, such beggars were said to inhabit dark hollows in copses by country lanes.[50]

Evidence of nefarious magic practices was to be found essentially at every step. One early nineteenth-century manuscript includes three Yiddish conjurations said to bring relief to people suffering from intense

[46] Lipiets, *Sefer matamim*, 105; Lilientalowa, 'Wierzenia, przesądy i praktyki', 151. Rashi saw the root of the custom of hiding hair trimmings in a passage in the book of Ezekiel; see his commentary on Ezek. 5: 3. Contemporary ethnography links this practice with indigenous European beliefs surrounding witches, female demons (Pol. strzyga), and phantoms; see Kolczyński, 'Jeszcze raz o upiorze (wampirze) i strzygoni (strzydze)', 211–46.

[47] Benczer, 'Jüdische Volksmedizin', 120–1; Silverman-Weinreich (ed.), *Yiddish Folktales*, 73; Cahan, 'Jewish Folk Tales' (Yid.), 229–30; 'Omens and Remedies' (Yid.), 291. See Mizish, 'Gentiles as Sorcerers' (Yid.), 147–71; Nigal, *The Hasidic Tale*, 125. According to legend, the tsadik Leib ben Sarah fought a kind of duel with Emperor Joseph II, who was said to be a great sorcerer; Even, *From the World of Hasidic Leaders* (Yid.), 77.

[48] Fayvushinski, 'The Folklore of Pruzhana' (Yid.), 200; Lilientalowa, 'Przesądy żydowskie', 279, 640. Cf. Moszyński, *Kultura ludowa Słowian*, 290. Evil was always about the person of the Catholic and the Orthodox priest. Particular caution was always exercised in the vicinity of churches of any denomination, which were colloquially referred to as 'unclean' (*beys-tome*, *tifle*).

[49] Wiener, 'Märchen und Schwänke', 104.

[50] Trunk, *Poland: Memories and Images* (Yid.), 30. Similar warnings were sometimes couched as lullabies; see Wiener, 'Aus der Russisch-Jüdischen Kinderstube', 49.

migraines, which were known as *heyptgeshpar* or *heybtshayn*. The language used in these formulas suggests a connection with the region of western Ashkenaz; in terms of their syntax and phraseology they are similar to texts printed in the German-speaking lands. Nonetheless, their presence in a source from eastern Europe is unequivocal proof that they were not alien to the therapeutic beliefs in this area of the diaspora. The ailment to which they referred may probably be identified as the German *Heuptschein*— the sense that one's head was splitting. It was usually treated using magic because in the popular conviction it was the result of a spell cast by a sorceress.[51] In the conjurations, this *heyptgeshpar* features in the form of an autonomous being, reminiscent of or a substitute for the she-demon Lilith —who was herself known as a sorceress—in dialogue with the prophet Elijah. As the incantation was being pronounced, the sufferer's head was to be girdled with a belt belonging to them, and the assurance uttered that in this way they were 'girding themselves' against indisposition. The incantation ran as follows:

The prophet Elijah was walking through a field when he came upon a *heyptgeshpar*. He asked: 'Where do you want to go?' It answered: 'I want to go to the house of X son of Y, to eat his flesh and drink his blood.' Elijah said: 'You shall not go, but you shall go to the abattoir, [where] a goat is standing by the block; eat its blood and flesh, so be it, in the name of God, *amen selah*.[52]

The conjurations for headaches in the pamphlet compiled by Israel Yudl Goldberg and Abraham Aba Eisenberg also included a version of the dialogue between Elijah and Lilith. This example is written in Yiddish typical of the east European diaspora, and although the name *heyptgeshpar* is not mentioned, it too requires the sufferer's head to be bound with a belt.[53]

It was extremely common for malicious magic to be associated with the practice of 'planting' illnesses.[54] Many sources warned that walking through dirty water or spilt froth would cause leprosy, pustules, or 'firefeather',[55] and thus if a man's wife was in the habit of pouring off the froth

[51] See 'Geschoss' in Hoffmann-Krayer and Stäubli (eds.), *Handwörterbuch des deutschen Aberglaubens*, 756.　　　[52] *Segulot urefuot*, Bibliotheca Rosenthaliana, HS. ROS. 444, 9*b*.

[53] Goldberg and Eisenberg, *Sefer laḥashim usegulot*, 7*b*.

[54] Lilientalowa's informants warned of the dangers of 'planted' objects, explaining that picking random items up off the street carried with it the danger of falling under a spell; 'Wierzenia, przesądy i praktyki', 151.

[55] Segel, 'Wierzenia i lecznictwo', 50; Lilientalowa, 'Wierzenia, przesądy i praktyki', 159. Dirty dishwater was said to harbour evil (ibid. 148). Infantile eczema, also known as

from the first cooking, he was advised to divorce her.[56] Sometimes rituals
would be enacted to establish whether there was a link between a given
complaint and magic. The vademecum *Rafa'el hamalakh*, which drew on
the kabbalistic pamphlet *Mifalot elokim*, recommended two methods in this
regard: to pour some oil into a glass, wrap the sides of the glass in black
paper, and have the sufferer try to discern their reflection in the oil (an
inverted reflection was an indication of an enchantment); or to sit them
down on an anthill and wait to see if the ants bit them (this suggested an
ordinary ailment) or ignored them (a spell).[57] The same source recommended as therapy against charms and demonic influence an extensive
range of apotropaics widely used for protection against spells. These included a little bag holding rue, hyssop, and deadly nightshade; walnut shells
filled with mercury, gastroliths taken from cockerels, and salt; parchment
amulets and *mezuzelekh* bearing the inscription *Shadai kera satan*; and
smudging the patient with smoke from a burnt fish heart, a cock's comb,
the brain of a white cockerel (or hen for a woman), or feathers from the
sufferer's bed.[58]

Demons and ghosts were believed to be beings of the dark, whose activity intensified after nightfall. There were a host of activities which by day
might seem innocuous, but performed after dark were considered very dangerous. When out walking in the street at night one should never whistle,[59]
in order not to attract anything evil; neither should one react to one's name
being called, in order not to be lured into danger.[60] Yet staying at home
alone, especially without the protection of a mezuzah, would also provoke
the demons to mischief, as would cursing one's children, making mention
of the dead without due cause (for instance when telling stories), and even

'firefeather' (Pol. *ognipiór*), fire, or cradle cap, was considered hard to cure. Among its presumed causes were scratching of scabs on the crown of the head (ibid. 173), sexual intercourse
during menstruation (Lilientalowa, *Dziecko żydowskie*, 21), and also the machinations of
unclean forces (Goldberg and Eisenberg, *Sefer laḥashim usegulot*, 5b–6a). Treatment of eczema
(like *plica*) was thought to cause blindness, and it was considered better for the child to let it
'stand'.

[56] Segel, 'Wierzenia i lecznictwo', 51.
[57] Halpern, *Mifalot elokim*, 27b; Rosenberg, *Rafa'el hamalakh*, 41.
[58] When performing a smudging ritual using the head of a cockerel, one should recite Ps.
119: 161 nine times; Rosenberg, *Rafa'el hamalakh*, 48; Plaut, *Likutei ḥever ben ḥayim*, 8a–b;
Berger, *Imrei yisra'el*, 10a–b.            [59] Elzet [Złotnik], 'Some Jewish Customs' (Heb.), 369.
[60] Fels, 'Zabobony lekarskie u Żydów', 4; Fayvushinski, 'The Folklore of Pruzhana' (Yid.),
199.

uttering the word 'cemetery'.[61] In the folk imagination, one of the few visible signs of the existence of unclean forces was the shade that formed in places where no light fell. Not only did this provide cover to evil spirits, which gave rise to the conviction that one should never sleep in the shade of trees or chimneys,[62] but further, inasmuch as the shadow cast resembled a human silhouette, this similarity would open up the possibility of anthropomorphization. Thus the shadow would be seen as a human but more powerful, and capable of luring its unfortunate victim into iniquity. People who stared at shadows would be warned that this could result in being haunted and even suffocated by those shadows in the night. It was also forbidden to poke fun at a shadow, make it perform lewd gestures, or throw stones at it; any such irresponsible behaviour might provoke revenge.[63] Similar beliefs surrounded one's reflection in the mirror. Looking in the mirror after dark was not something anyone should consider, and babies who had not yet cut their teeth should not be allowed to look into a mirror at all.[64]

The antidote for the dangers lurking in darkness or gloom was, naturally, light, which was associated with cleanliness. As a rule, it was not recommended to leave the house at night at all, but if the need did arise, for safety's sake it was wise to carry a candle, since this was 'as though there were two people walking together'.[65] 'A torch is sufficient for two [people], and the light of the moon for three' according to the Talmud, which added that evil spirits were only capable of harming people walking alone; to two people walking together they would do no more than show themselves, while to three they remained invisible.[66] Among the most risky times to journey by night was the end of the Jewish month, when the moon offered

[61] According to tradition, one could protect oneself from the negative consequences of saying this and other, similar words by adding the phrase *nit akegn nakht gedakht* ('not intended in connection with the night'); Buchbinder, 'Jewish Omens' (Yid.), 249; Bastomski, *At the Source: Jewish Proverbs* (Yid.), 102.

[62] Sperling, *Ta'amei haminhagim oyf ivri taytsh*, ii. 33; Segel, 'Materyały do etnografii Żydów', 319. *Sefer ḥasidim* stressed the importance of not sleeping under walnut trees, whose branches were inhabited by *mazikin* (harmful spirits); Judah Hehasid, *Sefer ḥasidim*, 476.

[63] Lilientalowa, 'Wierzenia, przesądy i praktyki', 150; Bastomski, *At the Source: Jewish Proverbs* (Yid.), 114.

[64] Lew, 'O lecznictwie i przesądach', *Izraelita*, 40, p. 381 (a child might get a 'twisted face' from looking in the mirror); Lilientalowa, 'Przesądy żydowskie', 280; Bastomski, *At the Source: Jewish Proverbs* (Yid.), 114; Sosnowik, 'Material on Jewish Folk Medicine in Belarus' (Yid.), 167; Rechtman, 'Some Customs and Their Folk Explanations' (Yid.), 261; Fayvushinski, 'The Folklore of Pruzhana' (Yid.), 204.

[65] Sperling, *Ta'amei haminhagim oyf ivri taytsh*, i. 108.                    [66] BT *Ber.* 43*b*.

no light.[67] Dawn put an end to the activities of unclean spirits, and the crowing of the cockerel, which heralded the new day, was believed to send the souls of the dead back to their graves, and evil fleeing to its lairs.[68]

Aside from the sun's rays, the other main source of light was fire, which differed from the other elements in its ability to consume both living beings and inanimate objects. In the Jewish tradition fire functioned as one of the manifestations of the Creator (the burning bush, the altar consuming burnt offerings). 'God is of fire', Lilientalowa noted in her ethnographic material,[69] and certain of his servants—angels, and in particular seraphim—were also endowed with similar properties. Fire served as an instrument of God's punishment; in popular conceptions of the other world, the fires of hell only went out for the duration of the sabbath. Nonetheless, as the Bible says, the Creator used flames not only to mete out punishment, but also to communicate with his people and lead them through the wilderness. This association of the fiery element with the figure of the Creator may have been the reason why the traditional Jewish community was mindful of the rule only to fan flames with an apron, and to extinguish a candle not by blowing it out but by putting it out with the fingers, as it was considered too holy to be extinguished with the help of sinful lips. This practice was also justified by the fear of accidentally articulating aloud, while blowing, the name of the evil angel Af, who ruled over death and was forged out of fire.[70] Fire was believed to hear everything and understand human speech. Indeed, it was able to speak, though only infants were able to understand it; they could also see various types of angels and ghosts.[71] In view of its link with the other world, fire also had a prophetic aspect. In certain circumstances it would reveal to the living matters which, in the natural course of events, were beyond their perception. Jews (in the Mława region, for instance) believed that when the fire in the hearth began to 'talk' it was a

[67] Friedlender, 'Jewish Life in the Shtetl' (Yid.), 125–6.
[68] Grunwald, 'Aus unseren Sammlungen. Teil I', 70.
[69] 'Wierzenia, przesądy i praktyki', 168.
[70] See Ginzberg, *Legends of the Jews*, i. 504–5; Lilientalowa, *Śmiecie*, fo. 25, no. 166. Blowing out a fire could cause leprosy, particularly in pregnant women; Segel, 'Materyały do etnografii Żydów', 321; An-sky, *The Yiddish Ethnographic Programme* (Yid.), 22; Lilientalowa, 'Wierzenia, przesądy i praktyki', 168; Rechtman, 'Some Customs and Their Folk Explanations' (Yid.), 261. At the same time, however, blowing up into the chimney flue was considered a tried and tested remedy for a sore throat; Lew, 'O lecznictwie i przesądach', *Izraelita*, 49, p. 476.
[71] Lilientalowa, *Kult ognia u starożytnych Hebrajczyków*, fo. 6v.

sign that one was being talked about in heaven. In such circumstances one should say: *Redn zol men guts* (Would that they were speaking well).[72]

When the challah was being baked for the sabbath or festivals, the law was to separate a small piece of the dough and burn it in the oven—a relic of the Torah obligation to give away a piece of bread for the needs of the priests in the Temple of Jerusalem (Num. 15: 20). Folk culture added secondary meanings to this imperative, which was one of the three *mitsvot* to be fulfilled by a woman. If a housewife threw this portion to the pigs or to a dog rather than burning it, someone in her family was bound to renounce the Jewish faith.[73] But if she gave it to a child who wet the bed at night as a result of playing with fire, she could expect the problem to go away.[74] One should never spit into a hot oven, or even onto a hotplate, as these carried the symbolic significance of a sacrificial pyre (and thus this was considered a sin that could cause sores on the tongue), or pour away the first froth on the soup as this could cause scabs or eczema. However, on occasion salt might be thrown into the oven as a way of neutralizing the harmful effects of libellous accusations by one's enemies.[75]

It is thus unsurprising that fire was probably the single most powerful apotropaic substance, considered capable not only of reversing but of physically annihilating evil. For this reason care would be taken not to remove a flame from the room of a woman in postnatal confinement, or from her house on the evening following the sabbath.[76] If alterations were being made to a house and the bread oven was taken out, care would usually be taken to leave some trace of it; obliterating all memory of its existence was thought to be a dangerous mistake. Fire was never lent, 'so that hell doesn't return it', and if somebody needed fire to start their own, the giver would say: 'I won't give it to you, and I don't want you to give it back to me. Take it yourself.' Neither did one thank the giver for fire. In this context, saying to someone: 'May your hearth grow cold' should be read as one of the most

---

[72] Yunis, 'The Old Homeland' (Yid.), 70.

[73] Fayvushinski, 'The Folklore of Pruzhana' (Yid.), 201.

[74] Lilientalowa, *Kult ognia u starożytnych Hebrajczyków*, fos. 8r–9v; ead., *Dziecko żydowskie*, 81.

[75] Lilientalowa, *Kult ognia u starożytnych Hebrajczyków*, fo. 8v; ead., 'Wierzenia, przesądy i praktyki', 152.

[76] Or indeed to remove it at all, which could cause eczema or sustained crying in the infant; Lew, 'O lecznictwie i przesądach', *Izraelita*, 38, p. 363; id., *Izraelita*, 40, p. 381; Lilientalowa, *Coitus, ciąża, poród*, fo. 3, no. 21; Elzet [Złotnik], 'Some Jewish Customs' (Heb.), 363; Zimmels, *Magicians, Theologians and Doctors*, 148.

malevolent curses in the Jewish repertoire.[77] The custom of burning candles at a dying person's bedside, like many similar practices forming part of other rituals, was intended as a means of protection from demons. What is more, the folk imagination carried over the properties of flames onto objects that either were associated with 'burning' (such as nettles) or had been in contact with fire, or had been made using fire. Water that had been used to quench red-hot metal (for example knife blades) was said to help with complaints including warts,[78] enlarged spleen (*ripkukhn*),[79] convulsions,[80] and insomnia.[81] In fact, folk medicine is full of testimonies to the apotropaic character of iron. In case of infantile convulsions, nine objects made from iron would be placed under the child's pillow or in its cradle.[82] During an attack of epilepsy, older children and adults would be given an item made of iron or steel—usually a knife—to hold.[83] A woman who had given birth to a son would keep a knife on her person not only until the day of his circumcision, but even until her first ritual bath after the birth. She would not leave the house without it, just as she would not go out without first having listened to a Torah reading.[84] A small pocket knife could prevent miscarriage if the woman had bought it without haggling on the night of her purification (following menstruation), taken it with her to the *mikveh*, and thereafter carried it with her constantly, even on the sabbath, until her newborn child was thirty days old.[85]

In curative practices, fire served to purify ingredients which could otherwise not be taken as medicine in view of either the *kashrut* laws (which, as shown above, were sometimes relaxed in connection with illness), or simply because they were unpalatable or off-putting. Jewish sources supply many examples of animal dung and body parts (such as hooves or placentas) being incinerated and subsequently added to wine or food. Other items,

[77] Lilientalowa, *Kult ognia u starożytnych Hebrajczyków*, fos. 5v, 6v.

[78] Rosenberg, *Der malekh refoel*, 45.

[79] In this case it would sometimes be drunk with caramel wine; see Berger, *Imrei yisra'el*, 13a; Rosenberg, *Rafa'el hamalakh*, 15, 38. Goldberg and Eisenberg (*Sefer laḥashim usegulot*, 16b) mention quenching hot steel in strong wine as a remedy for 'swelling coming from the belly'.

[80] Rosenberg, *Rafa'el hamalakh*, 69.      [81] *Refuot ha'am im darkhei yesharim*, 13.

[82] Rosenberg, *Rafa'el hamalakh*, 67; *Segulot urefuot*, JTS, MS 9862, 84; Lilientalowa, *Dziecko żydowskie*, 60; 'Aus unseren Sammlungen. II', 8.

[83] Fels, 'Zabobony lekarskie u Żydów', 4; Segel, 'Wierzenia i lecznictwo', 56.

[84] Lipiets, *Sefer matamim beḥadash*, 30; Lew, 'O lecznictwie i przesądach', *Izraelita*, 40, p. 382; Lilientalowa, *Coitus, ciąża, poród*, fo. 6, no. 24; Rosenberg, *Rafa'el hamalakh*, 42.

[85] *Sefer hatsadik r. yosef zundl misalant*, 68; Lilientalowa, *Dziecko żydowskie*, 25.

which derived their powers from the property of similarity, would also be used in the same way. One such example is a remedy recommended for incontinence: the soiled clothing of the sufferer burned to ashes and added to wine or food offered the hope of a rapid cure.[86] Fresh mare's dung caught before it fell to the ground could be used as a *segulah* for conception. It simply had to be rinsed and burned while held on a previously unused shovel. The material obtained in this way was to be ground up in a mortar and added to food or a beverage following a ritual bath for three successive nights during marital relations. The grounds for permission to consume such products were the rabbinic maxim: 'The ashes of all that has been burned are permissible.'[87]

Some illnesses that were perceived to be caused by unclean forces would be treated primarily with fire and actions with a symbolic link to that element. One such complaint was erysipelas, which was associated with flames in view of its colour and similarity to a burn. Primary treatment was *opbrenen a royz* (burning a rose), which involved covering the affected area with some kind of red material (this might be thick paper, flannel, a handkerchief, scarf, or other item of soft clothing, or a rye flour bag or one that had held an *etrog*, sprinkled with chalk, lead white, or lye), in order to 'draw out the weakness'.[88] If this did not help, offcuts of linen which had been laid on the wound would be set alight and sprinkled with amber, the flame turned three times towards the affected area.[89] In other cases a piece of paper inscribed with names or magic formulas known among Christians might be laid on the site;[90] sometimes the words of these formulas would be spoken together with Slavic and Yiddish exhortations to the 'dark rose' to 'flee into the field'.[91] Prayers might also be used that included biblical references to the burning properties of fire (Exod. 3: 5, Dan. 1–3), or which

[86] Plaut, *Likutei hever ben hayim*, 9b; Rosenberg, *Der malekh refoel*, 16.

[87] BT *Pes.* 26b; Kanarvogel, 'Hashmatah lebe'er mayim hayim', 1; Wellesz, 'Volksmedizinisches aus dem jüdischen Mittelalter', 119. See Jakobovits, *Jewish Medical Ethics*, 42.

[88] Rosenberg, *Rafa'el hamalakh*, 90; *Segulot urefuot*, JTS, MS 9862, 70; Lilientalowa, 'Wierzenia, przesądy i praktyki', 172; ead., *Dziecko żydowskie*, 68; Shabad, 'On Erysipelas' (Yid.), 53–4; cf. Haur, *Ekonomika lekarska*, 125.

[89] Segel, 'Wierzenia i lecznictwo', 55; Lilientalowa, *Dziecko żydowskie*, 68; Shlaferman, 'The Folklore, Customs, and Stories of Kazimierz' (Yid.), 173.

[90] These were usually formulas identical or very similar to non-Jewish conjurations imitating Latin, e.g. *Pila rosa afpa possa, Resi pete teti espesiesie*, etc.

[91] Kitri [Kronenberg], 'Feltsher', 140; *Segulot urefuot*, JTS, MS 9862, 10. This second source includes a Polish conjuration for erysipelas which begins: 'The Lord passed over the river Cedron.' Cf. Wereńko, 'Przyczynek do lecznictwa ludowego', 196.

symbolically annihilated the illness by gradually shortening the Hebrew words *hadaleket* (the inflammation), *hakadakhat* (the fever), *ha'adamut* (the redness), *hashet* (the tumour), *hashoshanah* (the erysipelas), or the Yiddish *hageshvilekhts* (the swelling).[92] After the end of this 'burning' or 'cauterizing' process, the wound would be dressed using any of a variety of ointments, honey, or other similar substances.[93] In some instances, the entire treatment process might be repeated several times over a period of three days.[94] Under no circumstances should the rash be wetted; if this happened, even stronger substances associated with fire had to be employed, in the first place liquor compresses (called *bronfn* or *yash*, from the Hebrew *yayin saraf*, fiery wine).[95] The exception to this was a dressing made from a cloth soaked in the (menstrual?) blood of a woman who had never given birth.[96]

Smudging was widely used in Jewish folk healing. Indeed, anthropologists believe that there is a close link between the application of compresses to the site of a complaint and its exposure to smoke.[97] Another significant aspect of the burning of herbs was its role in the struggle against unclean forces, whose presence was associated with unpleasant smells. In the popular imagination demons gave off a fetor (especially a sulphurous smell) and made their home in foul-smelling places. Jewish culture boasts a remarkable catalogue of warnings associated with their presence in such places. During a visit to the toilet it was ill advised to think about unclean creatures, because this would render one vulnerable to their whims.[98] On leaving the bathroom after relieving oneself one was obligated by halakhah to recite the 'Asher yatsar' blessing, thanking God for having equipped the human body with the vital openings. Anyone who failed to do so was doomed to danger according to folk belief. Sexual relations were forbidden for half an hour or an hour after leaving the toilet, because the demon that inhabited it would cling to one's person for that length of time.[99] And the

[92] *Segulot urefuot*, JTS, MS 9862, 8.

[93] Sperling, *Ta'amei haminhagim oyf ivri taytsh*, ii. 117; Rosenberg, *Rafa'el hamalakh*, 90. See Kitri [Kronenberg], 'Feltsher', 140.      [94] *Segulot urefuot*, JTS, MS 9862, 6.

[95] Rosenberg, *Rafa'el hamalakh*, 90; Cf. Haur, *Ekonomika lekarska*, 126. According to more recent sources, the tsadik Menahem Mendel of Kotsk was said to have recommended the use of oil left over from Hanukah for the treatment of erysipelas, citing the quotation from the song 'Maoz tsur': 'From the last little bottle [of oil] . . . a miracle for Israel [lit. a miracle for erysipelas]'. M. Kohen, *Leket hahanukah*, 424.

[96] *Segulot urefuot*, JTS, MS 9862, 10.      [97] Moszyński, *Kultura ludowa Słowian*, 210.

[98] Lilientalowa, *Złe duchy*, fo. 10. See BT *Ber.* 62a.

[99] BT *Git.* 70a. See Wilff, *Imrot shelomoh*, 54; Lilientalowa, *Dziecko żydowskie*, 20. According

first thing that one should do in the face of an epidemic was to purge one's house of all malodorous items, food remains, and faeces.[100] A variety of examples of smudging the sick and of prayers based on Bible quotations mentioning incense offerings (for instance Num. 17: 11–13) are discussed elsewhere in this book. In Moszyński's opinion the most efficacious were acrid smokes, and the Jewish sources abound in recipes with 'hell-related' references (deadly nightshade,[101] sulphur,[102] tar,[103] or juniper[104]). However, perhaps in view of the significance of spices in the religious tradition, in particular the burning of *bsomim* (spice mixture) to mark the closing of the sabbath, less pungent substances such as *levonah* (olibanum) were also used.

Bodies of water, streams, and springs were also thought to be the seat of demons, and similar motifs are to be found in the folklore of Ashkenazi Jews. According to many stories, the *lantukh*, a mischievous demon, inhabited damp places or riverbanks.[105] Pregnant women were forbidden to cross bridges, as this could cause miscarriage.[106] And Lilientalowa noted that when crossing a river it was considered wise to carry some form of protection, such as an iron knife, or at the very least a needle.[107] According to Jewish tradition, unclean forces were especially fond of gutters, and so one should not drink the rainwater that ran off them or take shelter beneath them from the rain, particularly during a storm.[108] In some places, includ-

to the *Kav hayashar*, every toilet space was inhabited by a demon. The unclean creature would alight on the fingers of anyone who went to relieve themselves, and it was thus recommended that a hand-washing vessel be placed in the immediate vicinity. It was strictly prohibited to start studying Torah without washing one's hands after using the toilet. See T. H. Koydanover, *Kav hayashar*, 36.

[100] Plaut, *Likutei hever ben hayim*, 7a; *Shemirot usegulot nifla'ot*, 31–2.

[101] Lilientalowa, 'Wierzenia, przesądy i praktyki', 171.

[102] Plaut, *Likutei hever ben hayim*, 9a.        [103] *Segulot urefuot*, JTS, MS 9862, 61.

[104] Both Jews and Christians burned juniper for its sharp, bitter smell; see Veynig, 'Medicaments and Remedies among the Jews' (Yid.), 28.

[105] Max Weinreich even suggested a link between this belief and Gallic-Roman mythology (Fr. *Lutin*, a water demon, from Lat. *Neptunus*), indicating a corrupted reading of the original old Romanic term transcribed in Hebrew characters (*tet* is similar to *mem*, *yod* is similar to *vav*, final *nun* similar to final *khaf*: *lutin—lamtukh*, *lantukh*); 'Lantukh: The History of a Jewish Demon' (Yid.), 231–4.

[106] An-sky, *The Yiddish Ethnographic Programme* (Yid.), 22; Fayvushinski, 'The Folklore of Pruzhana' (Yid.), 202; Friedlender, 'Jewish Life in the Shtetl' (Yid.), 126.

[107] Lilientalowa, 'Kult wody', 7.

[108] This warning was based on the suspicion that lightning was aimed at demons; Grunwald, 'Aus unseren Sammlungen. Teil I', 71; Buchbinder, 'Jewish Omens' (Yid.), 251; Bastomski, *At the Source: Jewish Proverbs* (Yid.), 104; Lilientalowa, 'Kult wody', 6. Demons lying in wait under gutters are mentioned as early as the Talmud (*Hul.* 105b).

ing Pruzhana, it was thought dangerous to go out to the well after dark.[109] If water was brought in in the dark, it might only be drunk after at least a few drops had been sprinkled on the ground. The same procedure was also advised before quenching one's thirst with a drink left uncovered at night, and if the vessel had been stowed under the bed, this advice should also be followed even if it had been covered.[110] According to Rashi's commentary, a demon was sure to have drunk from such 'bad water' first. The purpose of the sprinkling was thus to remove the evil, which might sometimes take the form of snake venom or worms.[111] Pouring off a little of the drink was also a way of protecting anyone who might want to drink after a sick person.[112] Protection from the potential dangers of drinking water drawn after dark was at hand in the form of words recommended by the Talmud—excerpts from Psalm 29 ('The voice of the Lord is over the waters; the God of glory thunders, the Lord, over the mighty waters'), warnings: 'X son of Y, I am thirsting for water', and the names Lul, Shafan, Anigron, and Anirada-fin, or the name of the demon Shabriri, gradually shortened (and thus destroyed).[113] Conversely, water considered especially useful for healing purposes was that drawn from the 'well of the prophetess Miriam', that is, drawn by a Jewess just after the end of the sabbath.[114]

In accordance with the precepts of Judaism, east European Jews used water for frequent ablutions. The customs surrounding the ritual purification of the body are of immense importance in the rabbinic interpretation of the Law. In their discussions of the meaning and ways of maintaining ritual cleanliness, the rabbis leave no doubt as to the vitality and currency of this aspect of their religion. In the most basic terms, purification by water falls into two categories: full immersion in an appropriately prepared body

---

[109] Bastomski, *At the Source: Jewish Proverbs* (Yid.), 102; Fayvushinski, 'The Folklore of Pruzhana' (Yid.), 200.

[110] BT *Pes.* 112*a*. However, it was believed that if one threw a piece of bread or bread roll into a watering can, the demons would not be able to get at it; Segel, 'Materyały do etnografii Żydów', 319.

[111] Sperling, *Ta'amei haminhagim oyf ivri taytsh*, ii. 11; Lipiets, *Sefer matamim*, 83; Grunwald, 'Aus unseren Sammlungen. Teil I', 981.

[112] Lipiets, *Sefer matamim*, 83; Schneersohn, *Sefer refuot*, 32, citing Shmelke of Nikolsburg.

[113] BT *Pes.* 112*a*.

[114] Sperling, *Ta'amei haminhagim oyf ivri taytsh*, i. 38; Lipiets, *Sefer matamim*, 124. Tradition had it that at this time water from the well of the prophetess Miriam flowed from all springs. According to the popular interpretation of Num. 21: 17–20, this water was said to have accompanied the Israelites in their wanderings through the desert. See Fayvushinski, 'The Folklore of Pruzhana' (Yid.), 204.

of water (*mikveh*, or ritual bath), and the washing of hands, which was crucial for removing uncleanliness before eating or performing rituals. The physical acts of immersion or washing were also to be accompanied by recital of the appropriate blessing. Spiritual and ritual imperatives also had a very clearly defined material aspect in the folk imagination: failure to observe any given ritual was associated with a host of potential bodily misfortunes, up to and including memory loss[115] and premature death,[116] which was particularly visible in the case of ablutions before crucial rituals. For instance, a scribe writing God's names without properly preparing by immersing himself in the *mikveh* committed an act of desecration. Purification by water was also mandatory for cooking and serving vessels, both new ones and those that had been used but had, for whatever reason, become unkosher. The same could be true of other objects of ritual importance, such as sabbath candlesticks if they had been lent out for a non-Jewish funeral.[117] The scale of the requirements involved increased with the intensification of contact with the Christian environment.

In the warm months of the year the Jewish residents of eastern Europe enjoyed bathing, more for recreation than for ritual purposes. It was a universal pastime, not regulated by social status, political views, or gender (though there were of course separate places for women). The quality of the water was of secondary significance, although many Jewish reminiscences contain expressions of regret at the pollutants which flowed into the rivers from private homes, public baths, and slaughterhouses.[118] For a long time the Jewish communities in the towns of eastern Europe maintained steam baths for use by men preparing for the sabbath; indeed, the Talmud forbade scholars to live in places where there was no bathhouse.[119] This institution should not be confused with the *mikveh*, or ritual bath, though they were often accommodated in the same building. Steam baths were also places where people with colds were sent, where controlled opening of veins was carried out, wet and dry cupping was performed, and other sudorific procedures were conducted. Jewish tradition regarded sweating as salutary,[120]

[115] Lew, 'O lecznictwie i przesądach', *Izraelita*, 46, p. 446.
[116] Weissenberg, 'Hygiene in Brauch und Sitte der Juden', 32.
[117] Blumental, *Reminiscences* (Yid.), 170.
[118] See Kotik, *My Memoirs* (Yid.), 61; 'The Steam Bath' (Yid.), 113; Nakhaliel, 'A Town There Was' (Yid.), 62; Shlaferman, 'The Folklore, Customs, and Stories of Kazimierz' (Yid.), 172.                                          [119] BT *San.* 17b.
[120] Three types of salutary sweating were distinguished: the sweat of a sick person,

and so on meeting someone who had just come out of the bathhouse it was customary to wish them *Tsu refue!* (To your cure!). Therapeutic baths were also widely used. In Budzanów the Jewish bathhouse attendant and his assistant offered sulphur-enriched baths as a remedy for rheumatism.[121] Wealthier citizens did not have to go to the bathhouse to take remedial baths. The highly popular bathtub (sitz bath) and footbath would often be prepared for them in the privacy of their own home as a tried and tested remedy for a plethora of ills. The recipe usually involved hot water with various types of herbs or other ingredients added to it. Sometimes the bath had a magical dimension, as illustrated by the recommendation that a child suffering from consumption should be bathed in the water in which nine pierogi had been cooked, for instance. This would reinforce the water's natural properties through the symbolic association of the dough with growing and gaining colour, which were, as shown above, indicators of health. For the most part, however, the views regarding baths tended to echo the tenets of medicine. The discomfort of rectal prolapse, for instance, might be relieved with a bath with the addition of oak 'skin' (bark) or acorns;[122] kidney stones would be treated with immersion in water with boiled oats or *herba equiseti* (horsetail);[123] and for mange, hard soap was added to the bath, and ointments containing corrosive sublimate (mercury(II) chloride), sulphur, petroleum, and Balsam of Peru were used concurrently.[124]

In the folk imagination water could take on the form of a living being, which was reflected in the description of its members, citing Genesis 2: 10: 'A river issued from Eden to water the garden, and it then divided and became four branches' (also read as 'heads', or 'legs'). In many towns in the Polish lands there was also a widespread conviction that water demanded regular sacrifices. 'It needs a man like the river in Dubno', the Jewish inhabitants of that particular region would say, though similar statements could

bathhouse sweat, and the sweat of labour (*Avot derabi natan*, 41: 4); see Hirshovitsh, *Minhagei yeshurun*, 226.

[121] Sulphur baths were thought to support the treatment of rheumatic diseases; Morgnshtern-Shifman, 'Budzanów as It Is' (Yid.), 25. See the extensive description of the bathhouse in Osherovitsh, 'According to Rubiezhevich Custom' (Yid.), 74.

[122] Rosenberg, *Rafa'el hamalakh*, 47, id., *Der malekh refoel*, 17. Cf. Haur, *Ekonomika lekarska*, 27. Baths in oak bark were also indicated for uterine pain; Rosenberg, *Rafa'el hamalakh*, 12–13.

[123] Rosenberg, *Rafa'el hamalakh*, 8; id., *Der malekh refoel*, 60. Cf. Haur, *Ekonomika lekarska*, 59.

[124] *Segulot urefuot*, JTS, MS 9862, 98. On the use of sulphur for mange, see Lilientalowa, 'Dziecko żydowskie', 155.

also be heard in other places.[125] One common way of sating the river's murderous desire was to throw live offerings into it, usually cats.[126] The general populace had no doubt that rivers could not only kill but could also point to where the body of a drowned person lay. In order to elicit this information, another sacrificial-type action had to be performed: a loaf of bread or a wooden bowl was to be floated out onto the water.[127] The cause of drowning was ultimately identified as the work of unclean forces, and thus it was natural that pronouncing magical formulas was the way to prevent it. One nineteenth-century manuscript recommended repeating seven times the names of the angels Tsuri'el and Patia before entering the water.[128]

At the same time, water also harboured dangers of another kind: it was inhabited by water folk (*vasermentshn*) and water maidens (*vasermoydn*), which were also known as mermaids (*rusalkes*). Tales of their half-human, half-fish bodies, golden or green hair and skin, the treasures they guarded in the murky depths of the water, and the singing with which they could lead a person to ruin were told and retold in many parts of eastern Europe.[129] The corpus of Jewish legends includes stories of the souls of sinners held captive in rivers, which, according to Isaac Luria, cited in *Ta'amei haminhagim*, attracted the errant souls of the damned. Anyone who drank from such a body of water, whether from cupped hands or from a vessel, was laying themselves open to danger.[130] One tale tells how, during a stay in Mogilev, a tsadik named Leib ben Sarah unravelled the mystery of a series of drownings: they were caused by the soul of a dissolute man who had once killed a woman. Now, bound in stone at the bottom of the Dnieper, his soul had to suffer penance, and took revenge on innocent people.[131] The presence in rivers of such *gilgulim* could have serious consequences. This was partly why it was ill-advised to gaze at one's reflection in water; it could cause one to become possessed.[132] Water drawn from a place where an expiating soul lay was said to seethe and moan as it boiled, and should be poured away into a deep hole in an unfrequented place.[133] A river could also make a

[125] Prilutski and Lehman, 'Jewish Proverbs' (Yid.), 25; Lilientalowa, 'Kult wody', 5.
[126] 'The River in Gliniany' (Yid.), 113; see Lew, 'O lecznictwie i przesądach', *Izraelita*, 37, p. 315. [127] Rosenberg, *Rafa'el hamalakh*, 41.
[128] *Segulot urefuot*, Bibliotheca Rosenthaliana, HS. ROS. 444, 4; perhaps the names are a perversion of Uriel and Peniel.
[129] Lilientalowa, 'Kult wody', 6. [130] Sperling, *Ta'amei haminhagim oyf ivri taytsh*, i. 111.
[131] Even, *From the World of Hasidic Leaders* (Yid.), 41–2.
[132] Lilientalowa, 'Kult wody', 6. [133] Ibid. 7.

claim on the descendant of anyone who had drowned another person or was
otherwise responsible for causing their death by water.[134]

All of this notwithstanding, the rabbinic sources stressed that water was
one of the main means of mitigating the effects of witchcraft, because 'the
unclean flee from the living water, at whose source is the *sitra dikedusha* [the
dimension of holiness]',[135] and 'all that on land is unclean, in the sea it is
clean'.[136] All forms of washing, spitting, licking, blowing, and similar were
applied in various types of medicinal practices as well as in the case of suspicion of use of the 'evil eye' or of fright. A peculiar washing ritual was performed if a child fell over when learning to walk; in order to alleviate the
pain, the floor where it had fallen should be doused with water or spat on.
One explanation for this action was that the water cancelled out the power
of the earth, which 'pulled the child down towards it'. Lilientalowa explains
it as a type of 'compensation' offered to the earth.[137] At the same time, this
custom also had an anti-demonic aspect, which, aside from the use of water,
would seem to be accented by the practice of blowing on the child three
times and ensuring for it angelic protection.[138]

The heightened magical potential of spaces associated with the presence of demons also offered the opportunity to use them in therapeutic
processes. One wooden bridge in the town of Pułtusk was a place where
many illnesses, including diphtheria, could be cured. A mother who walked
her sick child over this bridge and then encouraged it to cough up all the
mucus lingering in its airways could expect the problem to be solved.[139]
Similar examples of practices designed to stave off or send away illnesses—
float them away down the river, as it were—abound. The method of ridding
oneself of a complaint by cutting off hair or nails, described above, was
especially effective if carried out over running water. The sufferer would
bathe in the river (or wash their hands in it), or stand with their back to it
and cast mediatory objects into it over their shoulder (parents could do this
for their children by throwing the objects over the child's head).[140] Rituals
enacted on riverbanks were particularly common in the treatment of fever.
The use of water to alleviate this complaint (for example by dousing the
patient) has been discussed above. In fact, even simply crossing a river could

---

[134] Lilientalowa, 'Kult wody', 5.

[135] Zaler, *Yalkut yitsḥak*, 63.         [136] Sperling, *Ta'amei haminhagim umekorei hadinim*, 539.

[137] Lilientalowa, *Ziemia w wierzeniach żydowskich*, fos. 4r–5v; ead., 'Dziecko żydowskie', 150.

[138] Lilientalowa, *Dziecko żydowskie*, 47.         [139] Frost, 'The Wooden Bridge' (Yid.), 215.

[140] Lilientalowa, *Dziecko żydowskie*, 61; ead., 'Kult wody', 12.

help.[141] Another recommended method of treating fever was to throw seven (or nine, or thirteen) stones or dried peas over one's shoulder into water while saying: 'May all that is evil go away from me with this water.'[142] In case of illness caused by magic, one should buy a live pike for the first price asked, urinate into its mouth, and release it back into the river at the place where it was caught.[143] A woman prone to miscarriage who was in the ninth month of pregnancy should go to a place where a dog was giving birth, place her right foot on one of the puppies (selected in accordance with the presumed gender of her own foetus[144]) and repeat three times: 'Take this dead one and give me a live one.' She should then take the animal, place it on her belly with its head facing right, take it down to the river, and drop it into the water, repeating the same phrase three (or seven) times.[145]

In the popular imagination, the therapeutic properties of water could be carried over onto a variety of objects that had been in contact with it. One hugely popular way of warding off a cholera epidemic was to bury in the cemetery a sluice gate stolen from a non-Jewish mill. The idea behind this seems to have been to purify the site associated with death.[146]

Folk culture likewise attributed a demonic character to wind, which was consequently treated as the cause of certain illnesses. Although the word used in everyday speech was *vint*, Yiddish had also adopted from Hebrew the word *ruekh*, which was used to denote evil spirits, *beyze rukhes*. The natural phenomenon of eddying gusts of wind or gales was thought to be unclean forces at play (*In virbl zenen do sheydim*—There are demons in wind spirals). The Slavic populace, for its part, sometimes referred to the same phenomenon as a 'devil's wedding', while the Jews spoke of a demonic

[141] Tarlau, 'Volksmedizinisches aus dem jüdischen Russland', 144.
[142] Lilientalowa, 'Kult wody', 11. When one hasid from Dąbrowa Tarnowska sought help for his feverish daughter from the tsadik of Lublin, the holy man told him to bathe her in the nearby river Dunajec. See Bakon, 'Life of the Holy Rabbi Mordkhe David of Dąbrowa' (Heb.), 70.   [143] Rosenberg, *Rafa'el hamalakh*, 48.
[144] There were many folk beliefs regarding the signs indicating the gender of a foetus. In Mława and many other towns it was believed that if the expectant mother experienced heartburn it was a sign that she would give birth to a girl; a girl's hair—the symbol of her femininity—was said to start growing in her mother's womb, reach her heart, and irritate it; see Yunis, 'The Old Homeland' (Yid.), 71, Lilientalowa, *Dziecko żydowskie*, 22–4. Attempts to influence the gender of the foetus have been described in works including Klein, *A Time To Be Born*, 12–16.
[145] Halpern, *Toledot adam*, 93; Wilff, *Imrot shelomoh*, 101; *Segulot urefuot*, JTS, MS 9862, 101–2; Lifshits, *Berit avot*, 2b; Plaut, *Likutei hever ben hayim*, 7b.
[146] Veynig, 'Medicaments and Remedies among the Jews' (Yid.), 30.

dance, and took care not to say the word *khasene* (wedding) at night. If one were to thrust a knife into such an eddy of wind, one might expect to see the blood of demons dripping off it, but this would provoke their revenge.[147] The wind was thought to cause colds, which were treated by smudging with amber—a method of magical provenance.[148] Strong winds were also held responsible for symptoms such as dizziness and synaesthesia. The plague, which was often referred to as miasma, or 'bad air', was said to be heralded by howling dogs but also by wailing winds.[149] Another conviction held that if a strong wind had been blowing all day, it was a sign that an evil person had died (or someone had hanged themselves).[150]

There are many analogies in the beliefs of east European Jews with notions held by the Slavic peoples, which conceived the demons of the earth, fields, and woods to be responsible for 'windborne' diseases—those that came on suddenly and without warning.[151] The air, and wind in particular, were associated with paralysis, which was known in common parlance by a number of highly descriptive names, including *vind*, *luft* (*a guter luft*), and *tsug*. Along with apoplexy and sudden death, all these problems became fused into one concept of a 'clutching sickness' (*farkhapenish*, *oyskhapenish*). In the town of Tomaszów Lubelski it was believed that a person who was suddenly 'gripped', or who 'fell into the clutches' of such an illness, must have been provoking the demons. The partial paralysis that befell the son of a certain widow, for instance, was seen as punishment for lackadaisical breach of contract: he had failed to discharge his duty of bringing pails of water for washing the dead (he lived in the cemetery), and therefore angered the demons dwelling between the graves.[152] The popular curses

---

[147] Ch., 'Materiały do etnografii Żydów polskich', 437; Buchbinder, 'Jewish Omens' (Yid.), 252; Lilientalowa, *Złe duchy*, fo. 57. Cf. Moszyński, *Kultura ludowa Słowian*, 179–80 and 476.

[148] Lilientalowa, 'Dziecko żydowskie', 152.

[149] Rechtman, 'Some Customs and Their Folk Explanations' (Yid.), 261.

[150] Buchbinder, 'Jewish Omens' (Yid.), 258. Gales and the howling of dogs were perceived to presage pestilence; see e.g. 'Omens and Remedies' (Yid.), 280.

[151] See Libera, *Medycyna ludowa*, 80–1.

[152] Leybovitsh, 'One Patient, One Remedy', 450–1; Farber, 'Folk Healing' (Yid.), 181. Goldberg and Eisenberg's anthology *Sefer laḥashim usegulot* contains a lengthy mixed Hebrew and Yiddish formula (4*a*) for curing such 'air paralysis' (*luft*). It was to be pronounced while pouring wax, and it comprised quotations from the Bible, the names of angels, and even exhortations to Asmodeus. This is perhaps the origin of the custom of burning a candle containing a hair of a person suffering from 'air paralysis' at morning and evening prayers. See J. Ashkenazi, *Tsene urene fun harav hekhasid*, 3; Lilientalowa, *Choroby, lecznictwo*, fo. 46.

'I hope the *luft* enters you'[153] and 'May you be 'gripped'' made reference to this affliction.[154]

Notions surrounding lightning strikes also suggest a close affinity with windborne illnesses. The expression *shlag* or *shlak*, used in curses in both Polish and Yiddish (such as *A shlak zol zey trefn*, May they be struck [down]), might invite paralysis, epilepsy, or apoplexy. The causes of this misfortune were believed to be a sudden blow from the air[155] or from a bolt of lightning, which could also 'grab' or 'grip' its victim (*Khapt zey a duner*, I hope a bolt grabs them).[156] The custom of burying a paralysis victim up to their neck in the ground and leaving them there for a period of time (ten hours, or a whole day)—which was also widely practised in the case of people struck by lightning—seems natural in light of the fact that paralysis in Yiddish had certain connections with the earth: an apoplectic would often be termed *gelemt*, a word which also formed part of the expression *gelomt un gelemt* (lame and paralysed, in the sense of 'good for nothing'), which was in turn associated with the word *leym* (Yid. clay) and the insult *leymener goylem* (clay golem, someone stupid or clumsy).[157] Kalmen Marmor, in his memoirs, describes the magic attempted by his mother in her striving to restore the use of his legs, which he lost in infancy (the work of the wind, which suddenly gusted into the room). In the spring, when it started to get warmer, she would bury his limp legs in the sun-warmed sand.[158] Burying up to the shoulders in hot sand was also practised in the case of the 'English disease' (rickets), which presented as distortion of the limbs—the sand was said to be an excellent means of drawing out the disease.[159] Other methods for warming the body were also employed for apoplectics; these included mustard and juniper plasters, and rubbing with aqua vitae and concoctions used in early medicine (Venetian theriac or mithridate).[160]

---

[153] Lilientalowa, *Śmiecie*, fo. 24, no. 160.

[154] Ch., 'Materiały do etnografii Żydów polskich', 437.

[155] Linde, *Słownik języka polskiego*, v. 594.

[156] Y. Tsherniak, 'Linguistic Folklore in Yiddish' (Heb.), 101; Alexander Harkavy, *Yiddish–English–Hebrew Dictionary* (Yid.), 504; Stutshkov, *Thesaurus of the Yiddish Language* (Yid.), 410.

[157] *Segulot urefuot*, JTS, MS 9862, 46; Sosnowik, 'Material on Jewish Folk Medicine in Belarus' (Yid.), 166. Cf. Biegeleisen, *Lecznictwo ludu polskiego*, 157.

[158] Marmor, *My Life Story* (Yid.), 22. Hot sand compresses were said to help leg pain (ischias) and back pain (see Rosenberg, *Rafa'el hamalakh*, 88 and 18 respectively).

[159] Lilientalowa, *Dziecko żydowskie*, 65–6. In the town of Burshtin the local quack healer used hot bricks to treat rickets; see Schwarz, 'Characters and Personalities' (Yid.), 263.

[160] Plaut, *Likutei ḥever ben ḥayim*, 10a.

Procedures offering protection from demons often involved domestic animals. Essentially, the justification for this lay in the conviction that the sudden and unexpected death of such a creature could be interpreted as an auspicious sign suggesting that it had taken upon itself the misfortune which was to have befallen a human.[161] Before an infant was to be placed in its cradle for the first time, a cat, hen, or sometimes even a dog would be placed in it first, with the words: 'All bad dreams be on your head, your body, your life.'[162] The reasoning here was that the unclean force 'clung' to animals, in particular unkosher ones, and could thus be 'taken away' by them.[163] The author of *Shenei luḥot haberit* warned parents not to threaten their children with dogs or cats, because the very names of these animals were said to incorporate the names of demons capable of causing injury to their bodies and souls.[164] Anyone who, as a child, had played with a cat would later be cursed with a 'cat's mind'—a memory as poor as that of a 'cat in the attic'.[165] An important protective custom observed in many homes was *paslen di kats*: cutting off parts of a (black) cat's tail and ears. Black cats, especially those encountered after dark, were generally believed to be the incarnations of sorcerers or demons. There was a common conviction among the Slavs, undoubtedly shared at least to some extent by their Jewish neighbours, that a black cat (or in some versions a dog or a cockerel) in the home kept witches out. In order for the creature to be able to serve this purpose, however, it had to be shorn of any body parts that might attract or harbour unclean forces.[166] The blood from the tail of a black cat (male or

[161] Robinsohn, 'Tierglaube bei Juden Galiziens', 46.

[162] 'Aus unseren Sammlungen. II', 8; 'Jewish Omens' (Yid.), 255; Lew, 'O lecznictwie i przesądach', *Izraelita*, 40, p. 381 (and rock the animal for about half an hour); Bastomski, *At the Source: Jewish Proverbs* (Yid.), 105; Rechtman, 'Some Customs and Their Folk Explanations' (Yid.), 250; Fayvushinski, 'The Folklore of Pruzhana' (Yid.), 200.

[163] Sosnowik, 'Material on Jewish Folk Medicine in Belarus' (Yid.), 164.

[164] Horowitz, *Anaf ḥayim*, i. 46b. See Lerner, *Kuntres beit yisra'el*, 48.

[165] Charap, 'Sprichwörter galizischer Juden', 212; Pulner, 'Obryadi i povirya', 111; 'Omens and Remedies' (Yid.), 290–1; Rechtman, 'Some Customs and Their Folk Explanations' (Yid.), 263; Ben-Ezra, 'Customs' (Yid.), 175.

[166] Segel, 'Materyały do etnografii Żydów', 324; Lew, 'O lecznictwie i przesądach', *Izraelita*, 38, pp. 363–4 (there is a Polish testimony from the year 1700 confirming the existence among Jews of the custom of 'scraping' cats, 'not out of a desire to cause Christians any harm, but for their own health'); Sosnowik, 'Material on Jewish Folk Medicine in Belarus' (Yid.), 164; Ben-Ezra, 'Customs' (Yid.), 175. Cf. Gustawicz, 'Podania, przesądy, gadki', 130. Cats' tails were widely believed to contain poison, or to be a seat of evil or the devil; see Libera, *Medycyna ludowa*, 133. Evil forces were also said to take on the form of a black cat or dog to travel by night; see Robinsohn, 'Tierglaube bei Juden Galiziens', 48.

female, depending on the gender of the patient) featured repeatedly in descriptions of *segulot* in both printed and handwritten anthologies of therapeutic procedures. It was used to treat conditions including erysipelas, and rubbed on the gums of infants with teething problems. Aside from its deterrent function, it also had strong magical powers. In fact, the cat's tail was so strongly associated with demons, as a place where they liked to gather, that in some places (such as the town of Pińczów) only men would dare to use it as a therapeutic resource.[167] This same conviction also seems to have underlain several methods recommended in Jewish sources for relieving the symptoms of epilepsy, above all consuming the blood of a black cat or the dried placenta of a cat or pig.[168]

There were certain circumstances that mandated the performance of *paslen*. If a hen crowed like a cockerel, it should be slaughtered (*A hun vos kreyt muz men koylenen*), because it was surely possessed by an evil spirit.[169] At the very least, a diagnosis should be performed; if it landed tail first on the threshold three times when thrown, it could be allowed to live, with only its tail cut off. If it fell on its head, however, it should definitely be killed.[170]

A category apart were bats, creatures of a dual—and thus ambiguous and ambivalent—nature (reminiscent at once of birds and mice). Flying free, they were often considered dangerous, but if they flew inside or were caught, they would bring good luck. They could be attracted by white objects, which people would wave on seeing them. Bats might be nailed to the door above the threshold, inserted into the wall, or killed using a gold coin (or ring, or cord) and buried beneath the stove (or threshold), the central place in the house.[171] Moles, which 'swarm on the ground' (Lev. 11: 29),

---

[167] *Segulot vekameyot*, JTS, MS 10082, 6b; Lilientalowa, *Dziecko żydowskie*, 46, 68; Himmelblau, 'Medical Aid in Pińczów' (Yid.), 218. Cf. Haur, *Ekonomika lekarska*, 127.

[168] Rosenberg, *Rafa'el hamalakh*, 67; *Segulot urefuot*, JTS, MS 9862, 85; Plaut, *Likutei ḥever ben ḥayim*, 8a; Berger, *Imrei yisra'el*, 8a. Cf. Moszyński, *Kultura ludowa Słowian*, 214.

[169] Einhorn, 'Folk Proverbs' (Heb.), 346.

[170] An attribute typical of a cockerel that was present in a hen suggested a demonic aspect; Lilientalowa, 'Przesądy żydowskie', 644; Belova and Petrukhin, 'Demonologicheskiye syuzheti v krosskulturnom prostranstvie', 204.

[171] Robinsohn, 'Tierglaube bei Juden Galiziens', 48; Lilientalowa, 'Przesądy żydowskie', 643; Buchbinder, 'Jewish Omens' (Yid.), 250; Bastomski, *At the Source: Jewish Proverbs* (Yid.), 108; 'Omens and Remedies' (Yid.), 288; Taub, 'The Appearance of a Jewish Home' (Yid.), 278; 'Reminiscences: A Little Bit of Everything' (Yid.), 48. The same reason was given for hanging up horseshoes and old coins, though horseshoes were also said to provide protection from evil

were likewise ambivalent in nature, and were known in Yiddish by the name *moylvorm* or *multvorm* (vermin). In folk practice they were used in fighting epilepsy (advocated by authorities including the tsadik of Radzymin).[172] Not only bats but all kinds of animal body parts would often be buried under the threshold; a wolf's tail for keeping away flies, for instance (this might also be worn around the neck to guard against convulsions).[173] Many of these animals—cats, bats, and wolves—were predatory nocturnal creatures, which, by virtue of being active after dark (and in view of other attributes, such as eyes that shone in the dark), were associated with the world of demons.[174]

or mice; see e.g. *Segulot vekameyot*, JTS, MS 10082, 8*a*; Segel, 'Wierzenia i lecznictwo', 51; id., 'Materyały do etnografii Żydów', 323.

[172] See *Segulot urefuot*, Bibliotheca Rosenthaliana, HS. ROS. 444, 8*b*; '65-year-old Jewish woman' (Yid.), 5; Lew, 'O lecznictwie i przesądach', *Izraelita*, 41, p. 394.

[173] Rubinstein, *Zikhron ya'akov yosef*, 43*b*; Berger, *Imrei yisra'el*, 8*a*.

[174] On the subject of the 'gleaming' eyes of cats, dogs, and wolves, see Andrzej of Kobylin, *Gadki o składnosości członków człowieczych*, 21.

CHAPTER THIRTEEN

# THE EVIL EYE

A FUNDAMENTAL ROLE in Jewish beliefs surrounding medicine was played by the concept of the evil eye (*ayn-hore*). In biblical texts this originally denoted greed, envy, and antipathy towards others. In the book of Proverbs we read: 'A man with an evil eye hastens after riches' (Prov. 28: 22). This thought was popular as a subject for rabbinic sermons, though not specifically in connection with health. The far later notion of the evil eye that was in evidence in the talmudic period was largely consistent with the Slavic concept of *urok*, and denoted individuals who were in possession of eyes capable of casting spells, that is, of causing harm to others or damage to material objects, whether intentionally or not. This issue was discussed in detail by the early sages, who even claimed that out of every hundred deaths as many as ninety-nine were a result of the evil eye (BT *BM* 107*b*). The presence of such passages in the Talmud contributed to the spread of these beliefs across the Jewish diaspora. The preventative measures suggested by the rabbis, above all conjurations mentioning the name of Joseph (who was a righteous man, and whose moral integrity was proven by the many trials from which he delivered Israel in Egypt), became permanently fused with folk practices. They tended to include the quotation from Genesis 49: 22: 'Joseph is a wild ass, a wild ass by a spring—wild colts on a hillside.' According to the interpretation of this verse in *Berakhot* 20*a*, the text should be read not as 'by a spring', but as 'evading the [evil] eye', which was in turn supposed to offer evidence that Joseph's descendants were immune to the evil eye.[1] Later authorities likewise perpetuated beliefs connected with the *ayn-hore*, as did hasidism, perceiving both positive and

---

[1] This quotation forms part of the vast majority of Hebrew formulas designed to offer protection from the evil eye. As a preventative measure it might be inscribed on the tray on which the infant was laid during the ritual of redeeming the firstborn (Lilientalowa, *Dziecko żydowskie*, 37); on the *rimonim* decorating the Torah scroll (Schmid, 'Jüdische Amulette aus Osteuropa', 237); or on other types of amulets, either in its entirety, in abridged form, or as initials; see Schrire, *Hebrew Amulets*, 114.

negative aspects of the influence of the 'gaze'.[2] Among the beliefs mentioned by Joshua Trachtenberg is the conviction documented in the literature that an angry or jealous look spawned an evil angel and it was this angel that wreaked the damage attributed to the evil eye.[3] The kabbalistic explanation, taken from the hasidic work *Zera kodesh* by Naftali of Ropczyce (Ropshitz), sought the cause in the admiration that people, driven by worldly greed, afford a thing for itself, which severs it from its heavenly roots. For this reason, in order not to cast a glance that might have magical consequences, one should turn one's gaze to heaven.[4]

In a period of increasing influence of scientific thinking, this conviction was adapted to take account of new views on nature. Within the rationalistic vision of the world it was factored into explanations based on humoral theory and subordinated to views on physiology derived from that worldview. The author of the *Sefer haberit*, drawing on far earlier kabbalistic and ethical literature, described the power of the gaze as follows, using the example of an ostrich: 'Its females heat their chicks out of their eggs with their eyes; they stand by them and stare at them until the chicks crawl out. This shows us the power inherent in eyes. Human eyes harbour the same [power], that is: the *ayn-hore*.'[5] The soft matter of which human eyes are made was thought to allow noxious vapours to pass through: toxic fumes caused by the fermentation of the humours, poisoning, certain physiological traits, and the like. Unable to leave the body via any other route, they would rise upwards—as vapours do—and on reaching the head they could cause symptoms typical of hysteria, including migraine and lachrymation. The easiest way for them to leave the body was through the eyeballs, where they found reduced resistance. Even after their release they remained hazardous to the environment; they could poison living beings, causing serious health issues. On their passing through a window or other glass surface, the effect of these dangerous fumes/vapours was intensified, in the manner of sunbeams passing through a lens.[6] Such attempts at rationalization of the

---

[2] Zimmels, *Magicians, Theologians and Doctors*, 44–5; Trachtenberg, *Jewish Magic and Superstition*, 54–6.

[3] Trachtenberg, *Jewish Magic and Superstition*, 54–6. See also J. Ashkenazi, *Tsene urene*, 100–11.

[4] Sperling, *Ta'amei haminhagim oyf ivri taytsh*, ii. 15.

[5] Hurwitz, *Sefer haberit* (Yid.), 35. See Wolfson, *Through a Speculum That Shines*, 317–25.

[6] This section of text was not included in the Yiddish translation; see Hurwitz, *Sefer haberit hashalem*, 167–8, for the Hebrew original. Cf. Zimmels, *Magicians, Theologians and Doctors*, 45; Biegeleisen, *Lecznictwo ludu polskiego*, 237.

notion of the evil eye were nothing new. Andrzej of Kobylin, basing his arguments on the legacy of Aristotle, explained in his *Words on the Compositional Nature of Human Members* that a woman 'suffering vaginal discharge' could damage a mirror with her gaze.[7] The same vapours were also thought to be released from her body through an open mouth. The Jewish ethical literature even recommended the segregation of menstruating women at mealtimes, because 'the food left by her mouth on the spoon, and transferred from the spoon to the bowl, could place [others] in danger'.[8]

No less interesting for contemporary research than the speculations of rabbis, philosophers, and kabbalists is the interpretation of the beliefs and practices connected with the evil eye developed by Alan Dundes. According to this leading folklorist, some form of the evil eye was a typical feature of a number of cultures, from India, across the Middle East, to Europe. It was a belief founded on certain fundamental factors common to traditional Indo-European and Semitic cultures: ideas linking life with water and death with dryness; the limited availability of material goods; the concept that nature exists in a state of equilibrium, which is at the root of the envy of the poor and the suspicion of the rich; and the symbolism of the eyes (breasts, testicles), or the one eye (the phallus, vagina, and anus).[9] Naturally, folk culture did not reflect Dundes's model precisely; often only the broader context testified to the currency of certain ideas—hence a distanced approach is required, and a recognition of the heterogeneous character of customs surrounding the treatment of illnesses.

In accordance with Dundes's classification, the traditional Jewish community maintained that one was especially vulnerable to the effects of the evil eye when eating. A meal in itself can symbolize prosperity and well-being; it is also an intimate activity that has a direct impact on human health. At least partly for this reason it was considered unwise to converse at table, and also to eat outside the home. If a guest called while the evening meal was being eaten, they should be invited to the table, and one should eat less than usual; indeed, a little of every dish should be left on the plate, otherwise one might be at risk from a curse. The guest should greet those already seated, and wish them good health from their meal (*Est gezunterhayt!*). If they did not do so, they themselves might be at risk from the

---

[7] Andrzej of Kobylin, *Gadki o składności członków człowieczych*, 20–1.

[8] See T. H. Koydanover, *Kav hayashar*, 50.

[9] Dundes, 'Wet and Dry, the Evil Eye', 257–312.

*ayn-hore*, for it was written in the Talmud that anyone who did not eat in the company of others who were eating would experience sixty toothaches.[10] If food fell out of someone's mouth in the presence of another person, it was believed to be a sign that that person envied them their meal. Taking the last bite of a loved one's food was seen as taking their health; conversely, giving one's own last mouthful to a stranger would cause the death of an evildoer.[11]

Every sudden indisposition, according to Lilientalowa, was attributed to the influence of the evil eye. Symptoms which were a sure sign that one had fallen victim to it were a high temperature, headache, yawning, stretching, and drowsiness, but the list was an open one, and could also include various types of swelling, convulsions, vomiting, or accidents such as bone fractures or sprains.[12] This was indeed a prominent issue in Jewish culture. It is no coincidence that the phrase for banishing the evil eye, *keyn ayn-hore* (or *on an ayn-hore*, 'without the evil eye'), repeated whenever words about anyone or anything close to the speaker's heart were said, is mentioned in most ethnographic material from eastern Europe. More succinct or shorter sources often passed over the question of aetiology. In these cases the connection between particular problems and the evil eye only becomes clear when one studies not only the symptoms but also the remedies or remedial action recommended. Among the many treatments for a nosebleed given in home treatment guides, there is one that involves tying a red silk thread around the little finger of the patient's left hand. This was a method chiefly intended to offer protection from the evil eye, of which one of the many symptoms was profuse bleeding.[13] Elsewhere in Lilientalowa's material there is a note to the effect that hanging up a shell gives protection from swelling, while in An-sky's ethnographic survey this remedy was unequivo-

---

[10] BT *BK* 92*b*. This was partly because several sources warned that eating in the home of someone who subjected their guest to malevolent glances was bound to cause symptoms akin to those of food poisoning. The following quotation from Proverbs 23: 7 was given in support of this thesis: 'He is like one keeping accounts; "Eat and drink", he says to you, but he does not really mean it.' See T. H. Koydanover, *Kav hayashar*, 79; Lilientalowa, *Choroby, lecznictwo*, fo. 43.

[11] Choking on one's food was said to augur the arrival of a guest; see Lipiets, *Sefer matamim*, 83; Buchbinder, 'Jewish Omens' (Yid.), 258; Bastomski, *At the Source: Jewish Proverbs* (Yid.), 54, 102; Segel, 'Wierzenia i lecznictwo', 52; Lilientalowa, 'Wierzenia, przesądy i praktyki', 152; ead., 'The Evil Eye' (Yid.), 251. Animals and objects could also be affected by the evil eye—animals might fall ill, die, or stop giving milk, for instance, while objects would break.

[12] Lilientalowa, *Dziecko żydowskie*, 50; ead., 'The Evil Eye' (Yid.), 267; Farber, 'Folk Healing' (Yid.), 178; Rosenberg, *Rafa'el hamalakh*, 43.          [13] Plaut, *Likutei hever ben hayim*, 8*b*.

cally associated with the evil eye.[14] There are numerous other examples of similar ambiguities.

A perusal of the Jewish sources produces the impression that, while spells or curses usually affected adults, it was above all the young who fell victim to the 'good eye' (a euphemism for the evil eye). According to Lilientalowa, formulas for blocking its effects were most commonly sought for boys under the age of 13, that is, under the age of religious maturity. Similar precautions were taken in respect of girls, but these were far less common, and in the case of adults they were only deemed necessary in much more clear-cut situations.[15] In this regard, the language of the descriptions of methods for protecting pregnant or nursing women is telling: these texts always speak about the woman not in her own right but as an auxiliary to the baby. For example, one formula is 'for a pregnant woman so that she and her foetus are not possessed by the *ayn-hore*',[16] the implication being that the protection was only extended to the mother because her presence was vital to the child. Naturally, this was not an absolute rule. Young adults such as marriageable girls or talented yeshiva students were also prime targets for the evil eye. As hasidic sources testify, one of the grandsons of the rebbe of Kotsk, Barukh Mordecai, died at the age of 19 in spite of all his immense inherited and personal virtues—or perhaps precisely because of them. In hasidic circles the cause of his death was presumed to have been the *ayn-hore*.[17]

The power of the evil eye came not so much from otherworldly sources as from the free will—or lack thereof—of the person inflicting it. While the merits of one's ancestors and of holy men could restore one from a state of illness, they could not offer protection from the evil eye, especially if the victim was a child and 'slept it in', falling asleep before the conjuration process could begin.[18] It was believed that anyone who stared or pried too much, admired someone else's good fortune, or wondered at their numerous offspring, could unwittingly cause a tragedy, particularly if their gaze

---

[14] Lilientalowa, 'Wierzenia, przesądy i praktyki', 171; An-sky, *The Yiddish Ethnographic Programme* (Yid.), 50.                    [15] Lilientalowa, 'Dziecko żydowskie', 152.

[16] Wilff, *Imrot shelomoh*, 99; Rosenberg, *Rafa'el hamalakh*, 62. An expectant mother should recite eleven Bible verses beginning and ending with the letter *nun* every day; Lifshits, *Berit avot*, 1*b*; cf. T. H. Koydanover, *Kav hayashar*, 95. Folk wisdom advised a woman in postnatal confinement not to admit to feeling improvement in her condition, and to remain weak for as long as possible, as this was said to protect her from the evil eye; Lilientalowa, 'Additions: The "Evil Eye"' (Yid.), 433.

[17] Gliksman, *The Kotsker Rebbe* (Yid.), 112.                    [18] Lilientalowa, *Dziecko żydowskie*, 51.

was accompanied by words of admiration. In the folk imagination admiration held overtones of envy, and it was not only the wealthy or those who lived showily who were at risk of the envy of their environment; even poor families might be vulnerable to the evil eye if, for example, they had sons or their children were born healthy. Even staring for too long at a craftsman's hands as he worked could be seen as the reason for a botched job.[19] The blessings of good fortune should be enjoyed in the privacy of one's own home; boasting about them publicly was dangerous. If two sons of one man were being circumcised at once, a certain passage from the book of Genesis (Gen. 48: 16) should be recited for safety's sake.[20] Two brothers, or a father and son, could invite misfortune if they were both called up to read the Torah on the same occasion.[21] Children who were too beautiful or too clever provoked malicious looks wherever they went, and for fear of their life their face would be smeared with charcoal to make them look ugly and prevent them from attracting the evil eye.[22] Neither would they be praised in public; instead, they would be belittled with words such as: 'What a stupid, ugly child!' Prudent guests would themselves moderate the intensity of their gaze, using a variety of methods, including holding the child in their arms, taking three steps back, spitting, or reciting appropriate formulas, such as 'May the evil eye not harm him' or 'I won't give him beauty, I'll give him a wedding present instead.'[23] The following text, known in places including the Svislach region (present-day Belarus), was sometimes used as a prophylactic formula:

In balkn
Iz faran a shpaltn.
Dort vet zikh dem kinds
Ayn-hore bahaltn.[24]

In the ceiling
There's a crack.
There the child's own
*Ayn-hore* will find its home.

[19] Robinsohn, 'An ajen-hore oder Güt Auge' (Ger.), 20.    [20] Wilff, *Imrot shelomoh*, 107.
[21] Sperling, *Ta'amei haminhagim oyf ivri taytsh*, i. 29. The same applied when two brothers opened a business in the same place; Kaindl, 'Die Juden in der Bukowina', 159.
[22] Segel, 'Materyały do etnografii Żydów', 320; Lilientalowa, *Dziecko żydowskie*, 49.
[23] An-sky, 'Charm Reversals and Conjurations' (Yid.), 157; Bastomski, *At the Source: Jewish Proverbs* (Yid.), 54; Lilientalowa, *Dziecko żydowskie*, 50; Friedlender, 'Jewish Life in the Shtetl' (Yid.), 126.
[24] Ein, 'The Town of Sislevitsh' (Yid.), 65; Lilientalowa, 'The Evil Eye' (Yid.), 250.

Although anyone, even the most devout Jew, could unwittingly trans-
mit a curse caused by *ayn-hore*, some people were considered particularly
dangerous in this respect. This was the case when the community perceived
someone to be in possession of an attribute which suggested that they were
linked in some way to unclean forces. In fact, these could be signs also characteristic of witches and warlocks: advanced age, a hunchback, a missing
leg, or a missing eye among others. Aside from such physical features,
membership of any stereotypically defined group of 'others' was an indication that a person might have the power of the evil eye, and thus it was
commonly believed that such spells cast by non-Jews and those of the opposite gender were the strongest.[25] Moreover, powers of this nature were
intensified further if their holder was offended or angry; one popular saying
warned: *Az du host kinder in di vign, loz di layt tsufridn* (When you have
children in cradles, don't upset people).[26] According to Jewish tradition, as
among the Slavic peasantry, the point at which a person gained the power to
cast the evil eye (became an *ayn-hore-geber*, or an *ayn-horenik/ayn-horenitse*)
was around the time when they were weaned as a child. Once one had
started to feed a child solids, one should not return to feeding it breast
milk, because according to various sources this could cause problems with
its memory[27] or the evil eye.[28] As a preventative measure, on the day of
weaning (*antvoynung*) a protective pouch filled with coins, called an *antvoy-
nung-baytl*, would be hung around its neck.[29] This belief incorporates many
of the constitutive elements of the evil eye cited by Dundes—envy, nourish-
ment in the form of moist food, and the symbolic link between the eye and
the nipple. Other sources also stated that the ability to inflict curses via the
medium of the evil eye sometimes came as a result of rubbing one's eyes
with dirty or unclean hands. For this reason, when performing the morning

[25] Lilientalowa, 'Przesądy żydowskie', 320, and 'Wierzenia, przesądy i praktyki', 151.
Barukh Rotner published an interesting story of a tailor suffering from a headache brought on
by the evil eye because he had consorted with the wife of a non-Jew; *Sipurei nifla'ot*, 54. According to another folk theory, the evil eye caused headaches when cast by a man, and stomach
ache when cast by a woman (this belief was perhaps influenced by the societal roles of the two
genders: men as scholars and women as childbearers); Lilientalowa, 'Additions: The "Evil
Eye"' (Yid.), 433.
[26] Grunwald, 'Aus unseren Sammlungen. Teil I', 33. The husband of a woman in childbirth
should pay off all his debts; see BT *Shab.* 32b; Lifshits, *Berit avot*, 6b. Cf. Allerhand, 'Przysięga
kobiety ciężarnej u Żydów', 180–4.       [27] Bergner, *In the Long Winter Nights* (Yid.), 40.
[28] Lew, 'O lecznictwie i przesądach', *Izraelita*, 40, p. 382; Lilientalowa, 'Dziecko żydowskie',
150; Fayvushinski, 'The Folklore of Pruzhana' (Yid.), 203.
[29] 'Aus unseren Sammlungen. II', 8.

handwashing ritual to remove the unclean forces that had gathered on one's fingernails during the night, it was considered prudent also to rinse one's eyes with water.[30]

There was an extremely broad catalogue of preventative measures offering protection from the evil eye, and there were certain times in life when this protection should be redoubled, above all childhood, and early adulthood for both marriageable men and women. People would try to deflect the evil eye, which was most potent in the first glance, away from children, using brief formulas such as *keyn ayn-hore* or slightly more complex ones ('You're not in long trousers yet, so you can't take the evil eye'; 'Today is Wednesday [or another day of the week] so the evil eye won't cling to you'). Verbal attempts would be made to redirect the attention of the evil eye onto other objects, while guests and even people met on the street would be issued with warnings not to 'inflict the eye', to 'look at the lamp', or to 'count nine chimneys', otherwise their 'eyes would end up on the fifth house from here'.[31] If a person entering the room was suspected of having the power to do harm, one could always recite the following verse from the book of Numbers to be safe: 'As Balaam looked up and saw Israel encamped tribe by tribe, the spirit of God came upon him' (Num. 24: 2).[32]

A considerable range of common apotropaics was in widespread use in traditional society. Red threads, ribbons, or coral bracelets would be tied around infants' and children's wrists, and sometimes also around the little finger on one hand; sleeves might be hemmed with red thread. In the folk imagination, red was associated with fire, and protective objects of this colour attracted and then absorbed (and hence neutralized) the gaze of people with the evil eye; this was best evidenced by the phenomenon of tarnishing.[33] In addition to the many objects already discussed, a particular type of *baytele*, a red drawstring bag containing (presumably also red) mouse eyes, would be hung around the neck.[34] Animal bones (from beneath the

---

[30] Lilientalowa, 'Wierzenia, przesądy i praktyki', 152; Fayvushinski, 'The Folklore of Pruzhana' (Yid.), 203.

[31] An-sky, 'Charm Reversals and Conjurations' (Yid.), 157; Bastomski, *At the Source: Jewish Proverbs* (Yid.), 54; Lilientalowa, *Dziecko żydowskie*, 50; Herzog and Zborowski, *Life Is with People*, 317.          [32] Lilientalowa, 'Additions: The "Evil Eye"' (Yid.), 433.

[33] Rosenberg, *Rafa'el hamalakh*, 46; Lilientalowa, 'Dziecko żydowskie', 151; Segel, 'Wierzenia i lecznictwo', 60; id., 'Materyały do etnografii Żydów', 319; Elzet [Złotnik], 'Some Jewish Customs' (Heb.), 368.

[34] Also to guard against fever; Fels, 'Zabobony lekarskie u Żydów', 2; Tarlau, 'Volksmedizinisches aus dem jüdischen Russland', 144; Weissenberg, 'Südrussische Amulette', 369;

tail of a hen or a cockerel, preferably a black one) and teeth (of wolves or foxes) were widely used against the evil eye.[35] Twigs from besoms were also immensely popular among the Jews, both as an element of general therapeutic practices and as protection from the evil eye; they might be hung around a child's neck in a pouch, or suspended above the cradle (with some pepper and a stolen needle).[36] One object that would be placed in the confinement chamber, whether to distract attention from the child or to frighten unclean forces, was a cockerel's or hen's head (for a baby boy or baby girl respectively) impaled on a stick. If by some unforeseen circumstance a person who might cast a harmful glance at the infant did gain entry into the room, characteristic traps would be set for them, such as an inverted glass,[37] or a type of magic circle, created by filling a vessel with water, washing three sides of a table with it, then collecting the excess water and washing four corners of two windows with it, adding a little salt to the vessel, wetting a spoon in it, and washing the patient's (baby's) face with the wetted spoon.[38] Another variation of this ritual was for the oldest member of the family to sprinkle salt in the four corners of the chamber, then turn to face the child, shake their head, and spit three times in the opposite direction. One preventative measure, sometimes also used as an element of therapy, was to erase the footprints of the person who was thought to have cast the evil eye. Lumps of coal would be thrown out of the house after them (over the threshold), or salt sprinkled on their footprints;[39] and the infant's face would be washed in cold water.[40]

Robinsohn, 'Tierglaube bei Juden Galiziens', 48; Fayvushinski, 'The Folklore of Pruzhana' (Yid.), 203.

[35] Or even offal from these animals; Weissenberg, 'Südrussische Amulette', 368–9; Lilientalowa, *Dziecko żydowskie*, 49.

[36] Lilientalowa, 'Dziecko żydowskie', 151; ead., *Dziecko żydowskie*, 58. An old besom should never be thrown away; see ead., 'Wierzenia, przesądy i praktyki', 170.

[37] Segel, 'Wierzenia i lecznictwo', 60. Another explanation for this practice may have been the desire to reverse or 'overturn' the evil; see Moszyński, *Kultura ludowa Słowian*, 289.

[38] Sosnowik, 'Material on Jewish Folk Medicine in Belarus' (Yid.), 164.

[39] An-sky, 'Charm Reversals and Conjurations' (Yid.), 157. Pieces of coal would also be thrown after a pregnant woman whenever she left the house. This was said to be a way of 'keeping the mice away'; in other words, a way of protecting oneself from the loss of property which could ensue from refusing a pregnant woman something; Silverman-Weinreich, 'Beliefs' (Yid.), 33; Bastomski, *At the Source: Jewish Proverbs* (Yid.), 109. At the same time, there were other sources which stated that anyone who practised this custom had to accept responsibility if the woman died or her child fell ill; Lilientalowa, *Dziecko żydowskie*, 25.

[40] An-sky, 'Charm Reversals and Conjurations' (Yid.), 157; Lilientalowa, *Dziecko żydowskie*, 50.

Silver or tin discs or badges bearing the letter *he* and hence known in Yiddish as *heyele* would be placed around babies' necks. On the reverse they might have magic formulas, most commonly employing the words of Psalm 121: 5, 'The Lord is your keeper'. Although the *heyele* was unequivocally associated with the ineffable name of God (*he* symbolizes the Tetragrammaton), some sources have drawn attention to the custom of using this method to place a mark on firstborn boys who were exempt from the redemption requirement (*pidyon haben*; the letter *he* stands for the five silver coins with which the baby was to be redeemed).[41] There were other, similar amulets, bearing the Hebrew inscription 'May this child mature to the Torah, to marriage, and to good deeds' on one side, and on the other 'May it be Your will, O Eternal One, our God and the God of our fathers [this invocation would be written as an abbreviation], to protect the offspring of Your people Israel from the *ayn-hore*, that diphtheria may not attack it, and to bring it up for the Holy Order—by Your mercy, amen.'[42] The means by which the materials for this and other popular amulets were obtained also had a symbolic dimension. Various sources advised that the silver, tin, or copper should be collected from nine couples whose parents were still alive but who themselves had not brought children into the world (or from nine women), in the form of various items, such as tableware, keys, or similar. After melting them down, the metal thus obtained could be used to make a necklace or ring (which would be worn on a string) engraved with the names of God.[43]

In addition to the *heyelekh*, ordinary silver coins could also be used as amulets if they had been gifted by a tsadik with this purpose in mind. Sickly boys would grow up wearing them, and, according to Samuel Weissenberg, would continue to do so 'often until their wedding'.[44] Acolytes of the descendants of Rebbe Israel Friedman of Ruzhin, most of whom lived in the Bukovina region and in eastern Galicia (present-day western Ukraine), would wear such coins throughout their lives, in special pouches, might melt them down to make ornamental religious utensils (such as Kiddush

[41] Lipiets, *Sefer matamim*, 47, which cites *Shulḥan arukh*, 'Yoreh de'ah', 305: 15; Rosenberg, *Rafa'el hamalakh*, 46; Lilientalowa, *Dziecko żydowskie*, 75–6; Rechtman, 'Some Customs and Their Folk Explanations' (Yid.), 250. See Schmid, 'Jüdische Amulette aus Osteuropa', 348–9.
[42] Lilientalowa, *Dziecko żydowskie*, 75–6. Cf. JT *Ta'an*. 4: 3.
[43] *Segulot urefuot*, Bibliotheca Rosenthaliana, HS. ROS. 444, 6b; Berger, *Imrei yisra'el*, 5a–b (as a remedy for convulsions).          [44] Weissenberg, 'Kinderfreud', 316.

cups), and were even buried with them.[45] As mentioned above, scraps of parchment inscribed with passages from the Torah would also be hung up, usually inside mezuzot. Amulets drawn on parchment or paper were not uncommon in the context of the evil eye. Examples of magic formulas used in such pieces are to be found in manuscripts,[46] and then there are also those featured on printed sheets of popular conjurations or spells (in both Hebrew and Yiddish), which not only served as 'crib sheets', but were also hung up in people's homes as protective measures.[47] In most cases, the sources seem to suggest that amulets in widespread use as protection from the she-demon Lilith and from spells were also employed against the *ayn-hore*.[48]

One extremely popular method of deflecting the evil eye, which was also known in other cultures, was to make the 'fig sign'. In its earliest form (the gesture of concealing the thumb of one hand in the other hand) it was known to Jews even in the talmudic period.[49] It tended not to be made overtly, but behind the addressee's back, often after taking three steps backwards, or with one's hands in one's pockets (especially when wearing new clothes), or as the person was leaving the room. In some cases it would be accompanied by a whispered curse, such as 'May your eyes fall out.' The fig sign as phallic motif (the most evident symbol of vitality, or simply of life) would sometimes also take on the form of a red amulet, to be hung around the neck of a child or other person at risk from the evil eye.[50] Another popular practice offering protection from envious glances was that of wearing one's shirt, yarmulke, or underwear inside out (as a way of 'reversing' the ill will),[51] or, in another variant, wearing clothes that had been gifted rather than bought (to deflect envy).[52] Whenever one put a new (or even simply clean) shirt on a child, it was important to spit into it three times and recite a preventative formula, such as: *A hemdele arop, a gezunt in kop; a*

[45] Rothstein [Nisnzohn], *Dos malkhesdike khsides*, 122, 208. The custom of placing coins in graves as a type of amulet was undoubtedly widespread beyond hasidic circles; see Fijałkowski, 'Obrządek pogrzebowy Żydów polskich', 25–42.

[46] *Segulot urefuot*, Bibliotheca Rosenthaliana, HS. ROS. 444, *6b, 7a*.

[47] Schmid, 'Jüdische Amulette aus Osteuropa', 204–5.

[48] Lilientalowa, 'The Evil Eye' (Yid.), 254.          [49] BT *Ber.* 55*b*.

[50] Lipiets, *Sefer matamim*, 14; Segel, 'Wierzenia i lecznictwo', 60; Buchbinder, 'Jewish Omens' (Yid.), 251; Bastomski, *At the Source: Jewish Proverbs* (Yid.), 111; Lilientalowa, 'The Evil Eye' (Yid.), 251; Ben-Ezra, 'Customs' (Yid.), 175.

[51] Lilientalowa, 'Dziecko żydowskie', 151; ead., 'The Evil Eye' (Yid.), 250.

[52] An-sky, 'Charm Reversals and Conjurations' (Yid.), 156; Ben-Ezra, 'Customs' (Yid.), 175.

*hemdele aruf—a gezunt in guf* (Shirt down for a healthy head, shirt up for a healthy body).[53] In addition to all of the above, various kinds of religious artefacts were also used in prophylactic contexts.

Despite the existence of such vast numbers and types of protective measures, it was widely believed that 'the most common cause of illness . . . was the *ayn-hore*'.[54] When signs of affliction by the evil eye became apparent, a series of steps were taken, firstly to confirm the suspicion, then to establish who had cast the curse, and finally to neutralize its negative impact. Magic was used to combat the effects, which did not, of course, rule out the concurrent use of other methods to alleviate symptoms. Such practices were rather complex, and some of their elements might be omitted, while others were selected according to individual habit and experience. Since these actions were performed within a short time of each other, usually one after the other, their individual functions often became blurred or unclear, though not to such an extent that it is impossible to recreate them, at least to some degree.

There were several basic ways of diagnosing the evil eye. These were sometimes the same as the methods used to identify spells, though the latter usually required the initiative of the patient, and as such tended to be used mainly for adults. One widespread belief was the perception that yawning was a symptom of enchantment. At the first sight of a child yawning, the appropriate steps were taken, which included spitting three times into its open mouth and tapping it on the lips ('May they not remain open for ever').[55] Another highly popular reaction was to lick its forehead, eyelids, or temples (according to Lilientalowa, its pulse[56]), again usually three times, and then to spit the same number of times, and to recite any one of a plethora of magic formulas, such as: *Mir far dir, mir far dayne beyner* (Me instead of you, me instead of your bones). If the child's mother or a servant—as they were the ones who most often performed these actions—discerned a salty taste on licking, this was clear proof that the child had come under a curse.

[53] Elzet [Złotnik], 'Some Jewish Customs' (Heb.), 368. Lilientalowa also gives other variants: *Dziecko żydowskie*, 48.          [54] Neumann, 'Our Town' (Yid.), 423.

[55] Lilientalowa, 'Przesądy żydowskie', 640; ead., *Dziecko żydowskie*, 67; Benczer, 'Volksglaube', 274; 'Aus unseren Sammlungen. II', 7. Cf. Wuttke, *Der deutsche Volksaberglauben der Gegenwart*, 391; Hovorka and Kronfeld (eds.), *Vergleichende Volksmedizin*, 706.

[56] Taking the pulse was one of the tasks reserved largely for physicians, medical orderlies, or other practitioners conversant with the concepts of anatomy, whether early or contemporary. On occasion, however, the pulse was used as an indicator of detrimental demonic activity; see T. H. Koydanover, *Kav hayashar*, 201–2.

According to some sources the very act of licking might be either preventative (if the child was asleep, or about to go to sleep, because it would 'do no
harm') or therapeutic in character.[57] It would also be employed in case of a
fright.[58] Another method of diagnosing a curse caused by the evil eye was
to lay a new knife on the pillow by the sick child's head, sometimes without
their knowledge, and to check whether the blade turned black or went
rusty. If it did, the knife should be used to cut a slice of bread from a new
loaf, and a fingernail clipping from the patient should be inserted into the
slice, which should then be fed to a male or female dog (depending on
the patient's gender). According to a manuscript from Dieveniškės, in such
cases a conjuration by rabbi Hayim Joseph David Azulai (known as Hida)
would also be recited. After this process had been repeated for three days,
the child was safe.[59] According to yet another variant, the knife would be
thrown to the ground, and if the blade lodged in the earth, that was proof of
the presence of a curse.[60]

In contrast to cases of misfortune caused by demons, knowledge about
the person who had cast the evil eye was significant inasmuch as it enabled
others to take added precautions and implement counter-measures. 'The
first thought was always that it was a curse, and the family would start to
think back over who had been in the house that day and who could have cast
the *ayn-hore*', one resident of the town of Tomaszów Lubelski remembers.[61]
It was commonly believed that the person who had cast the evil eye had the
best chance of lifting it. One method considered immensely effective was
smudging the victim with items connected with the source of the curse
(*ayn-hore-geber/in*), such as elements of their clothing (even individual
threads) or hairs, which usually had to be procured—and this was not
always easy, since even if it did prove possible to identify the culprit unequivocally, they were not always willing to co-operate. On the other hand,
pulling threads out of a guest's clothes was often treated as a standard
prophylactic measure, and on occasion was even initiated by the guest.[62]

[57] Buchbinder, 'Jewish Omens' (Yid.), 252; Lilientalowa, *Dziecko żydowskie*, 50; Yoffie,
'Popular Beliefs and Customs', 382; Friedlender, 'Jewish Life in the Shtetl' (Yid.), 126.

[58] Segel, 'Materyały do etnografii Żydów', 319; Yoffie, 'Popular Beliefs and Customs', 377.

[59] Szymon ben Abraham z Dziwieniszek, *Varia*, Warsaw, ŻIH, MS no. 771, 20*a*; Plaut,
*Likutei ḥever ben ḥayim*, 7*b*; An-sky, 'Charm Reversals and Conjurations' (Yid.), 158; Lilientalowa, *Dziecko żydowskie*, 50.               [60] Segel, 'Wierzenia i lecznictwo', 60.

[61] Leybovitsh, 'One Patient, One Remedy' (Yid.), 449.

[62] Segel, 'Wierzenia i lecznictwo', 60; id., 'Materyały do etnografii Żydów', 319; Lilien-

Testing for the evil eye by 'quenching coals' (*koyln opleshn, opleshn an ayn-hore*) took a more ritualized form; at the same time as diagnosing a curse, this procedure also incorporated alleviation of its effects.[63] Seven or nine lumps of coal would be dropped into a glass or other vessel containing 'silent water' (usually drawn after sunset or before sunrise—meaning that the ritual itself also had to take place around the same time). While performing the ritual, the devout healer should focus their mind on the sacred name Agla (acronym of *Atah gibor le'olam adonai*, 'You, O God, are eternally powerful'). As the coals were hot, they would be carried from the kitchen on the point of a knife. On the sabbath, when lighting a fire was prohibited, pieces of the sabbath challah, or even of ordinary bread, would be used in their place. If the coal sank or sizzled (according to some sources) on being thrown into the water, the patient had evidently been bewitched. In such a case some were of the opinion that not only was the presence of the evil eye beyond doubt, but also the sinking of the coal was a sign that the person who had cast it was a man. This was not the end of the ritual, however, which then proceeded to the therapy phase. The coals were counted as they were thrown into the water, and conjurations were recited. If the person performing the curative rite knew Hebrew, the following quotation from the book of Numbers played an important role (sometimes in abbreviated form): 'Moses prayed to the Lord, and the fire died down' (Num. 11: 2). This would be repeated three times, with the healer circling the patient, holding a handful of salt, which would then be thrown into a hot oven, or into the water; this would later be used to wash the child's face, chest, and sometimes also other parts of its body. It might also be given small quantities of the same water to drink. Its face would then be wiped dry with its own or its mother's shirt. After the ritual was completed, kabbalists would also whisper the names of angels into the patient's ear, while the water would be poured away into as many different corners of the house as possible—into the four corners of the room, over the door hinges, beneath the threshold, and into the oven—or taken out to a little-frequented place.[64]

talowa, 'The Evil Eye' (Yid.), 261; Shlaferman, 'The Folklore, Customs, and Stories of Kazimierz' (Yid.), 170; Friedlender, 'Jewish Life in the Shtetl' (Yid.), 126.

[63] Rosenberg, *Rafa'el hamalakh*, 49.

[64] *Segulot urefuot*, Bibliotheca Rosenthaliana, HS. ROS. 444, 6b; Rosenberg, *Rafa'el hamalakh*, 72; Segel, 'Wierzenia i lecznictwo', 58; Lilientalowa, *Dziecko żydowskie*, 51; ead., 'The Evil Eye' (Yid.), 258; Friedlender, 'Jewish Life in the Shtetl' (Yid.), 126–7; 'Obergloybns un folks-vertlekh', 327. Cf. Biegeleisen, *Lecznictwo ludu polskiego*, 241.

It went without saying that the patient should be quite literally cleansed of the influence of the evil eye. Methods for doing this included spitting or blowing in their face, usually three times, which was to be done ideally by a firstborn (usually a boy under 13 years of age, on an empty stomach).[65] Moszyński was of the opinion that this ritual spitting was similar to that of sucking out poison.[66] The child's face might also be wiped with another child's hand (usually likewise that of a firstborn son, three times), its mother's apron, or the inside of its own or its mother's wetted shirt (dashed with wine, spat on, or licked). For added efficacy if the curse was of a more serious nature, the item of clothing used to wipe the child should be appropriate to its gender.[67] Urine was also used as a rinse in some instances, as in the 'revulsion' method described in Chapter 11 above.[68] Another popular measure was to enact a traversing ritual by having the victim walk, step, or otherwise pass over a significant object or natural feature. Among such items or features cited in the Jewish sources were a ditch (filled with water),[69] a knife blade (if the evil eye had caused problems with walking),[70] and a trouser leg. Another method was to have the child walk between the legs of a firstborn (or better still, three firstborns in a row). Sometimes this ritual was carried out at a fork in the road or a crossroads,[71] and it might be accompanied by the licking of the child's forehead and spitting—in the town of Kazimierz on the Vistula, it was customary to spit three times to the left and three to the right.[72] Stepping over a child, in turn, could have negative consequences, inhibiting its growth. Anyone who did so by mistake should step back again.[73]

Smudging was widespread, and all manner of items with ritual significance were used: earth from beneath three thresholds, a splinter from the

[65] Segel [Schiffer], 'Alltagglauben', 273; id., 'Materyały do etnografii Żydów', 319; id., 'Wierzenia i lecznictwo', 60; Lilientalowa, 'Dziecko żydowskie', 152. Cf. Szukiewicz, 'Wierzenia i praktyki ludowe', 269; Talko-Hryncewicz, *Zarys lecznictwa ludowego*, 207.

[66] Moszyński, *Kultura ludowa Słowian*, 202.

[67] Segel, 'Wierzenia i lecznictwo', 60; Lilientalowa, 'Wierzenia, przesądy i praktyki', 151; ead., *Dziecko żydowskie*, 51; Sosnowik, 'Material on Jewish Folk Medicine in Belarus' (Yid.), 165; Yoffie, 'Popular Beliefs and Customs', 376.         [68] Segel, 'Wierzenia i lecznictwo', 60.

[69] Lilientalowa, 'Wierzenia, przesądy i praktyki', 151.

[70] Rosenberg, *Rafa'el hamalakh*, 45; Tarlau, 'Volksmedizinisches aus dem jüdischen Russland', 144; Lilientalowa, 'Dziecko żydowskie', 150; ead., *Dziecko żydowskie*, 47.

[71] The latter is described in Lilientalowa, 'The Evil Eye' (Yid.), 260.

[72] Shlaferman, 'The Folklore, Customs, and Stories of Kazimierz' (Yid.), 171.

[73] Fels, 'Zabobony lekarskie u Żydów', 4; Spinner, 'Zur Volkkunde', 96. Cf. Moszyński, *Kultura ludowa Słowian*, 283.

threshold of the synagogue, the front hooves of a goat, a 'devil's finger' (fossilized belemnite), an umbilical cord—which would have been kept and dried for this very purpose—and herbs used in incense intended for protection from demons.[74] On occasion the patient's scalp would be smeared with a clove of garlic prepared while reciting a conjuration based on the dialogue between the prophet Elijah and the she-demon Lilith.[75] In Belarus the victim would be given water containing crumbs from a thrice-scraped bread paddle to drink. The bread paddle was of immense magical significance in Slavic culture; it could protect the house from the hordes of lightning-wielding demons that inhabited the earth.[76] Some woman healers (Pol. *szeptucha*, whisperer) would cover their patient's head during the ritual, and when they began to suffocate, they would interpret this as a sign that the unclean forces were leaving the body.[77] Others would crush a spider over the patient's heart. Spiders were often associated with demons, and as such would be placed inside amulets made from nutshells, killed, or immobilized with wax ('As this spider is powerless to move, so let my enemies be powerless when they want to harm me').[78]

There were several types of incantation for warding off the evil eye, and each one functioned in a range of variants, none of which differed markedly from the basic form.[79] The simplest of them, which were relatively short and were usually pronounced while spitting, dispatched the charm to places that were inaccessible to humans. They adjured the misfortune to leave the immediate environment (the house, farmstead, or community) and relocate to any one of several places believed to be the home of unclean forces.[80]

---

[74] *Segulot urefuot*, Bibliotheca Rosenthaliana, HS. ROS. 444, 2*b*; Spinner, 'Zur Volkkunde', 96; Lilientalowa, 'Dziecko żydowskie', 151; ead., *Dziecko żydowskie*, 51; ead., 'The Evil Eye' (Yid.), 259–60.     [75] Rechtman, 'Some Customs and Their Folk Explanations' (Yid.), 261.
[76] Sosnowik, 'Material on Jewish Folk Medicine in Belarus' (Yid.), 165. The recommendation to eat bread as protection from being struck by lightning was probably an echo of this belief in Jewish medicine; Fayvushinski, 'The Folklore of Pruzhana' (Yid.), 200.
[77] Harkavy and Gesik, 'Medical Care in Our Town' (Heb.), 42.
[78] Segel, 'Wierzenia i lecznictwo', 60; id., 'Materyały do etnografii Żydów', 323; 'Omens and Remedies' (Yid.), 293–4.
[79] Basic actions and formulas for warding off charms were taught in traditional Jewish communities from childhood, at home, at school, and in the *beit hamidrash*. This 'education' in preventing the harm that could be done by the evil eye was given to both boys and girls, and was usually of an informal character. See Tuszewicki, 'Żydowska medycyna ludowa', 38.
[80] According to one interpretation, the Hebrew word *shed* (demon) denoted a creature that lived in the field (*sadeh*); see Sperling, *Ta'amei haminhagim oyf ivri taytsh*, ii. 11. On the subject of the relationship between *orbis interior* and *orbis exterior* (one's own, familiar, human space vs

In this respect there are clear and close parallels, if not relationships, between Yiddish phrases (*oyf puste felder un velder, in alde drerdn, in farlozene krenitses*; in deserted fields and woods, deep in the ground, in abandoned springs)[81] and Slavic ones ('Go into the hills, go into the woods, go to dry roots, where none can set foot'[82]). Lilientalowa recorded a rhyming formula to ward off charms, which began with the words *orene, vorene, dembene, korene, veytsene klayen* (*orene, vorene*, oak, rye, wheat bran),[83] and was very similar to that described by Yehudah Leyb Cahan: *Nie hore, nie more, nit veyts un nit klayen*.[84] In both versions there are evident borrowings from Slavic phrases such as *na góry, na bory* (into the hills, into the woods), which also feature in other Jewish sources in forms closer to the original (*Ny hory, ny bory, ny denbyny kory*[85] or *Nie hora nie bora nie kiki liki nie hora nie bora nie dzisiaj nie wczoraj*[86]). The Jewish extension *veytsene klayen* (wheat bran) in some of these rhymes may have been a consequence of a misinterpretation of the word *korzenie* (roots) (as the Yiddish word *korene* means rye). This example merely testifies to traces of the coexistence, in the catalogue of Jewish magical texts, of elements both vernacular and extrinsic; it does not offer any clues to the origins of folk exorcisms formulated in this way.

Among the most popular magical formulas, aside from the 'dialogues' between the prophet Elijah and Lilith, the angel Ashtruvi (also identified as Striga, a witch or Lilith herself), or the angel Dumah (the angel of silence), was a passage about three (more rarely two[87]) maidens (more rarely sisters,[88] or Jewesses[89]). Its distinguishing characteristic was the image of three women sitting (or standing) on a stone or at the pinnacle of a rock, one of whom said: '[he] has a hex' (or: '[he] is sick'); the second responded with 'no', and the third stated: '[it] will return whence [it] came' (or: '[he] is not, and will not be, sick'). This image calls to mind the conjuration banishing charms in which the leading roles were played by the three daughters of

foreign, unfamiliar, savage space) and its significance for east European folk culture, see e.g. Stomma, *Antropologia kultury wsi polskiej*, 82–4.

[81] Ganuzowicz (Ganuz), 'Methods and Charms for Banishing Fright' (Heb.), 219.

[82] See e.g. Kotula, *Znaki przeszłości*, 199, 423.

[83] Lilientalowa, *Dziecko żydowskie*, 56; ead., 'The Evil Eye' (Yid.), 268.

[84] Cahan, 'Parallels of Jewish Customs and Remedies' (Yid.), 277.

[85] Robinsohn, 'An ajen-hore oder Güt Auge' (Ger.), 20.

[86] Meler, *Besorot tovot*, 50.          [87] Fels, 'Zabobony lekarskie u Żydów', 2.

[88] The sisters figure in Yiddish variants recorded in manuscripts dating from around 1800; *Segulot urefuot*, Bibliotheca Rosenthaliana, HS. ROS. 444, *6a–6b*; *Segulot vekameyot*, JTS, MS 10082, *5b*.          [89] M. Kohen, *Leket haḥanukah*, 112.

St Ottilie (or St Sophia) in German and Polish folklore, and even has overtones of the persons of the Christian Trinity.[90] In the Jewish text the maidens are positioned on a rock, which to a certain degree reflects the biblical
scene in which Moses wrought miracles from an elevated mountain site.
One variant of the incantation seems to reinforce this impression, starting
as it does with the words: *In der midber shteyt a groyser shteyn, oyf im zitsn
dray vayber* (In the desert stands a great rock, and on it three women are
seated).[91] Moreover, in folk topology the rock (mountain) is a symbol of the
boundary between two worlds, on which figures with the power to perform
magic may have their seat.[92] The motif of a white rock in the middle of
the sea, or of rocks in a white sea, may be associated with the notion of the
centre of the world, and indeed functioned as such in Slavic folklore. It also
occurs in Jewish conjurations for banishing nosebleeds, another category of
ailment attributed to the evil eye.[93]

The next part of the passage about the three women took a variety of
forms. In the Yiddish version, as opposed to the Hebrew one, the text was
sometimes supplemented by a formula for banishing the evil eye 'into all
the empty fields, into all the empty woods, where people do not go, and
where wild animals live', or by spitting (three times) and yawning.[94] Some
wise women could tell from the type of yawn they emitted by the end of
the ritual whether the *ayn-hore-geber* had been a man or a woman.[95] The
Hebrew-language version, attributed to the tsadik Shmelke of Nikolsburg
(Mikulov), included a bid to reverse the charm and send it back to the person who had cast it: 'If it was a man who did the evil, may he lose the hair
from his head and beard; if it was a woman who did you wrong, may her
teeth fall out and her cheeks sink in.'[96] At the end, extra effect was added by
the use of biblical quotations connected with the descendants of Joseph
(Gen. 49: 22), water, and Miriam's wandering well (Exod. 15: 1, Num. 21:
17–20), which were preceded by the words: 'Just as the sea has no path, and
the fish in the sea do not fall ill, so too may nothing, neither weakness nor

[90] Biegeleisen, *Lecznictwo ludu polskiego*, 243.
[91] Fried, 'Volksmedizinisches und Diätetisches aus Ostgalizien', 168.
[92] Bartmiński (ed.), *Słownik stereotypów*, i. 356–7.
[93] Rosenberg, *Rafa'el hamalakh*, 104; Avida [Złotnik], 'Incantations and Remedies in Arabic
and Yiddish' (Heb.), 3. Cf. Bartmiński (ed.), *Słownik stereotypów*, 381–2.
[94] Lilientalowa, *Dziecko żydowskie*, 55; Rechtman, *Jewish Ethnography and Folklore* (Yid.),
293.                                   [95] Stern, 'A Translation School in Tishevits' (Yid.), 268.
[96] Lilientalowa, 'Dziecko żydowskie', 152.

the evil eye, cling to X.' In addition to some closing formulas (amen, *selah*, *netsaḥ va'ed*), magical names might also feature at this point, usually Agla[97] or Agaf Nagaf Sagaf.[98]

Another method of removing a charm was connected with the belief in the possibility of destroying something by counting it. The fear of counting people, discussed in both the written and the oral Torah, was ubiquitous in the folk culture of the Jews, and certainly influenced the customs of this community more strongly than it did those of their non-Jewish neighbours.[99] The conviction of the danger inherent in such ways of checking or controlling reality, like the fear of even numbers, had ancient roots. When the Creator made his covenant with Abraham, he assured him that he would have countless descendants (Gen. 13: 16; 15: 5). In the book of Exodus (30: 12) we read: 'When you take a census of the children of Israel according to their enrolment, each shall pay the Lord a ransom for himself on being enrolled, that no plague may come upon them by being enrolled.' In the second book of Samuel (24: 1–3), when God orders David to make a count of the nation, the king's nephew, Joab, is overcome with terror. These fears remained very real in the Ashkenazi world, and this was reflected in folk sayings such as *Az me tseylt nisht, kumt arayn di brokhe* (When you don't count, a blessing comes).[100] If a count was unavoidable for some reason, the Hebrew letters were usually used instead of numbers (*alef, beys, giml*), or the successive numbers were preceded by the word 'not' (*nisht-eyns, nisht-tsvey, nisht-dray*).[101] When teachers in Polish public schools counted their pupils, Jewish children would protect themselves from harm by whispering *Oyf di tseyn!* (On my teeth).[102] Counting was one element of various magic

---

[97] Rosenberg, *Rafa'el hamalakh*, 105; An-sky, 'Charm Reversals and Conjurations' (Yid.), 161; Lilientalowa, *Dziecko żydowskie*, 56.

[98] According to other sources, the three biblical quotations cited here made up the whole of the ritual, and these were recited over a mug of 'silent water', which at the end was given to the patient to drink and wash their face in, and the rest was poured out at a crossroads (and the mug placed under the patient's bed). On occasion these same quotations were also combined with the names of angels. See Plaut, *Likutei ḥever ben ḥayim*, 7b; *Tehilim im sefer mishpat tsedek*, 8a; Avida [Złotnik], 'Incantations and Remedies in Arabic and Yiddish' (Heb.), 6; Ganuz, 'Snippets of Jewish Folklore' (Heb.), 25.

[99] Country boys would tease Jewish children by counting them out loud and pointing at them; Lew, 'O lecznictwie i przesądach', *Izraelita*, 37, p. 316.

[100] Landau, 'Sprichwörter und Redensarten', 360.

[101] Lilientalowa, 'The Evil Eye' (Yid.), 249.

[102] 'Reminiscences: A Little Bit of Everything' (Yid.), 49. If a child was bored and had nothing to do, their mother would tell them to 'count [their] teeth'; Elzet [Złotnik], 'Some Jewish

formulas used against demons. It features, for instance, in a method for drawing out worms, known also to the Slavic population, which included a reference to the biblical Job.[103] In such cases the numbers were not preceded by negation; on the contrary, their use guaranteed the efficacy of the procedure.

According to An-sky, warding off the evil eye was more reminiscent of a sacred practice than the drawing out of illnesses, which was often performed in the local language. Texts used to lift charms were intended to resemble Hebrew prayers, and the ritual itself resembled a religious act.[104] An-sky's opinion would seem to be supported by the fact that numerous texts of conjurations are to be found in religious literature intended for Hebrew speakers. These formulas were reproduced in collections of works by rabbinic scholars and hasidic masters, and were also appended to prayer books, psalters, books of ethics, and other writings. Many such texts incorporated extensive quotations from the Bible and Aramaic phrases typical of yeshiva jargon, which was peppered with talmudic-style figures of speech. Removing charms was not only the domain of medical practitioners from the less educated strata of Jewish society; it was also practised by *soferim*, whose main line of work was writing and correcting sacred texts,[105] and by rabbis who devoted themselves to study,[106] not to mention hasidic leaders, for whom such forms of assistance were one of the duties they were expected to perform for their communities. One of the most popular conjurations was that by the above-mentioned Rabbi Azulai, which took the form of a kind of anti-litany: 'I expel you, all manner of evil eyes: black eye, heavy eye, narrow eye, wide eye, straight eye, crooked eye, eye of man, eye of woman, eye of mother and her daughter, eye of daughter-in-law and her mother-in-law, eye of young bachelor, old man's eye.'[107] The many versions invariably include the quotation from the book of Psalms (121: 4), 'See, the Guardian of Israel neither slumbers nor sleeps', and the statement

Customs' (Heb.), 376; Avida [Złotnik], 'Incantations and Remedies in Arabic and Yiddish' (Heb.), 5; Gilad, 'Wise Words' (Heb.), 146.

[103] *Segulot urefuot*, Bibliotheca Rosenthaliana, HS. ROS. 444, 7*b*. Cf. Talko-Hryncewicz, *Zarys lecznictwa ludowego*, 339; Vietukhov, *Zagovory*, 443.

[104] An-sky, 'Charm Reversals and Conjurations' (Yid.), 164.

[105] Sokołów, *My Father* (Yid.), 132. In Szydłowiec the local *sofer*, Zelikl, tackled erysipelas with pseudo-Latin formulas; Rosenzweig-Blander, 'Lifestyle, Customs, Remedies' (Yid.), 155.

[106] Fishteyn, 'Rabbi Ben-Tsiyon Fraylikh' (Yid.), 205; Belova, *Narodnaya magiya*, 118.

[107] Rechtman, *Jewish Ethnography and Folklore* (Yid.), 302.

that the eyes have no power, 'either by day or by night', over any one of the 248 members of the sufferer's body, nor over any of their 365 veins and other organs. One factor in the popularity of Rabbi Azulai's formula may have been the fact that some knowledge of Aramaic was necessary to recite it.

Samples of other popular conjurations with additional kabbalistic motifs would seem to confirm An-sky's thesis of the link between the sacred tongue and the magical potency ascribed to Hebrew incantations. An example attributed to the tsadik Menahem Mendl of Rymanów began with three repetitions of the following excerpt from the book of Psalms: 'As for me, may my prayer come to You, O Lord, at a favourable moment; O God, in Your abundant faithfulness, answer me with Your sure deliverance' (Ps. 69: 14). Next, one should address the Creator in Hebrew:

Ruler of the world, Lord of the names that were created from the verse 'But I, through Your abundant love, enter Your house; I bow down in awe at Your holy temple' [Ps. 5: 8], from the first letters and the last letters and the middle letters, expel the evil eye from X son/daughter of Y, amen. And may Your will be done, for I have acquired [in thought] all the intentions [*kavanot*] from Rav Huna, may he rest in peace.

This conjuration was to be said with one's face turned to the east, as an element of the morning prayers, without looking back, and placing one hand on the patient's head or forehead. After it was completed, or while saying it, the healer should yawn, and at the end wish the patient a full recovery (*tsu refue*).[108]

The examples given in various parts of this book clearly show that both women and men whose knowledge of Hebrew was poor did not hesitate to offer their services in curing the effects of the evil eye. At this point I will briefly mention one further type of conjuration, which involved an item associated unequivocally with women—the scarf. This was to be folded and wound around one finger, to the accompaniment of a 'negated count': 'not one, not two, not three' (and then the same count in reverse). Folds, like certain types of knots, were perceived in traditional culture as places inhabited by unclean forces, and smoothing or shaking out folds and counting

---

[108] Sperling, *Ta'amei haminhagim oyf ivri taytsh*, ii. 101; Berger, *Imrei yisra'el*, 13*b*; Rubinstein, *Zikhron ya'akov yosef*, 71*a*; Lilientalowa, 'The Evil Eye' (Yid.), 269. Slightly different variants are given in Rosenberg, *Rafa'el hamalakh*, 106–7; J. Ashkenazi, *Tsene urene fun harav hekhasid*, 3–4; Lilientalowa, *Dziecko żydowskie*, 57.

them was one way of neutralizing the power of a charm. In place of a Hebrew quotation here, a popular formula in Yiddish was used: 'Just as the evil eye had no power over Joseph, so may the evil eye have no power over X son/daughter of Y.'[109] Here the ambiguity characteristic of traditional culture renders it difficult to draw a clear distinction between sickness brought about by natural processes and that imposed by magic. In both cases, however, the role of the healer could be played by people without a religious education. The prayerful character of the conjurations for the evil eye described by An-sky was determined not by what was to be exorcized from the patient's body, but by who was performing the ritual. Devout rabbis and kabbalists tended to focus more on lifting charms than on curing illnesses, but in both fields they faced unscholarly competition.

[109]  Segel, 'Wierzenia i lecznictwo', 60.

CHAPTER FOURTEEN

# FRIGHT

OLK MEDICINE tended to credit strong emotions with having a significant influence on the physical aspects of human life. Death could
be caused by an overload of all types of passion, from fear to joy to desire.[1]
The phrases *Kh'gey oys fun libshaft* (I'm dying of love) or *fun benkshaft*
(of longing) reflected attitudes that were entirely absent from the ascetic
mindset of the rabbis, but any anthology of Jewish folk songs overflows
with them. In addition to such extreme examples, there are also numerous
illustrations of belief in the detrimental character of excessive emotions,
which was rooted in equal measure in natural and magical approaches to
traditional medicine. One should not sit down to a meal in a fury, or one
would suffer digestive problems.[2] Having sexual intercourse when angry or
scared could cause health issues in the child conceived from the act, such as
scrofula.[3] It was believed that if a husband gave his pregnant wife a fright,
their child would be prone to choking (*kaykhn zikh*), and would suffer in
other ways.[4] At least some of these convictions may be linked to rationalist
theories of the humours and temperaments.

Sources do not always indicate exactly what kind of experience is associated with a person acquiring this or that symptom. The strongest feeling
mentioned in this context was fear, an emotion that stimulates the most
primal mechanisms of our psyche and may result in shock or long-lasting
trauma. Fear was the reason for the belief in the dangerous consequences of
a fright—a term used to describe various forms of ailment usually caused by
a sudden, unexpected, and unpleasant encounter. In most cases the direct
triggers of the ailment were 'terrible' characters, animals, and demons.
However, fear was not the sole cause of such calamities. The innate greed of
the victim or their curiosity may also lead to situations no less hazardous

[1] Zelkovitsh, 'Death and Its Accompanying Moments' (Yid.), 156.
[2] Rosenberg, *Rafa'el hamalakh*, 12.
[3] Lilientalowa, *Dziecko żydowskie*, 21.
[4] Lilientalowa, 'Dziecko żydowskie', 144.

to both adults and children. The negative consequences of frightening experiences were treated primarily with the help of magical means—an important indication that this was a phenomenon that went beyond what was called 'natural'.

Like the Slavic population, Jews sometimes perceived crying in babies to come under the category of conditions brought on by unclean forces. Persistent crying for which it was difficult to find an evident reason gave rise to mythical explanations. And because children typically react to fear with tears, it seemed natural that their state could be caused by fear of unclean forces. This conviction was particularly strong in cases where the infant could not be soothed by any natural methods such as cuddling, blowing in the mouth, or giving it poppyseed infusion.[5] Among the methods believed to be effective for calming babies there were a vast number of 'anti-demonics', including amulets, biblical quotations (Isa. 30: 19; Pss. 8 and 9), sometimes used as accompaniments to other actions such as massaging with oil,[6] and remedies using anti-demonic ingredients (plasters with earth from beneath the threshold boiled in milk,[7] or bathing in a stock made from onions, garlic, and a comb, to be poured out at a crossroads after the procedure[8]). According to another method, which was based on the notion that disease entered the body from outside, the frightened child should be beaten with a switch, which was immediately thereafter to be discarded (as the cause of the complaint) by being thrown onto a passing cart or into the river.[9] Sacred books and a knife were placed under the pillow not only of women experiencing a difficult birth, but also of crying infants.[10] All these methods are clear evidence of the belief in the demonic aetiology of crying in babies. A similar type of belief applied to screaming babies. Known as *krikses* (from Blr. *kriksa*, raucous), they would be treated with methods familiar from the ethnography of the Slavs: as one person was cooking millet, a second was to ask her in Yiddish, from across the threshold: 'What are you cooking?' The answer, 'I'm cooking *krikses*', elicited the response: 'Then cook them well.' The whole dialogue was to be

---

[5] Lew, 'O lecznictwie i przesądach', *Izraelita*, 41, p. 395.

[6] Rosenberg, *Rafa'el hamalakh*, 42–3.

[7] *Segulot urefuot*, Bibliotheca Rosenthaliana, HS. ROS. 444, 1*b*.

[8] Segel, 'Materyały do etnografii Żydów', 327.

[9] Segel, 'Wierzenia i lecznictwo', 56; Lew, 'O lecznictwie i przesądach', *Izraelita*, 41, p. 395; Lilientalowa, 'Dziecko żydowskie', 149.

[10] Lew, 'O lecznictwie i przesądach', *Izraelita*, 41, p. 395.

repeated three times.[11] In one manuscript, an ailment referred to as *kriske* was listed among advice for treating epilepsy. A child suffering from this problem was to be soothed by having its face, hands, and feet washed in water that had run off the porch roof.[12]

A closer look at fright yields further interesting findings. Like in the case of the evil eye, its connection with children was strongly emphasized. In some instances both misfortunes would be tackled with the same types of action, one of which was to trickle sand around the outline of the child's hand.[13] Children have always been associated with innocence, and this was why it was they who usually fell victim to such afflictions. Their vulnerability to fright persisted more or less as long as the danger from the evil eye, that is, until religious maturity. Only boys born in the caul were free from the threat of fright, as well as from all natural forms of fear.[14] Fright caused by unclean forces was one reason for regularly checking the mezuzah.[15] Potential threats lurked everywhere from conception onwards, and the entire pregnancy was a sensitive period. In particular the mother's behaviour and what she experienced on her return from the *mikveh* would almost literally leave their mark on her child's health and appearance. If a woman experienced a fright, whatever the cause, she should not touch any part of her body with her hand; instead, she should keep both hands well away from her, for any site that she touched on her own body while under the influence of a fright would be marked on her child's body by a blemish. The most frequent cases of such problems occurred if she noticed a conflagration or other dangerous type of fire, which, according to folklore, would cause infantile eczema or 'firefeather' (*ogniopiór*, a red birthmark, especially on the face). Other, no less widespread, cautions warned against mice (or sometimes bears), which were said to cause hairy moles, also known as 'mice'. Even seemingly innocent things could have a detrimental effect if touched, such as raspberries, as they allegedly imprinted themselves on

[11] Rubinstein, *Zikhron ya'akov yosef*, 105*b*; Goldberg and Eisenberg, *Sefer laḥashim usegulot*, 6*a*. In the Polish sources *kryksa* denotes the *nocnica*, or night maiden, who robbed children (and *płaksy*, or 'cry-babies') of their calm and took the shrieking children themselves. Cf. Biegeleisen, *Matka i dziecko*, 272; Karłowicz, Kryński, and Niedźwiedzki (eds.), *Słownik języka polskiego*, ii. 584; Libera, *Medycyna ludowa*, 172.

[12] *Segulot urefuot*, Bibliotheca Rosenthaliana, HS. ROS. 444, 8*b*.

[13] Ganuz, 'Snippets of Jewish Folklore' (Heb.), 26.

[14] *Segulot urefuot*, JTS, MS 9862, 26. The caul (known as a 'cap' in Polish) also offered protection from fright; see the Vienna edition of the *Book of Medicaments* (Heb.), 29; Segel, 'Materyały do etnografii Żydów', 323.    [15] Lilientalowa, *Dziecko żydowskie*, 57.

the skin in a raspberry-coloured blemish (strawberry mark). Having been caused by magic, these birthmarks could be removed by adding three lumps of coal to the infant's first bath.[16]

In extreme cases, fright could even cause the deformation of the foetus and lead to it being born a humpback, a dwarf, with a limp, or as an animal. This was mainly the case when the cause of the deformation was linked to distracted staring. Because it was a common belief in patriarchal culture that curiosity was a trait typical of women, a pregnant woman's gaze was said to be characterized by insatiable desire, which inevitably affected the foetus in one way or another, particularly if her eyes rested on something terrifying. For this reason, it was widely believed that on leaving the *mikveh* before the child was even conceived she should turn her gaze heavenwards, and only lower her eyes once she was sure that she would see something pleasant.[17] Another form of protection from distracted gazing (and most likely also from fright) was for her to keep her right thumb hooked under her belt.[18]

Fright was also a standard explanation for rabies, and one that was prof-fered independently of other aetiologies, including the one according to which the disease was caused by the bite of a mad dog or wolf. The sympto-matic fear of water (hydrophobia) observed in those infected was attributed to the shock elicited by the bite. Sufferers were thought to perceive the shadows of little dogs in drinks offered them, and even, according to early modern medicine, to have nightmares of dogs barking and attacking them. It was thus recommended that the sufferer be given water through a funnel, in such a way that they could not see it.[19] Similar beliefs existed concern-ing wild dogs, especially wolves. In the latter case, fear seemed to play a fundamental role. Since ancient times wolves had been ascribed the power to render humans dumb—hence the advice in Jewish sources that a wolf will only flee from a human if it is the human who sees the wolf first and thus will not be taken by surprise; wolf tails were also worn as a form of protection.[20]

---

[16] Elzet [Złotnik], 'Some Jewish Customs' (Heb.), 362; Lilientalowa, 'Dziecko żydowskie', 143; Pulner, 'Obryadi i povirya', 104; Bastomski, *At the Source: Jewish Proverbs* (Yid.), 109; Lew, 'O lecznictwie i przesądach', *Izraelita*, 38. Cf. S. Udziela, 'Materiały etnograficzne', 84–5.
[17] Herzog and Zborowski, *Life Is with People*, 312–13.
[18] Lilientalowa, *Dziecko żydowskie*, 24.
[19] Hurwitz, *Sefer haberit* (Yid.), 59; Wilff, *Imrot shelomoh*, 69. Cf. *Compendium medicum*, 501.
[20] Segel, 'Materiały do etnografii Żydów', 323; Cf. Andrzej of Kobylin, *Gadki o składności*

Symptoms of fright were similar to the effects of the evil eye,[21] and like-wise the folk therapy was reminiscent of the procedures used to lift charms, and ranged from sluicing with water,[22] through smudging with *lulav*,[23] to throwing a piece of bread to a dog.[24] One sequence of actions, also known from Slavic sources[25] and undertaken whenever a victim of fright (usually a child) started to show symptoms, was particularly widespread. This was to spit or blow into the child's face three times, rip its shirt, or at least the hem of it, and give it three sips of water to drink.[26] Often it would also be made to urinate, probably in order to cleanse its body of the poison that had flooded it as a result of the fright.[27] Urinating on the shirt and then wiping the child's face with it might also serve as protection from the consequences of fright.[28] Another ubiquitous method was smudging with 'cobwebs taken from four corners'.[29] One specifically Jewish remedy was to encourage the victim—if male—to recite the Shema.[30]

In the case of fright, as in that of the evil eye, it was deemed important to find the source of the problem. Here too, the investigation involved the use of 'silent water', though lead or wax was usually used rather than coals, in a procedure known as pouring (*blay/vaks gisn*). According to instructions scattered across various ethnographic collections, a bowl of water would be placed by the patient's head or on their belly, and the substance would be melted on a teaspoon and poured over the twigs of a besom onto the surface of the water three times. The pouring action would be accompanied by a variety of magical formulas, often derived from the local language. One such formula was a Belarusian conjuration beginning with the words: 'A bee

---

*członków człowieczych*, 35. Some sources advised hanging 'a laurel branch or wolf's tooth and goat's beard' above the child's bed to ward off fright; Khotsh, *Segulot urefuot*, 9.

[21] e.g. convulsions; see Berger, *Imrei yisra'el*, 5a.

[22] *Segulot urefuot*, JTS, MS 9862, 93; Segel, 'Materyały do etnografii Żydów', 320.

[23] Lilientalowa, *Dziecko żydowskie*, 57.        [24] Segel, 'Materyały do etnografii Żydów', 320.

[25] See e.g. Wereńko, 'Przyczynek do lecznictwa ludowego', 210.

[26] Segel, 'Wierzenia i lecznictwo', 58; Lilientalowa, 'Wierzenia, przesądy i praktyki', 175; ead., 'Kult wody', 12; Bastomski, *At the Source: Jewish Proverbs* (Yid.), 114.

[27] Herzog and Zborowski, *Life Is with People*, 345. The speechlessness caused by wolves was also described as 'cold and poisonous air which comes to a person's mouth on the wind, and one draws it into oneself by breathing'; Andrzej of Kobylin, *Gadki o składności członków człowieczych*, 35.        [28] Segel, 'Materyały do etnografii Żydów', 320.

[29] Lilientalowa, 'Wierzenia, przesądy i praktyki', 175. Among Christians, the cobwebs were to be taken from the four corners of the cross; cf. Wereńko, 'Przyczynek do lecznictwa ludowego', 210.        [30] Herzog and Zborowski, *Life Is with People*, 345.

was flying over an open field, collecting wax.'[31] The shape formed by the substance when it cooled down (usually interpreted as a non-Jew, a dog, a horse, a cat, etc.), was an indication as to the source of the fright. According to a testimony from the town of Kazimierz on the Vistula, it was sufficient to show the child the shape for it to recover,[32] but the cure was not always this simple. After the performance of the ritual the water was to be poured out at a crossroads, and the bowl or glass that was used had to be placed under the patient's bed or cradle.[33] This image is supplemented by a description of wax-pouring from a nineteenth-century manuscript, which recommended the use of eight lots (4 oz) of lead and 'silent water'. The first melt was a preliminary measure; the metal was cooled rapidly and the angelic names Atina Batina written on its surface. It was then reheated, the patient was covered up from head to foot, and the molten metal poured onto the water three times, once above their head, once above the middle of their body, and once at their feet, to the accompaniment of the appropriate incantation (*Avginets ferdinets altar atar*). The vessel should then be left under the patient's bed for three days, and only after that time were its contents to be poured out at a crossroads.[34] A very similar custom, known also to the Slavs, was to encircle the patient's head three times with an egg, then break the shell and pour out the egg (sometimes over the twigs of a besom) into a bowl of water placed at the patient's head. After the source of the fright was identified, the water should be poured out over the fence.[35] If this ritual failed to produce the desired effect, the next recommended course of action was to obtain hairs from the person or dog that was the cause of the fright, and rub the victim with these or use them in a smudging ritual.[36]

The anthology *Rafa'el hamalakh* offered various methods of protection from sudden fright, all of them with their roots in biblical tradition. One of these was the recitation of Proverbs 3: 25: 'You will not fear sudden terror

[31] Maggid, 'Inoyazichniye zagavori', 585.

[32] Shlaferman, 'The Folklore, Customs, and Stories of Kazimierz' (Yid.), 172.

[33] Segel, 'Wierzenia i lecznictwo', 58; Lilientalowa, *Dziecko żydowskie*, 58; Ganuz, 'Snippets of Jewish Folklore' (Heb.), 25.

[34] *Segulot vekameyot*, JTS, MS 10082, 2*b*. The rhyming words of this magical incantation are reminiscent of pseudo-Latin conjurations in traditional European therapeutic magic and those for curing erysipelas.

[35] Segel, 'Wierzenia i lecznictwo', 58; Lilientalowa, 'Przesądy żydowskie', 320.

[36] Lilientalowa, 'Dziecko żydowskie', 152; Sosnowik, 'Material on Jewish Folk Medicine in Belarus' (Yid.), 164. Cf. Hovorka and Kronfeld (eds.), *Vergleichende Volksmedizin*, 686; Wereńko, 'Przyczynek do lecznictwa ludowego', 210.

or the disaster that comes upon the wicked', as well as eleven other Bible verses, all beginning and ending with the letter *nun*, to be followed by an excerpt from the prayers for the first day of the week (*ma'amadot*). The same source also recommended kosher amulets containing names, worn around the neck, or a *mezuzele* with the added words 'tear Satan apart'.[37] Another method that could help was wearing a pouch containing rue, belladonna, and the white excrement of a pigeon.[38]

To conclude the subject of fright, and the related problem of crying in children, it is worth taking a brief look at insomnia. The traditional Jewish community invested considerable effort in getting their offspring to sleep and keeping them asleep. Among the measures suggested for achieving this were not hanging nappies up to dry outside the house or in the attic, not leaving the confinement chamber too soon, not throwing the baby's bath water out, and not lending objects to anyone who did not live in the same home. In all of these cases, performing the action after dark was deemed particularly dangerous.[39] As a cure, tradition proposed a range of anti-demonic methods similar to those employed against the evil eye and fright, and in fact it sometimes treated sleeplessness as a clear symptom of these afflictions. In this context, a recommended remedy was to wind a lock of hair belonging to someone who was a frequent guest in the house—and hence the most likely source of the problem—around a piece of cloth and place it under the child's head.[40] Items sometimes placed under the pillow included a comb,[41] a linen pouch containing salt,[42] and even a set of objects which might comprise nine items made of iron, a Havdalah candle, and some hair from a female dog.[43] If the child's insomnia was thought to be caused by the evil eye, the recommended course of action was to circle it three times while holding salt in one's right hand, and then throw the salt into the oven.[44] Natural remedies were used in tandem with magic. The standard was poppyseed infusion, or application of a poppyseed compress with egg white or milk (also mother's milk) and a cereal (barley groats, oats, or wheat bread) to the forehead and temples.[45] The pulse or upper lip might

---

[37] Halpern, *Toledot adam*, 12; Rosenberg, *Rafa'el hamalakh*, 79.

[38] Rosenberg, *Rafa'el hamalakh*, 79.

[39] Segel, 'Wierzenia i lecznictwo', 56–7, 60; Lilientalowa, 'Dziecko żydowskie', 148–9.

[40] Segel, 'Wierzenia i lecznictwo', 56.          [41] Lilientalowa, *Dziecko żydowskie*, 39.

[42] Rosenberg, *Rafa'el hamalakh*, 91.          [43] *Refuot ha'am im darkhei yesharim*, 13.

[44] Lilientalowa, 'Wierzenia, przesądy i praktyki', 151; ead., *Dziecko żydowskie*, 51.

[45] Lilientalowa, *Dziecko żydowskie*, 39. In the nineteenth century white poppyseed oil mixed

be smeared with nutmeg oil,[46] water, and grated horseradish,[47] or with rose extract blended in the mother's milk.[48] Placing pine cones, or *shlofkepelekh* ('sleeping heads', recorded by Lilientalowa as *shlofepelekh*, 'sleep apples'), under or inside the child's pillow was also counted as a natural method of inducing sleep.[49]

with milk or another type of oil and given orally or laid on the temples was still in widespread use as a soporific; see *Refuot ha'am im darkhei yesharim*, 13; Schneersohn, *Sefer refuot*, 22–3. Empty poppyseed heads under the pillow were another insomnia remedy; Fayvushinski, 'The Folklore of Pruzhana' (Yid.), 201.

[46] *Refuot ha'am im darkhei yesharim*, 13; Cf. Haur, *Ekonomika lekarska*, 60.

[47] Sperling, *Ta'amei haminhagim oyf ivri taytsh*, ii. 107; Rosenberg, *Rafa'el hamalakh*, 91; *Segulot urefuot*, JTS, MS 9862, 111.     [48] Berger, *Imrei yisra'el*, 13a.

[49] Lilientalowa, *Dziecko żydowskie*, 39; 'Omens and Remedies' (Yid.), 297.

# CONCLUSION

IN THE UNITED STATES during the tragic Spanish influenza pandemic of 1918–19, Polish and Russian émigré peasants believed that cupping would protect them from death. In their search for specialists willing to perform these procedures they encountered complete bewilderment from American physicians, who had long since abandoned such methods and considered them relics of the distant past. It was Jewish barbers who eventually came to their aid: they not only knew how to perform cupping procedures, apply leeches, and let blood, but were also well aware of the significance of such auxiliary treatments.[1]

This brief anecdote—which I took from Moyshe Weissman's mid-twentieth-century Yiddish memoir—may be treated as a methodological pointer. Although it is not particularly detailed, and concerns a phenomenon that was observed on a continent distant from the centre of Ashkenazi culture, it tells us a lot about Jewish folk medicine and potential motifs to pursue in recreating and representing it. The beliefs and practices of the Jews of eastern Europe surrounding health issues and their treatment are a fascinating though difficult subject for research. On the one hand they are indicative of the richness of Ashkenazi culture, which sustained contact both with other centres of the diaspora and with the renascent national home in the Land of Israel. On the other, they offer proof of the impossibility of teasing out 'truly Jewish' elements from the mass of popular natural therapies, old women's cures, and therapeutic customs, theories, and magic. The body of questions that arise in the course of research in this field increases rather than decreasing. How should one approach folk medicine when the 'folk' population under study is not an essentially illiterate rural community dependent on the agricultural calendar? How should one interpret the presence in the therapeutic catalogue of procedures derived from ancient medical thought? The above story cited by Moyshe Weissman, despite not providing any clear answers, motivates us to strive for the fullest possible description of this aspect of Jewish life.

One of my fundamental intentions in working on the analyses which comprise this book was to recreate the picture of the folk medicine

[1] Weissman, *A Half-Century in America* (Yid.), 80–1.

practised by the Ashkenazim of eastern Europe around 1900: to showcase the plethora of health-related beliefs and practices current at that time both within the traditional Jewish community and in the host society. This undertaking necessitated the expansion of my perspective sufficiently to take account not only of uniquely Jewish approaches but also of others, influenced by the broader historical and social contexts of eastern Europe. At the same time, however, it was vital to find a cohesive method that permitted the clear examination of details while preserving the succinct character of both individual chapters and the book as a whole. In order to achieve all these aims, it proved necessary to go beyond the narrow understanding of 'folk-type medicine' to encompass the whole spectrum of convictions, views, methods, and actions considered crucial for health within the traditional world-view. This also meant employing a diverse catalogue of sources, not restricted to collections of folklore or stereotypical folk texts.

Jewish folk medicine represented a body of beliefs and practices many of which were known to the ethnography of both eastern Europe and its western, Slavic-Germanic borderlands. Around 1900 it was still firmly embedded in the tradition of early medicine, mixed with an attachment to a premodern mindset that sought supernatural explanations for the origins of disease and other afflictions. It was not distinguished by any one particular approach to health issues, nor did it draw exceptionally frequently on magic. It perpetuated a model of the treatment process in which the patient's own opinion played a central role, both with regard to the nature of the illness and in terms of the choice of remedy. In accordance with traditional norms, contact with a practitioner was only sought in extreme cases. Consultation with a variety of 'specialists' was accepted, and the scale and hierarchy of options (wise woman, medical orderly, quack healer, doctor, or tsadik) was not fixed. By the end of the nineteenth century even the most conservative Jewish circles had begun to open up to biomedicine. Previously this process had been hindered by a suspicion of new ideas and those who disseminated them, as they were associated with deviation from faith and tradition. From the 1880s onwards, however, printed material composed by authors with links to hasidism began to circulate which openly praised the work of 'professors', and even shared contemporary recommendations and prescriptions. Pharmacists, not necessarily Jewish, became important figures in the catalogue of practitioners, and in addition to supplying remedies they also offered advice and diagnosis. Journeys to large urban centres for hospital treatment, and to fashionable spa and health resorts, gradually became acceptable among the Orthodox.

The Jews of eastern Europe, like their Christian compatriots, perceived health to be a matter of vitality. In the folk imagination physical strength and robustness long remained inalienably associated with the absence of disease and with happiness; conversely, misery was synonymous with illnesses and a general susceptibility to them. The traditional Ashkenazi community sustained a belief in parallels or similarities connecting the human body (the microcosm) and the world (the macrocosm); it was this belief that formed the basis of their notions of the aetiology, symptoms, and treatment of diseases. The importance and depth of this layer of myth in the context of health are difficult to overestimate. The human body held associations with the earth, with plant life, with animals, and with all manner of man-made objects. Each relationship or connotation of this nature provided an angle from which to approach healthcare and take entirely rational and logical prophylactic or remedial action. If growth was linked to the waxing of the moon and dying with its waning, reservations about taking action at the time of the new moon or full moon acquired a new dimension. If a horse had patches of dry, scaly skin, contact with a place where it had been rolling was bound to carry the risk of contagion. At the same time, the Jews in this region also held views that had their roots in humoral pathology and astrology, in particular the belief in the influence of the seven planets. Visions of the structure and functioning of the world that originated in previous eras retained their currency thanks to the approval given to them in the rabbinic literature. Other ideas constituted a point of reference partly because of the popularity of works based on natural philosophy and partly because they replicated advice found in early modern and even ancient medicine, in particular the works of Hippocrates and Galen. In Ashkenazi folklore these beliefs had undergone popular simplification and interpretation processes, and there was often an interplay with myth.

Members of the traditional Jewish community were united in their views on sin and the belief in the ubiquity of demons, sorcery, and the evil eye, a legacy of previous generations. While from the twentieth-century perspective these may have seemed idiosyncratically Jewish, essentially they were not; they were in fact one of the last manifestations of a world-view that was intrinsic to the beliefs of all or many of the societies of premodern Europe. Jewish ethical literature, which continued to be a major source of influence, sustained this belief in the extrasensory sources of misfortunes afflicting the human body. In parallel with natural aetiologies, this discourse invariably painted a harsh picture of the severe judgements passed by the divine tribunal, which was nonetheless capable of granting mercy and healing to creation. Authors warned of the far-reaching consequences of violating the Torah commandments, and offered interpretations ranging from the perception of a direct relation between various aspects of human anatomy and the number of religious injunctions and prohibitions to visions of myriads of unclean beings. Indeed, the presence of demons was an inherent element of the folk world-view. Largely averse to humans and capable of wreaking harm and damage, they were nonetheless also bound by the rigours of the Law, and could on occasion prove important allies by helping a craftsman or bringing sudden wealth. Some illnesses and afflictions were also believed to be demonic in character, and were treated using magic or by trying to negotiate a mitigation of symptoms. Some, such as the heartworm or the *plica*, were so deeply invasive that any attempt to evict them from the body was considered more dangerous than resignation to a form of symbiosis.

The intrigues of sorcerers and the evil eye were also considered a significant threat, and much energy was expended on putting in place measures providing protection from misfortunes of this nature, and no less on their diagnosis and rectifying their consequences. The belief in witches was characterized by a certain ambivalence: while they were portrayed as invariably evil and malevolent, and the obligation to annihilate them was inferred from the Torah itself, those with the power to perform witchcraft were afforded considerable respect, and were sometimes treated as healers and quacks, or wise women and seers, who were equally capable of doing harm and of offering treatment. Those who were believed to cast the evil eye could not be assured of such balanced judgement, the more so because their victims were far more likely than in the case of enchantments to be infants and small children. In view of the supernatural character of these afflictions, magic was used as a way of alleviating the effects of both enchantment and the evil eye. The problems of inconsolable crying or screaming in babies, insomnia, and other similar issues were also linked in folk culture to the negative effects of the evil eye.

Jews' beliefs surrounding the treatment of illness were set apart from those of other populations of the region by the influence of Jewish religious and mystical tradition. This relationship was most in evidence in practices employing objects of cult or ritual, such as Passover matzah or the Sukkot *lulav* bundle. Cures of this type had a popular dimension, and were used irrespective of a given patient's experience of talmudic study or kabbalah. The religious tradition was sometimes drawn on directly, and it supplied elements of treatment rituals (such as quotations from psalms) and quite specific solutions to various health issues. The latter included kabbalistic manipulations using numerical techniques and sacred names, but also natural recommendations based on views regarding the correspondence of the microcosm and the macrocosm found in the rabbinic literature from the Talmud onwards. Naturally, access to these methods and treatments required at least a good knowledge of Hebrew, and in some cases also the skill of writing or calligraphy (for amulets).

A broad treatment of the subject of Jewish folk medicine is of greater than merely educational value. Because health-related notions and actions cannot be separated from the overall world-view to which a person or social group subscribes, they can serve as a type of sounding mechanism enabling us to plumb the fullness of Ashkenazi culture. We cannot research folk medicine without also mentioning what are ostensibly unrelated matters, such as Jewish ritual life, astrology, and ethics. The aetiologies of misfortunes besetting the body, the circumstances of their intensification or abatement, and more or less efficacious ways of combating them—all these were the combined products of factors rooted in very different and seemingly unrelated areas of culture. Of course the subjects of health and sickness are the central focus of this work, but through them we are able to access details of the Ashkenazi world-view of which we were previously unaware, or whose significance was previously underestimated.

A close examination of that dimension of Jewish culture connected with physicality and health reveals important details of intercultural contact, above all aspects of the relations between the Jews and their predominantly Slavic environment. It offers proof of the existence of a broad shared heritage, which had, in some areas, grown out of the same roots, and was, in others, the outcome of mutual influence. The purpose of the observations recorded in this book was not to cast doubt on the distinctness of the Jews as a religious and ethnic group. Nonetheless, the numerous parallels and testimonies to the intermingling of cultures offer proof of strong links between the Jewish community and the other groups inhabiting the same region, and more widely with the societies of the countries into which the unexpected turns of history had flung them. The members of An-sky's ethnographic expedition in the 1910s were astonished by the fact that, despite the Jews' considerable ignorance of and antipathy towards the non-Jewish world, it was such an important point of reference in terms of folk medicine.[2] This seems the more understandable in light of the fact that Jews had for centuries been active participants in the medical culture of Europe, which was reflected in their relations with both its elite strata and the wider populace. Historical research has confirmed, for example, the presence of Jewish physicians at east European royal and aristocratic courts, and of increasing numbers of Jews in the medical departments of Russian and Austrian universities in the nineteenth century. Little has been written in the context of health on the subject of contacts between the lower strata of Jewish society and neighbouring groups. Yet the sources reveal that such contacts were far from rare, and were sufficiently diverse in character as to warrant more detailed distinction than the collective categories 'influences' or 'borrowings'.

There were a number of important though not always appreciated factors that smoothed and promoted relations between Jewish and Christian inhabitants of the provinces. Notwithstanding the relatively high level of literacy within the Jewish community, a considerable proportion of its members could read only prayer books or were entirely illiterate. Historians (such as Yohanan Petrovsky-Shtern) have noted that this was to a large degree an oral culture, and in this it did not differ much from its environment. The question of language and employment may be approached from a similar angle. The traditional Jewish community in eastern Europe was primarily Yiddish-speaking until the 1930s, but any knowledge of the local and official languages was useful, and, if not sufficient for direct communication, it was at least enough for the negotiation of an intermediate 'dialect'. Jewish society maintained lively trade relations with the Slavic (or, where relevant, Romanian and Lithuanian) residents of the countryside. There was also a broad spectrum of other forms of interaction: wealthier Jews would employ Christian domestic staff and farmhands, while poorer ones became door-to-door artisans, farmers, shepherds, smugglers, and in extreme cases even members of mixed-religion robber bands. The Jewish

[2] Rechtman, *Jewish Ethnography and Folklore* (Yid.), 294.

districts of larger towns and cities might seem to have functioned as en-
claves, meeting almost all the needs of their residents with minimum cause
for engagement with the wider environment, yet these same cities also
attracted people from the provinces, who in this period on the threshold of
modernity were to form a dynamic, multi-ethnic proletariat.

Taking a broad approach to the issue of folk medicine facilitates a more
confident discussion of those elements of east European folk medicine
which did not, or at least not entirely, have their roots in myth. Perhaps,
as we rediscover the importance of Jewish artisans for rural culture, we
should think about re-examining the question of how Jews functioned in
the context of rural healthcare, for they were a major presence, not only as
Others—quack healers, and holy rabbis who were approached for help
in expectation of remedies involving magic—but also as barber-surgeons
and feldshers, innkeepers and door-to-door salesmen, and practitioners
of many other trades who were also capable of setting broken limbs, admin-
istering natural remedies, and even recommending procedures invested
with the authority of early medicine. The consequences of the importance
in Jewish circles of vademecums and other medical publications that drew
on medieval and early modern thought, and of the Jews' widespread activity
as barber-surgeons, almost certainly extended beyond the boundaries of
their own community. The role of the Jews in the overall mosaic of east
European treatment modes and methods is thus unlikely to have been
limited to the reproduction of models sourced from kabbalah or gematria,
or of Hebrew magic formulas.

# BIBLIOGRAPHY

## ARCHIVAL SOURCES

**Biblioteka Publiczna Miasta Stołecznego Warszawy, Spuścizna Reginy Lilientalowej (Warsaw Public Library, Papers of Regina Lilientalowa)**

*Choroby, lecznictwo* [Sicknesses, Treatment], acc. no. 2377.1.5.1.
*Coitus, ciąża, poród* [Coitus, Pregnancy, Birth], acc. no. 2375 A.2.
*Kult ognia u starożytnych Hebrajczyków i szczątki tego kultu u współczesnego ludu żydowskiego* [The Cult of Fire among the Ancient Hebrews and the Vestiges of that Cult in the Contemporary Jewish Folk], acc. no. 2375.A.4.
*Obrzędy pogrzebowe* [Funeral Rites], acc. no. 2377.1.2.1.
*Śmiecie* [Debris], acc. no. 2377.1.1.
*Ziemia w wierzeniach żydowskich* [Earth in Jewish Beliefs], acc. no. 2375.A.10.
*Złe duchy* [Evil Spirits], acc. no. 2377.1.9.2.

**Bibliotheca Rosenthaliana, Amsterdam**

*Segulot urefuot* [Remedies and Medicaments], HS. ROS. 444.

**Jewish Theological Seminary, New York (JTS)**

*Segulot urefuot* [Remedies and Medicaments], JTS, MS 9862.
*Segulot vekameyot* [Remedies and Amulets], JTS, MS 10082.

**Żydowski Instytut Historyczny (Jewish Historical Institute, Warsaw)**

GOLDSTEIN, YONAH, *Halikhot olam*, Warsaw, ŻIH, MS no. 73.
SZYMON BEN ABRAHAM Z DZIWIENISZEK, *Varia*, Warsaw, ŻIH, MS no. 771.

## PRINTED SOURCES

'65-year-old Jewish woman who treated patients with traditional remedies charged with conducting treatment without diploma' (Yid.), *Haynt*, 297 (1931), 5.
AARON BERAKHYAH OF MODENA, *Ma'avar yabok* (Vilna, 1895/6).
ABRAHAMS, BERNARD, *My Seventy Years: An Autobiography* [Mayne zibetsik yor. Otobiografye] (Johannesburg, 1953).
AGNON, SHMUEL YOSEF, *The Bridal Canopy*, trans. I. M. Lask (Syracuse, NY, 2000).

AKALOVICH, ELENA, 'Zamietki o yevrieiskoy narodnoy demonologii (po materi-alam folklora na idishe)', in Olga Belova et al. (eds.), *Mezhdi dvuma mirami* (Moscow, 2002), 136–62.

AKERMAN, MENDL, *Oysgeloshene shtern* (Buenos Aires, 1960).

ALFABET, F., 'Material for the Study of Idiom from the Town of Piaski, Lublin Region' (Yid.), *Yidishe filologye*, 1 (1924), 61–72.

ALLERHAND, MAURYCY, 'Przysięga kobiety ciężarnej u Żydów' [The Vow Taken by the Pregnant Woman among the Jews], *Lud*, 4 (1898), 180–4.

ALMI, A. [ELIOHU CHAIM SHEPS], *A Reckoning and Summary: Chapters from the Book of My Life* [Khezhbn un sakh-akl: kapitlen fun mayn seyfer hakhayim] (Buenos Aires, 1959).

ALTMANN, ALEXANDER, 'Astrology', *Encylopaedia Judaica* (Detroit, 2007), ii. 616–20.

*A naye shas tkhine* (New York, 1942).

ANDRZEJ Z KOBYLINA, *Gadki o składności członków człowieczych* [Words on the Composition of the Parts of the Human Body] (Kraków, 1893).

AN-SKY, S., 'Charm Reversals and Conjurations of the Lithuanian-Ruthenian Jews' (Yid.), in id., *Collected Writings*, xv. 153–67.

—— *Collected Writings* [Gezamlte shriftn], 15 vols. (Vilna, 1922–5).

—— 'Khane the Cook' (Yid.), in id., *Collected Writings*, vii. 7–58.

—— 'A Letter from the Other World' (Yid.), in id., *Collected Writings*, viii. 81–119.

—— *The Yiddish Ethnographic Programme* [Dos yidishe etnografishe program] (Petrogrod, 1914).

*Apteka domowa i podróżna doznawana lekarzami* [The Domestic and Travelling Medicine Chest as Advised by Physicians] (Leipzig, c.1810).

ARAMA, ISAAC, *Akedat yitshak* (Lemberg, 1868).

ARENDS, JOHANNES, *Volkstümliche Namen der Drogen, Heilkräuter, Arzneimittel und Chemikalien* (Berlin, 2005).

ASHKENAZI, JACOB, *Tsene urene* (Yid.) (Vilna, 1889).

—— *Tsene urene fun harav hekhasid mahar'r yitshak zal mik'k yanov im hosafot rabot* (n.p., n.d., early 20th c.); unpaginated.

ASHKENAZI, SOLOMON, 'The Evil Eye' (Heb.), *Yeda am*, 22 (1984), 100–11.

*Atarat tsadikim* (Warsaw, 1925/6).

AUERBACH, ISRAEL MATITYAHU, *Shomer yisra'el* (Sighet, 1939).

AXENFELD, ISRAEL, *The Kerchief* [Dos shterntikhl] (Buenos Aires, 1971).

AYZLAND, REUVEN, 'In the City of Torah Scrolls' (Yid.), in Itshok Turkov-Grudberg and Hilel Harshoshanim (eds.), *Radomyśl Wielki and Its Surroundings. Memorial Book* [Groys radomishle un svive, izker-bukh] (Tel Aviv, 1971).

AYZNBUND, MOYSHE, *The Jews of Nesvizh: Stories* [Niesvizher yidn, dertseylungen] (Melbourne, 1965).

BAKON, HAYIM DAVID, 'Life of the Holy Rabbi Mordkhe David of Dąbrowa' (Heb.), *Kerem hahasidut*, 3 (1986), 65–86.

—— *The Rabbi of Sieniawa* [Der shinover rov] (New York, 1987).

BAŁABAN, MAJER, *Dzieje Żydów w Galicyi i w Rzeczypospolitej Krakowskiej 1772–1868* [A History of the Jews in Galicia and in the Kraków Republic 1772–1868] (Lwów, 1916).

—— *Żydzi w Krakowie i na Kazimierzu* [The Jews in Kraków and Kazimierz], 2 vols. (Kraków, 1936).

BALAKIRSKY KATZ, MAYA, 'Rebbishe Representation: Pre-War Polish Photography of Hasidic Leaders', in Jerzy Malinowski, Renata Piątkowska, and Tamara Sztyma-Knasiecka (eds.), *Jewish Artists and Central-Eastern Europe* (Warsaw, 2010), 363–70.

BANASIEWICZ-OSSOWSKA, EWA, 'Warunki życia i stan zdrowia Żydów polskich w świetle czasopism polskich i żydowskich z drugiej połowy XIX i pierwszej połowy XX wieku' [The Living Conditions and Health of the Polish Jews as Reflected in Polish and Jewish Periodicals of the Second Half of the Nineteenth and First Half of the Twentieth Centuries], in Bożena Płonka-Syroka and Andrzej Syroka (eds.), *Studia z dziejów kultury medycznej: Życie codzienne w XVIII–XX wieku i jego wpływ na stan zdrowia ludności* [Studies in the History of Medical Culture: Daily Life in the Eighteenth to the Twentieth Centuries and Its Effect on the State of Public Health] (Wrocław, 2003), 234–45.

BANDTKIE, JERZY SAMUEL, *Nowy słownik kieszonkowy polsko-niemiecko-francuzki* [A New Pocket Polish-German-French Dictionary] (Wrocław, 1827).

BANK, C., 'Reb Yoysef Glikman' (Yid.), in Avraham Levita (ed.), *The Brzozów Memorial Book* [Sefer zikaron kehilat breziv (bzhozov)] (n.p., 1984), 221.

BARILAN, YECHIEL MICHAEL, *Jewish Bioethics: Rabbinic Law and Theology in their Social and Historical Contexts* (New York, 2014).

BAR-ITZHAK, HAYA, 'Introduction: Folklore and Jewish Folklore', in Raphael Patai and Haya Bar-Itzhak (eds.), *Encyclopedia of Jewish Folklore and Traditions* (New York, 2013), pp. xiii–xvi.

BARTMIŃSKI, JERZY (ED.), *Słownik stereotypów i symboli ludowych* [Dictionary of Stereotypes and Folk Symbols], 2 vols. (Lublin, 1996–2017).

BARUKH OF SHKLOV, *Derekh yesharah* (The Hague, 1779).

BASTOMSKI, SHLOYME, *At the Source: Jewish Proverbs, Maxims, Sayings, Expressions, Comparisons, Blessings, Wishes, Swearwords, Curses, Signs, Remedies, Superstitions, and Others* [Bam kval: yidishe shprikhverter, vertlekh, glaykhvertlekh, rednsartn, farglaykhenishn, brokhes, vintshenishn, kloles, kharomes, simonim, zgules, zabobones, un andere] (Vilna, 1920).

BAUMGARTEN, JEAN, *Introduction to Old Yiddish Literature*, ed. and trans. Jerold C. Frakes (Oxford, 2005).

BEILIN, S., 'Jüdische Sprichwörter und Redensarten aus Russland', *Mitteilungen zur Jüdischen Volkskunde*, 3 (1910), 131–9.

—— 'Sprichwörter und Redensarten aus Russland', *Mitteilungen zur Jüdischen Volkskunde*, 1 (1910), 39–40.

BELOVA, OLGA, 'Narodnaya magiya v regionakh etnokulturnikh kontaktov slavian i yevrieyev', in Olga Belova et al. (eds.), *Narodnaya meditsina i magiya* (Moscow, 2007), 110–36.

—— and VLADIMIR PETRUKHIN, 'Demonologicheskiye syuzheti v krosskulturnom, in Olga Belova et al. (eds.), *Mezhdi dvuma mirami* (Moscow, 2002), 196–216.

BEN-AMOS, DAN, and DOV NOY (eds.), *Folktales of the Jews*, vol. ii (Philadelphia, 2007).

—— and JEROME MINTZ, *In Praise of the Baal Shem Tov: The Earliest Collection of Legends about the Founder of Hasidism* (New York, 1970).

BENCZER, BENJAMIN, 'Jüdische Volksmedizin in Ostgalizien', *Am Ur-Quell*, 4 (1893), 120–1.

—— 'Volkglaube galizischer Juden', *Am Ur-Quell*, 4 (1893), 273–4.

BENET, MEIR, *Sheloshah sefarim niftaḥim . . . likutei me'ir* (New York, 1958/9).

BEN-EZRA, AKIVA, 'Customs' (Yid.), in Akiva Ben-Ezra (ed.), *Horodets: History of a Town* [Horodets: a geshikhte fun a shtetl] (New York, 1949), 172–6.

—— 'The Book of Psalms—A Book of Remedies' (Heb.), *Yeda am*, 24 (1988), 54–8.

BENIN, STEPHEN D., 'A Hen Crowing Like a Cock: "Popular Religion" and Jewish Law', *Journal of Jewish Thought and Philosophy*, 8 (1999), 261–81.

BERGER, MEIR, *Imrei yisra'el* (Sasfala, 1911/12).

BERGMAN, MOSES AARON, *Ma'asiyot nora'im* (Piotrków, 1913/14).

BERGMAN, SAMUEL HUGO, 'The Tsadik of Wolnica (a Hasidic Tale from Przemyśl)' (Yid.), in Aryeh Mencher (ed.), *The Book of Przemyśl* [Sefer pshemishl] (Tel Aviv, 1964), 490–1.

BERGMAN, YEHUDAH, *Jewish Folklore: The Folk Knowledge, Faith, Character, and Customs of the People of Israel* [Hafolklor hayehudi: yedi'at am yisra'el, emunotav, tekhunotav uminhagav ha'amamiyim] (Jerusalem, 1953).

BERGNER, HINDE, *In the Long Winter Nights* [In di lange vinternekht] (Montreal, 1946).

BERLIN, ADELE, and MARC ZVI BRETTLER (eds.), *The Jewish Study Bible* (Oxford, 1985).

BERLINSKI, S., *The First Generation* [A dor fun breyshis] (Munich, 1947).

BERNSTEIN, AARON, *Bernstein's Popular Books on the Natural Sciences* [Bernsteins natur-visnshaftlekhe folks-bikher], 21 vols. (London, 1910).

BERNSTEIN, BEN-ZVI, *Memories and Personalities* [Zikhroynes un geshtaltn] (London, 1962).

BERNSTEIN, G., 'Expressions and Proverbs from Rizhin' (Yid.), *Yidishe Shprakh*, 23 (1963), 54.

BERNSTEIN, IGNATZ, *Jewish Proverbs and Sayings* [Yidishe shprikhverter un rednsartn] (Warsaw, 1908).

BERNSTEIN, MORDECAI, 'Two Remedy Books in Yiddish from 1474 and 1508', in Raphael Patai, Francis Lee Utley, and Dov Noy (eds.), *Studies in Biblical and Jewish Folklore* (Bloomington, 1960), 289–305.

BIEGELEISEN, HENRYK, *Lecznictwo ludu polskiego* [Polish Folk Medicine] (Kraków, 1929).

—— *Matka i dziecko w zwyczajach, obrzędach i praktykach ludu polskiego* [The Mother and Child in the Customs, Rites, and Practices of the Polish Folk] (Lwów, 1927).

BILU, YORAM, 'The Taming of the Deviants and Beyond: An Analysis of "Dybbuk" Possession and Exorcism in Judaism', in Matt Goldish (ed.), *Spirit Possession in Judaism: Cases and Contexts from the Middle Ages to the Present* (Detroit, 2003), 41–72.

—— and BENJAMIN BEIT-HALLAHMI, 'Dybbuk-Possession as a Hysterical Symptom: Psychodynamic and Socio-Cultural Factors', *Israeli Journal of Psychiatry and Related Sciences*, 3 (1989), 138–49.

BIN WOLF, GANIA, 'Memories from My Father's House' (Heb.), *Yeda am*, 17 (1974), 149–50.

BLOCH, JOSEF SAMUEL, *Erinnerungen aus meinem Leben* (Vienna, 1920).

BLUMENFELD, L., 'Characters from Bygone Days' (Yid.), in Zvi Yashiv, *Olkusz (Elkish): Memorial Book of a Community Annihilated in the Holocaust* [Sefer zikaron likehilah shehukhḥadad basho'ah] (Tel Aviv, 1972), 240–8.

BLUMENTAL, NAKHMEN, *Reminiscences* [Tsurikblikn], (Tel Aviv, 1973).

BODEK, MENAHEM MENDEL, *Mifalot hatsadikim* (Lublin, 1927).

BOHAK, GIDEON, *Ancient Jewish Magic: A History* (Cambridge, 2008).

*Booklet on the Use of Psalms* [Kuntres shimush tehilim] (Łódź, 1931).

BOS, GERRIT, 'Ḥayyim Vital's Practical Kabbalah and Alchemy: A 17th Century Book of Secrets', *Journal of Jewish Thought and Philosophy*, 4 (1994), 55–111.

BRIKMAN, PLATIEL, 'Jewish Charitable Institutions in the Town' (Yid.), in M. S. Geshuri and Gershon Zilberberg (eds.), *The Book of Ostrowiec: In Memory and Testimony* [Sefer Ostrovtse: lezikaron ule'edut] (Tel Aviv, 1971), 227–8.

BROD, A., 'Judendeutsche Sagen und Schnurren', *Der Urquell*, 1 (1897), 344–6.

BRÜCKNER, ALEKSANDER, *Literatura religijna w Polsce średniowiecznej* [Religious Literature in Medieval Poland] (Warsaw, 1902).

BUCHBINDER, AVROM YITSHOK, 'Jewish Omens (Zabobones)' (Yid.), *Hoyz-fraynd*, 2 (1909), 249–58.

BUCK, MICHAEL RICHARD, *Medicinischer Volksglauben u. Volksaberglauben aus Schwaben* (Ravensburg, 1865).

BUCZKOWSKI, ADAM, *Społeczne tworzenie ciała: Płeć kulturowa i płeć biologiczna* [The Social Creation of the Body: Cultural Gender and Biological Gender] (Kraków, 2005).

BURTON, ROBERT, *The Anatomy of Melancholy* (London, 1838).

CAHAN, YEHUDAH LEIB, *The Jew on Himself and Others in His Proverbs and Sayings* [Der yid vegn zikh un vegn andere in zayne shprikhverter un rednsartn] (New York, 1933).

—— 'Jewish Folk Tales (Gathered from Oral Testimonies)' (Yid.), *Pinkes*, 1 (1927/8), 217–34.

—— 'Parallels of Jewish Customs and Remedies' (Yid.), in Y. L. Kahan, *Studies in Jewish Folklore* [Shtudies vegn yidisher folksshafung] (New York, 1952), 275–8.

—— ['Production and Reproduction in Folklore'] (Yid.), in id., *Studies in Jewish Folklore* [Shtudies vegn yidisher folksshafung] (New York, 1952), 222–7.

CH., 'Materiały do etnografii Żydów polskich' [Material for the Ethnography of the Polish Jews], *Lud*, 4 (1898), 436–8.

CHAJES, JEFFREY HOWARD, *Between Worlds: Dybbuks, Exorcists and Early Modern Judaism* (Philadelphia, 2011).

'Characters Among the Jews of Gliniany' (Yid.), in Henokh H. Halpern (ed.), *The Gliniany Scroll: Reminiscences and Experiences from an Annihilated Community* [Megiles Gline: zikhroynes un iberlebungen fun a khorev gevorener kehile] (New York, 1950), 169–84.

CHARAP, J. A., 'Sprichwörter galizischer Juden', *Am Ur-Quell*, 4 (1893), 212–13.

—— 'Zum Volksglauben der Juden in Polen', *Am Ur-Quell*, 3 (1892), 18–19.

CHMIELNICKI, M., 'Y. L. Peretz's Popular Medical Brochure' (Yid.), *YIVO bleter*, 28 (1946), 146–53.

*Compendium medicum auctum to iest krótkie zebranie i opisanie chorób* [*Compendium medicum auctum* i.e. a Concise Collection and Description of Illnesses] (Częstochowa, 1789).

CRATO, JOHANNES, *Johannis Cratonis . . . ausserlesene Artzney-Künste vor alle des menschlichen Leibes Zufälle, Gebrechen und Kranckheiten* (Frankfurt am Main, 1690).

CULPEPER, NICHOLAS, *Culpeper's Complete Herbal* (London, 1814).

DAN, DEMETER, 'Die Juden in der Bukowina', *Zeitschrift für Österreichische Volkskunde*, 7 (1901), 169–79.

DAN, JOSEPH, 'Raziel, Book of', *Encyclopaedia Judaica* (Detroit, 2007), xvii. 129.

DANZIG, ABRAHAM, *Ḥokhmat adam* (Jerusalem, 1967/8).

DAVID BEN ARYEH LEIB, *Sod hashem* (Berlin, 1708/9); unpaginated.

DIK, AYZIK MEYER, *Old Jewish Sayings* [Alte yidishe zogn] (Vilna, 1876).

DIMOND, BENJAMIN, 'Reminiscences and Historical Research' (Yid.), in Benjamin Dimond (ed.), *Husiatyn: The Podolia Guberniya* [Husiatin: podolier gubernie] (New York, 1968), 5–42.

DINARI, NATAN, 'When Jewish Zelów was alive' (Yid.), in Avraham Klushiner (ed.), *Memorial Book of the Zelów Community* [Sefer zikaron likehilat zelov] (Tel Aviv, 1976), 115–25.

DIOSCORIDES, *De materia medica*, trans. Tess Anne Osbaldeston, 5 vols. (Johannesburg, 2000).

DUNDES, ALAN, 'The J. A. P. and the J. A. M. in American Jokelore', *Journal of American Folklore*, 98 (1985), 456–75.

—— 'Wet and Dry, the Evil Eye', in Alan Dundes (ed.), *The Evil Eye: Casebook* (Madison, Wis, 1992), 257–312.

DYNNER, GLENN, *Men of Silk: The Hasidic Conquest of Polish Jewish Society* (New York, 2006).

DŹWIGOŁ, RENATA, *Polskie ludowe słownictwo mitologiczne* [Polish Folk Mythological Vocabulary] (Kraków, 2004).

EIN, AVRAHAM, 'The Town of Sislevitsh' (Yid.), *YIVO bleter*, 24 (1944), 47–66.

EINHORN, SHIMON, 'Folk Proverbs' (Heb.), *Reshumot*, 5 (1927), 338–48; 6 (1930), 398–407.

—— 'Folk Proverbs in Yiddish' (Heb.), *Reshumot*, NS 5 (1953), 196–208.

ELIASBERG, YEHUDAH BETSALEL, *Marpe le'am*, Part I (Vilna, 1834).

ELIOR, RACHEL, *Dybbuks and Jewish Women in Social History, Mysticism and Folklore* (Jerusalem, 2011).

EMIOT-GOLDWASSER, Y., 'Reb Mordecai Leyb Goldwasser z'l (Grandfather and Healer)' (Yid.), in Aba Gordin, M. Gelbart, and Aryeh Margalit (eds.), *Memorial Book of the Ostrów Mazowiecka Community* [Sefer zikaron likehilat ostrov-mazovietsk] (Tel Aviv, 1960), 209.

EPSTEIN, LISA, 'Caring for the Soul's House: The Jews of Russia and Health Care 1860–1914', Ph.D. diss. (Yale University, 1995).

ESTERZON, S. [SHEMUEL ASHKENAZI], *500 Rhyming Proverbs and Sayings* [500 gegramte shprikhverter un rednsartn] (Jerusalem, 1962/3).

ETKES, IMMANUEL, *The Besht: Magician, Mystic, and Leader* (New York, 2005).

*Ets ḥayim vehu sefer kitsur shenei luḥot haberit* (Vilna, 1889).

EVEN, ISAAC, *From the World of Hasidic Leaders* [Fun der gut-yidisher velt] (New York, 1917).

FARBER, J., 'Folk Healing' (Yid.), in Akiva Ben-Ezra (ed.), *Horodets: A History of the Town* [Horodets: a geshikhte fun a shtetl] (New York, 1949), 178–80.

FAYVUSHINSKI, A., 'The Folklore of Pruzhana' (Yid.), in Mordkhe W. Bernstein and Dovid Forer (eds.), *Pinkas Pruzhana, Bereze, Maltsh, Shershev, Selts: Their Establishment, History, and Destruction* [Pinkes pruzhene, bereze, maltsh, shershev, selts: zeyer oyfkum, geshikhte un umkum] (Buenos Aires, 1958), 199–205.

FELS, IZRAEL, 'Zabobony lekarskie u Żydów' [Medical Superstitions among the Jews], *Wschód*, 31 (1906), 2–6.

FENSTER, HERSH, 'Characters from the Shtetl' (Yid.), in Nakhmen Blumental (ed.), *The Memorial Book of Baranów* [Sefer yizkor baranov] (Jerusalem, 1964), 152–61.

FERDERBER-ZALTS, BERTA, 'Of Events and People' (Yid.), in Israel M. Brider-
man (ed.), *The Pinkas of Kolbuszowa* [Pinkes kolbushov] (New York, 1971),
341–84.

FIJAŁKOWSKI, PIOTR, 'Obrządek pogrzebowy Żydów polskich w świetle badań
archeologicznych' [The Funeral Rite of the Polish Jews in Light of Archaeo-
logical Research], *Biuletyn Żydowskiego Instytutu Historycznego*, 3 (1989),
25–42.

FISHTEYN, LEYBELE, 'Rabbi Ben-Tsiyon Fraylikh' (Yid.), in Barukh Kaplinski
(ed.), *The Book of Kozienice: Twenty-Seven Years on from the Terrible Destruction
of Our Former Home* [Sefer kozhenits: tsum 27-tn yor-tog nokh dem groyza-
men khurbn fun undzer gevezener heym] (Tel Aviv, 1969), 204–15.

FOLMER, MARGARETHA, 'A Jewish Childbirth Amulet for a Girl', *Studies in
Jewish Thought*, 12 (2007), 41–56.

FOUCAULT, MICHEL, *The Order of Things: An Archeology of the Human Sciences*
(London, 2002).

FRANASZEK, PIOTR, *Zdrowie publiczne w Galicji w dobie autonomii (wybrane prob-
lemy)* [Public Health in Galicia in the Period of Autonomy (Selected Issues)]
(Kraków, 2002).

FRIED, MOSES, 'Volksmedizinisches und Diätetisches aus Ostgalizien', *Mitteilungen zur Jüdischen Volkskunde*, 13 (1910), 167–8.

FRIEDLÄNDER, EMIL, 'Volksmedizin', *Der Urquell*, 2 (1898), 33–4.

FRIEDLENDER, SHIMON, 'Jewish Life in the Shtetl' (Yid.), in Natan Mark and
Shimon Friedlender (eds.), *Memorial Book Devoted to the Jews of the Cities that
Were Destroyed in the Shoah in the Years 1939–1944: Linsk, Istrik, Baligrod, Litovisk, and the Surrounding Areas* [Sefer yizkor mukdash liyhudei ha'ayarot
shenisepu basho'ah beshanim 1939–1944: linsk, istrik, baligrod, litovisk veha-
sevivah] (Tel Aviv, 1964/5), 122–7.

FRIEDMAN, FILIP, 'Dzieje Żydów w Galicji (1772–1914)' [A History of the Jews
in Galicia (1772–1914)], in Ignacy Schipper, Arie Tartakower, and Aleksander
Hafftka (eds.), *Żydzi w Polsce odrodzonej* [The Jews in Restituted Poland]
(Warsaw, 1932), i. 377–412.

FRIMER, PETACHIA, 'A Podolian's Observations on the Language in *Genarter
Velt*' (Yid.), *Yidishe shprakh*, 4 (1944), 44–9.

FROM, LEYB, 'The Doctor and Domestic Remedies' (Yid.), in Shimon Kants
(ed.), *The Memorial Book of Wojsławice* [Sefer zikaron voyslavitse] (Tel Aviv,
1970), 344–6.

'From the Folklore of Parysów' (Yid.), *Yidishe filologye*, 4–6 (1924), 396–7.

FROST, SORE, 'The Wooden Bridge' (Yid.), in Itzhak Ivry (ed.), *Pułtusk: Memorial
Book* [Pultusk: sefer zikaron] (Tel Aviv, 1971), 214–16.

FRUMKIN, L., *Eternal Sources: Folk Creativity* [Eybike kvaln: folksshafung] (Warsaw, 1953).

GANUZ, YITSHAK [YITSHAK GANUZOWICZ], 'Methods and Charms for Banishing Fright and Neutralizing the Effects of the Evil Eye' (Heb.), in Aleksander Manor, Yitshak Ganuzowicz, and Aba Lando (eds.), *The Book of Lida* [Sefer lida] (Tel Aviv, 1970), 219.

—— 'Snippets of Jewish Folklore' (Heb.), *Yeda am*, 15 (1971), 25–6.

—— 'Thirty-Six Righteous in the Towns of Lithuania and Belarus' (Heb.), *Yeda am*, 43–44 (1976), 28–31

GANZ, MEIR, *Maḥzor mikol hashanah, minhag polin* [festival prayer book] (Altona, 1825/6).

GANZFRIED, SOLOMON, *Keset hasofer* (Ungvar, 1871).

—— *Kitsur shulḥan arukh* [abridged code of law] (New York, 2012).

GARBUZ, ANDRZEJ, and RADOSŁAW TUMIEL (eds.), *Obraz wsi sokólskiej połowy XIX wieku w rękopisie Adama Baćkiewicza* [The Image of Mid-Nineteenth-Century Rural Sokółka in the Manuscripts of Adam Baćkiewicz] (Sokółka, 2011).

GAY, RUTH, *Unfinished People: Eastern European Jews Encounter America* (New York, 2001), 6–9.

GELBARD, SAMUEL PINHAS, *Otsar ta'amei haminhagim* [A Treasury of Reasons for the Customs] (Petah Tikvah, 1995).

GEVAT, TSEVI, 'Thousands of Memorial Candles' (Heb.), in Mosheh Tamari (ed.), *The Rise and Fall of Zamość* [Zamosc bigenonah uveshivrah] (Tel Aviv, 1952/3), 279.

GILAD, HAYIM, 'Wise Words from the Mouth of My Grandfather, R. David Sofer' (Heb.), *Yeda am*, 17 (1974), 144–6.

GINGOLD, HENEKH, 'The Ostrołęka that Is No More' (Yid.), in Yitshak Ivry (ed.), *The Book of the Ostrołęka Community* [Sefer kehilat ostrolenka] (Tel Aviv, 1963), 214–17.

GINZBERG, LOUIS, *Legends of the Jews*, 4 vols. (Philadelphia, 2003).

GINZBURG, SAUL, 'How Our Forefathers Fought Cholera' (Yid.), in S. Ginzburg, *Historical Works* [Historishe verk] (New York, 1937), i. 229–37.

—— and PEYSAKH MAREK (eds.), *Yevrieyskaya narodnaya piesni v Rossiyi* (St Petersburg, 1901).

GLIKSMAN, PINHAS ZELIG, *The Kotsker Rebbe* [Der kotsker rebe] (Piotrków, 1937).

GLOGER, ZYGMUNT, 'Zabobony i mniemania ludu nadnarwiańskiego tyczące ptaków, płazów i owadów' [Superstitions and Beliefs of the Narev Folk Regarding Birds, Reptiles, and Insects], *Zbiór Wiadomości do Antropologii Krajowej*, 1 (1877), 101–7.

GLÜCKEL OF HAMELN, *The Life of Glückel of Hameln, Written by Herself*, trans. Beth-Zion Abrahams (Philadelphia, 2010).

GOLDBERG, ISRAEL YUDL, and ABRAHAM ABA EISENBERG, *Sefer laḥashim usegulot vegoralot umazalot* [Book of Incantations, Remedies, Lots, and Constellations] (Jerusalem, 1880/1).

GOLDBERG-MULKIEWICZ, OLGA, *Ethnographic Topics Relating to Jews in Polish Studies* (Jerusalem, 1989).

—— 'Obrzędy żałobne i pogrzebowe Żydów polskich' [Mourning and Funeral Rituals of the Polish Jews], *Polska Sztuka Ludowa*, 40 (1986), 103–8.

GOLENPOL, AKIVA, *Lexicon of Hebrew Folklore* [Leksikon hafolklor ha'ivri] (Kaunas, 1936).

GORDIS, ROBERT, *The Dynamics of Judaism: A Study in Jewish Law* (Bloomington, 1990).

GORDON, BENJAMIN, *Between Two Worlds: The Memoirs of a Physician* (New York, 1952).

GOTTESMAN, ITZIK N., *Defining the Yiddish Nation: The Jewish Folklorists of Poland* (Detroit, 2003).

GRĄCIKOWSKI, PIOTR, 'Kobieta żydowska w badaniach Reginy Lilientalowej' [The Jewish Woman in the Research of Regina Lilientalowa], in Joanna Lisek (ed.), *Nieme dusze? Kobiety w kulturze jidysz* [Mute Souls? Women in Yiddish Culture] (Wrocław, 2010), 379–400.

GRAVES, ROBERT, and RAPHAEL PATAI, *Hebrew Myths: The Book of Genesis* (Manchester, 2005).

GREEN, ARTHUR, 'The Zaddiq as Axis Mundi in Later Judaism', *Journal of the American Academy of Religion*, 45 (1977), 327–47.

GRIMM, JACOB, *Deutsche Mythologie*, 2 vols. (Göttingen, 1854).

—— and Wilhelm Grimm, *Deutsches Wörterbuch*, online edn.

GROER, FRANCISZEK, 'Szpital Starozakonnych w Warszawie' [The Jewish Hospital in Warsaw], *Tygodnik Lekarski*, 12 (1847), 89–91.

GRUNWALD, MAX, 'Aus Hausapotheke und Hexenküche II (Forts.)', *Mitteilungen zur Jüdischen Volkskunde*, 4 (1907), 118–45.

—— 'Aus Hausapotheke und Hexenküche III', *Jahrbuch für Jüdische Volkskunde* (1923), 178–226.

—— 'Aus unseren Sammlungen. Teil 1', *Mitteilungen der Gesellschaft für Jüdische Volkskunde*, 1 (1898), 1–116.

—— 'Aus unseren Sammlungen. II', *Mitteilungen der Gesellschaft für Jüdische Volkskunde*, 1(3) (1899), 4–40.

—— *Die Hygiene der Juden* (Dresden, 1911).

—— and KAUFMANN KOHLER, 'Bibliomancy', *Jewish Encyclopedia* (New York, 1903), iii. 202–5.

GRZYBOWSKI, KONSTANTY, *Galicja 1848–1914: Historia ustroju politycznego na tle historii ustroju Austrii* [Galicia 1848–1914: The History of the Political System in the Context of the History of the Austrian System] (Kraków, 1959).

GUSTAWICZ, BRONISŁAW, 'Podania, przesądy, gadki i nazwy ludowe w dziedzinie przyrody' [Folk Tales, Superstitions, Sayings, and Names in the Field of Nature], *Zbiór Wiadomości do Antropologii Krajowej*, 5 (1881), 102–86.

HABERMAN, JACOB (ed.), *The Microcosm of Joseph Ibn Saddiq* (Danvers, Mass., 2003).

HAKOHEN, TUVYAH, *Ma'aseh tuvyah* (Kraków, 1907/8).

HALKOWSKI, HENRYK, *Żydowski Kraków: Legendy i ludzie* [Jewish Kraków: Legends and People] (Kraków, 2009).

HALPERN, JOEL, *Mifalot elokim* (Lemberg, 1858).

—— *Toledot adam* (Lemberg, 1872); unpaginated.

'A Handful of Beliefs from Zhitomir' (Yid.), *Yidisher folklor*, 3 (1962), 63.

HARKAVY, AHARON, and YEHUDAH GESIK, 'Medical Care in Our Town' (Heb.), in Michael Valtser-Fas and Moshe Kaplan (eds.), *The Turzec and Jeremicze Communities: Memorial Book* [Kehilot turts veyeremits: sefer zikaron] (Tel Aviv, 1978), 41–5.

HARKAVY, ALEXANDER, *Yiddish–English–Hebrew Dictionary* [Yidish–english–hebreisher verterbukh] (New Haven, 2006).

HAUR, JAKUB KAZIMIERZ, *Ekonomika lekarska albo domowe lekarstwa* [Medical Economics; or, Domestic Medicines] (Berdyczów, 1793).

HELLER, SAMUEL, *Medicaments and Remedies* [Refuot usegulot] (Jerusalem, 1906/7).

HERZOG, ELIZABETH, and MARK ZBOROWSKI, *Life Is with People* (New York, 1962).

HIMMELBLAU, FRIDA, 'Medical Aid in Pińczów' (Yid.), in Mordkhe Shner (ed.), *The Memorial Book of the Pińczów Community* [Sefer zikaron likehilat pintshev] (Tel Aviv, 1970), 212–20.

HIRSHOVITSH, ABRAHAM ELIEZER, *Minhagei yeshurun* (Vilna, 1898/9).

HOFFMANN-KRAYER, EDUARD, and HANNS BÄCHTOLD STÄUBLI (eds.), *Handwörterbuch des deutschen Aberglaubens*, 10 vols. (Berlin, 1974).

HOLENDER, YOSEF MENAKHEM, 'A Kaddish for You, My Town' (Yid.), in Nakhmen Blumental (ed.), *The Memorial Book of Baranów* [Sefer yizkor baranov] (Jerusalem, 1964), 36–57.

HOROWITZ, HAYIM HAKOHEN, *Anaf ḥayim* (Jerusalem, 1925).

HOVORKA, OSKAR, and ADOLF KRONFELD (eds.), *Vergleichende Volksmedizin*, 2 vols. (Stuttgart, 1908).

HUFFORD, DAVID J., 'Medicine, Folk', in Charlie T. McCormick and Kim Kennedy (eds.), *Folklore: An Encyclopedia of Beliefs, Customs, Tales, Music, and Art* (Santa Barbara, 2011).

HURVITS, S., 'My Mother's Sayings' (Yid.), *Lebn un visnshaft*, 8–9 (1912), 120–3; 10 (1912), 90–2.

HURWITZ, PINHAS ELIYAHU, *Sefer haberit* (Yid.) (Warsaw, 1898).

HURWITZ, PINHAS ELIYAHU, *Sefer haberit hashalem* (Piotrków, 1904).

IDEL, MOSHE, *Hasidism: Between Ecstasy and Magic* (Albany, NY, 1995).

ISAAC BEN ELIEZER, *Refuah vehayim miyrushalayim* (Jerusalem, 1892).

ISSERLES, MOSES, *Torat ha'olah* (Prague, 1569).

'Items' (Heb.), *Reshumot*, 1 (1918), 381.

JACOBUS, HELEN R., '4Q318: A Jewish Zodiac Calendar at Qumran?', in Charlotte Hempel (ed.), *The Dead Sea Scrolls: Text and Context* (Leiden, 2010), 365–95.

JAGUŚ, INGA, *Lecznictwo ludowe w Królestwie Polskim na przełomie XIX i XX wieku* [Folk Healing in the Kingdom of Poland at the Turn of the Nineteenth and Twentieth Centuries] (Kielce, 2002).

JAKOBOVITS, IMMANUEL, *Jewish Medical Ethics* (New York, 1975).

JESZKE, JAROMIR, *Lecznictwo ludowe w Wielkopolsce w XIX i XX wieku: Czynniki i kierunki przemian* [Folk Healing in Greater Poland in the Nineteenth and Twentieth Centuries: Factors in and Areas of Change] (Wrocław, 1996).

'Jewish Festivals in the Shtetl' (Yid.), in Henokh H. Halpern (ed.), *The Gliniany Scroll: Reminiscences and Experiences of an Annihilated Community* [Megiles Gline: zikhroynes un iberlebungen fun a khorev gevorener kehile] (New York, 1950), 56–67.

JUDAH HEHASID, *Sefer hasidim* (Lwów, 1934/5).

KAC, ALBIN (TOBIASZ), *Nowy Sącz, miasto mojej młodości* [Nowy Sącz, Town of My Youth] (Kraków, 1997).

KACYZNE, ALTER, *Shtarke un shvakhe* [The Strong and the Weak], 2 vols. (Buenos Aires, 1954).

KAINDL, RAIMUND FRIEDRIECH, 'Die Juden in der Bukowina, II (Schluss)', *Globus*, 80/10 (1901), 157–61.

KANARVOGEL, ABRAHAM ABELE, *Be'erot hamayim, mahadurah tinyanah . . . be'er lehai ro'i* (London, 1957).

—— 'Hashmatah lebe'er mayim hayim', in id., *Be'erot hamayim, mahadurah tinyanah . . . be'er lehai ro'i* (Szatmárnémeti, 1942); unpaginated.

—— *Ta'amei mitsvot . . . im sefer be'erot hamayim* [Reasons for the Commandments] (Przemyśl, 1888); unpaginated.

KAPLAN, ARYEH, *Sefer Yetzirah: The Book of Creation* (Boston, 1997).

KARŁOWICZ, JAN, *Słownik gwar polskich* [A Lexicon of Polish Dialects], 6 vols. (Kraków, 1900).

——ADAM KRYŃSKI, and WŁADYSŁAW NIEDŹWIEDZKI (eds.), *Słownik języka polskiego* [Dictionary of the Polish Language], 8 vols. (Warsaw, 1902).

KASTRINSKI, E., 'Two Grandmas' (Yid.), in Akiva Ben-Ezra (ed.), *Horodets: A History of the Town* [Horodets: a geshikhte fun a shtetl] (New York, 1949), 182–4.

KATSENELSON, YEHUDAH LEIB, *The Talmud and Medical Knowledge* [Hatalmud vehokhmat harefuah] (Berlin, 1928).

'Katzensporn: Eine Umfrage', *Am Ur-Quell*, 3 (1892), 77–8, 139, 168–9, 206–7, 227–8, 252, 296.

KAZDAN, K. S., 'Imagery in Jewish Folk Language' (Yid.), *Yidishe shprakh*, 9 (1949), 34–50.

*Keter shem tov hashalem* (New York, 2004).

KH. S., 'Childhood Years in Boyberke' (Yid.), in Shraga Fayvel Kalai (ed.), *In Memory of the Community in Bobrka and the Surrounding Area* [Lezekher kehilat bobrka uvenoteiha] (Jerusalem, 1964), 176.

KHAYES, HAYIM, 'Death-Related Beliefs and Customs' (Yid.), *Filologishe shriftn*, 2 (1928), 281–328.

KHAZAN, M., 'Wedding in the Cemetery' (Yid.), in Hayim Rabin (ed.), *Shumsk: A Memorial Book for the Martyrs of Shumsk Killed by the Nazis in the Year 1942* [Shumsk: sefer zikaron likdoshei shumsk shenisepu besho'at hanatsim bishnat 1942] (Tel Aviv, 1968), 382–6.

KHOTSH, TSEVI HIRSH, *Segulot urefuot* [Remedies and Medicaments] (Amsterdam, 1703).

KINDLER, DOVID, 'Jewish Philanthropic Organizations and Institutions in Sokal' (Yid.), in Avraham Khomel (ed.), *The Book of Sokal, Tartaków, Warȩż, Stojanów, and the Surroundings* [Sefer sokal, tartakov, varenzh, stoyanov vehasevivah] (Tel Aviv, 1968), 205–11.

KING, HELEN, 'Once Upon a Text: Hysteria from Hippocrates', in Helen King, *Hippocrates' Woman: Reading the Female Body in Ancient Greece* (London, 2014), 205–46.

KIPNIS, ITSIK, *My Town Sloveshne* [Mayn shtetele sloveshne], 2 vols. (Tel Aviv, 1971).

KIRSHENBLATT-GIMBLETT, BARBARA, 'Folklore, Ethnography, and Anthropology', *The YIVO Encyclopedia of Jews in Eastern Europe*, online edn. (accessed 27 Jan. 2015).

KITRI, A. [ABRAHAM KRONENBERG], 'The Feldsher' (Yid.), in Abraham Kronenberg (ed.), *The Destruction of Biłgoraj* [Khurbn bilgoraj] (Tel Aviv, 1956), 139–41.

KLAGSBRUN, SHELOMOH, *Jews of Mielec* [Mieltser yidn] (Tel Aviv, 1979).

KLEIN, MICHELE, *A Time To Be Born: Customs and Folklore of Jewish Birth* (Philadelphia, 1998).

KLEINMAN, ARTHUR, *The Illness Narratives: Suffering, Healing, and the Human Condition* (New York, 1988).

KLEMENTINOVSKI, DOVID, *Dr Yosef Khazanovitsh: Idealist, Nationalist, and Man of the People* [Dr yosef khazanovitsh: der idealist, natsyonalist un folksmentsh] (New York, 1956).

KLING, Y., 'The Unwritten Book of My Mama's Remedies' (Yid.), in Yoyne Boym (ed.), *Felsztyn: A Collection Commemorating the Felsztyn Martyrs* [Felshtin: zamlbukh tsum ondenk fun di felshtiner kdoyshim] (New York, 1937), 547–62.

Klots, Pinkhes, 'A Kaddish for You, My Shtetl' (Yid.), in Yitshak Berglas and Shelomoh Yaholomi (Diamant) (eds.), *The Book of Strzyżów and the Region* [Sefer strizov vehasevivah] (Tel Aviv, 1969), 291–3.

Klus, Jerzy, *Neues Taschenwörterbuch deutsch–polnisch und polnisch–deutsch* (Třebíč, 1917).

Knapheys, Moyshe, *A Boy from Warsaw* [A yingl fun varshe] (Buenos Aires, 1960).

Kohen, David, *Shpola: A Chapter on the Life of the Jews in the Town* [Shpola: masekhet ḥayei yehudim ba'ayarah] (Haifa, 1965).

Kohen, Menasheh, *Leket haḥanukah zikhron david* (Jerusalem, 2009/10).

Kolberg, Oskar, *Dzieła wszystkie* [The Complete Works], 86 vols. (Wrocław, 1962).

Kolczyński, Jarosław, 'Jeszcze raz o upiorze (wampirze) i strzygoni (strzydze)' [The Phantom (Vampire) and the *Strzygoń* (*Strzyga*) Revisited], *Etnografia Polska*, 47 (2003), 211–46.

Kopff, Wiktor, *Wspomnienia z ostatnich lat Rzeczypospolitej Krakowskiej* [Reminiscences from the Last Years of the Kraków Republic] (Kraków, 1906).

Kositsa, Rokhl Ene, *Reminiscences of a Woman from Białystok* [Zikhroynes fun a bialistoker froy] (Los Angeles, 1964).

Kosofsky, Scott-Martin, *The Book of Customs* (San Francisco, 2004), pp. xv–xxx.

Kosover, Mordkhe, 'Jewish Sayings and their Origins: An Anthology' (Yid.), in Shemuel Rozhanski (ed.), *Yiddish Ideologies in the Twentieth Century* [Yidish-lekhe ideologyes in 20stn yorhundert. Antologye] (Buenos Aires, 1982), 196–228.

Kossoy, Edward, and Abraham Ohry, *The Feldshers: Medical, Sociological and Historical Aspects of Practitioners of Medicine with Below University Level Education* (Jerusalem, 1992).

Kotik, Yehezkel, *My Memoirs* [Mayne zikhroynes], 2 vols. (Berlin, 1922).

Kotula, Franciszek, *Znaki przeszłości: Odchodzące ślady zatrzymać w pamięci* [Signs of the Past: Capturing Fading Traces in the Memory] (Warsaw, 1976).

Kowalski, Piotr, 'Wanda, Ofelia i inne topielice. Kilka uwag o znaczeniach motywu śmierci w wodzie' [Wanda, Ophelia, and Other Drowned Women: A Few Remarks on the Meanings of the Motif of Death in Water], in Piotr Kowalski, *O jednorożcu, Wieczerniku i innych motywach mniej lub bardziej ważnych* [On the Unicorn, the Upper Room, and Other More or Less Significant Motifs] (Kraków, 2007), 209–30.

Koydanover, Aaron Samuel, *Emunat shemuel* (Lemberg, 1884/5).

Koydanover, Tsevi Hirsh, *Kav hayashar* (Stettin, 1864/5).

Krausz, Asher Anshl, *The Life of the Ba'al Shem Tov* [Dos lebn fun ba'al shem tov] (New York, 1967).

KUPER, MORDKHE, *The Jews of My Nostalgia* [Di yidn fun mayn benkshaft] (Buenos Aires, 1968).

KVARTIN, ZAVEL, *My Life* [Mayn lebn] (Philadelphia, 1952).

KVITNI, YEHUDAH, 'Sayings Including "Hand" and Parts Thereof' (Yid.), *Shriftn*, 1 (1928), 305–20.

LAMM, NORMAN, *The Religious Thought of Hasidism* (Hoboken, 1999).

LANDAU, ALFRED, 'Notes and Comments on *Yidishe Filologye*, 1–3' (Yid.), *Yidishe filologye*, 4–6 (1924), 323–37.

—— 'Sprichwörter und Redensarten', *Jahrbuch für Jüdische Volkskunde* (1923), 335–61.

LANDAU, MARCUS, 'Zur Geschichte der jüdischen Vornamen', *Mitteilungen der Gesellschaft für Jüdische Volkskunde*, 1 (1902), 1–9.

LEBEDA, AGNIESZKA, 'Gwiazdy' [Stars], in Zygmunt Kłodnicki (ed.), *Komentarze do polskiego atlasu etnograficznego* [Commentaries on the Polish Ethnographic Atlas], vi: *Wiedza i wierzenia ludowe* [Folk Knowledge and Beliefs] (Wrocław, 2002), 62–76.

LEFIN, MENAHEM MENDEL, *Folk Medicine* [Refuot ha'am] (Lemberg, 1851); unpaginated.

LEHMAN, SHEMUEL, 'The Prophet Elijah in Folk Imagination: Stories and Legends Recorded from Oral Testimonies' (Yid.), in Noyekh Prilutski and Shemuel Lehman (eds.), *Archive of Jewish Linguistics, Literary Studies, and Ethnology* [Arkhiv far yidisher shprakhvisnshaft, literaturforshung un etnologye] (Warsaw, 1926–33), i. 115–78.

LEICHT, REIMUND, 'The Planets, the Jews and the Beginnings of "Jewish Astrology"', in Gideon Bohak, Yuval Harari, and Shaul Shaked (eds.), *Continuity and Innovation in the Magical Tradition* (Leiden, 2011), 271–88.

—— 'The Reception of Astrology in Medieval Ashkenazi Culture', *Aleph*, 13/2 (2013), 201–34.

LERNER, ISRAEL ABRAHAM, *Kuntres beit yisra'el al hasefer ḥokhmat adam* (Jerusalem, 1967/8).

'Letter Box' (Yid.), *Folksgezunt*, 1923–6.

LEVIN, GERSHON, *From the Good Old Days (A Cholera Excursion)* [Fun di alte gute tsaytn (a rayze oyf di kholera)] (Warsaw, 1925).

—— 'Z pamiętnika lekarza' [From a Physician's Diary], in Jan Kirszot (ed.), *Safrus, Książka zbiorowa poświęcona sprawom żydostwa* [Safrus: A Collective Book Relating to Jewish Matters] (Warsaw, 1905), 231–4.

LEVIN, JACOB, *Ḥotam kodesh* (Kraków, 1892).

LEVINE, B., *Memories Tell Stories* [Zikhroynes dertseyln] (New York, 1967).

LEVINSKI, YOM-TOV (ed.), *Book of Festivals* [Sefer hamo'adim], 8 vols. (Tel Aviv, 1946–55).

LEVINSKI, YOM-TOV (ed.), 'Learned Women: Women from Zambrów Who Read the Sacred Books' (Yid.), in Yom-Tov Levinski (ed.), *The Book of Zambrów* [Sefer zambrov] (Tel Aviv, 1963), 295–301.

——'In the Quarter of the Kabbalists: Tu Bishvat—The New Year of Trees' (Heb.), in Yom-Tov Levinski, *The Book of Festivals* [Sefer hamo'adim] (Tel Aviv, 1956), v. 329–33.

——'Silent Water (From a Collection of Folk Medications and Remedies)' (Heb.), *Yeda am*, 1/3–4 (1949), 3–5.

LEVITA, AVRAHAM, 'A Stroll Around the Town' (Yid.), in Avraham Levita (ed.), *The Brzozów Memorial Book* [Sefer zikaron kehilat breziv (bzhozov)] (n.p., 1984), 163–77.

LEW, HENRYK, 'Lecznictwo i przesądy lecznicze ludu żydowskiego' [Jewish Folk Remedies and Treatment-Related Superstitions], *Izraelita*, 47 (1898), 493–4; 48 (1898), 505; 50 (1898), 530.

——'O lecznictwie i przesądach leczniczych ludu żydowskiego' [On Jewish Folk Remedies and Treatment-Related Superstitions], *Izraelita*, 35 (1896), 296; 36 (1896), 305–6; 37 (1896), 315–16; 38 (1897), 362–4; 40 (1897), 381–3; 41 (1897), 394–5; 42 (1896), 364–5; 42 (1897), 406–7; 46 (1897), 446–7; 49 (1897), 475–6.

——'Z ludoznawstwa. Śmierć i obrzędy pogrzebowe u Żydów' [From Folk Studies: Death and Funeral Rituals Among the Jews], *Izraelita*, 17 (1899), 186–7; 18 (1899), 196–7; 22 (1899), 238–9.

LEWIN, GERSZON, *Ochrona zdrowia i eugenika w Biblii i Talmudzie* [Health Care and Eugenics in the Bible and the Talmud] (Warsaw, 1934).

LEWIS, JUSTIN JASON, *Imagining Holiness: Classic Hasidic Tales in Modern Times* (Montreal, 2009).

LEYBOVITSH, S., 'One Patient, One Remedy' (Yid.), in S. Likht (ed.), *The Tomaszów Lubelski Memorial Book* [Tomashover Lub. izker bukh] (New York, 1965), 448–54.

LIBERA, ZBIGNIEW, *Medycyna ludowa: Chłopski rozsądek czy gminna fantazja?* [Folk Medicine: Peasants' Common Sense or Community Fantasy?] (Wrocław, 1995).

——*Mikrokosmos, makrokosmos i antropologia ciała* [Microcosm, Macrocosm, and the Anthropology of the Body] (Tarnów, 1997).

——*Znachor w tradycjach ludowych i popularnych XIX–XX wieku* [The Quack Healer in Folk and Popular Traditions of the Nineteenth and Twentieth Centuries] (Wrocław, 2003).

LIBERMAN, HAYIM, 'Discussion: Remarks on Shloyme Nobel's Article "Reb Yechiel Mikhel Epstein—an Educator and Fighter for Yiddish in the 17th Century"' (Yid.), *YIVO bleter*, 36 (1952), 305–19.

LIEBES, YEHUDA, *Studies in Jewish Myth and Jewish Messianism*, trans. Batya Stein (New York, 1993).

LIFSHITS, SHABETAI, *Sefer haḥayim hanikra segulot yisra'el* (Munkács, 1905).

—— *Sefer sharbit hazahav heḥadash hanikra berit avot* (Munkács, 1913/14).

LILIENTALOWA, REGINA, 'Additions: The "Evil Eye"' (Yid.), in Noyekh Prilut-ski and Shemuel Lehman (eds.), *The Archive of Jewish Linguistics, Literary Studies, and Ethnology* [Arkhiv far yidisher shprakhvisnshaft, literaturforshung un etnologye] (Warsaw, 1926–33), i. 433–4.

—— 'Dziecko żydowskie' [The Jewish Child], *Materyały Antropologicno-Archeologiczne i Etnograficzne Akademii Umiejętności*, 7 (1904), 141–73.

—— *Dziecko żydowskie* [The Jewish Child] (Warsaw, 2007).

—— 'The Evil Eye' (Yid.), trans. Nekhame Epstein, *Yidishe filologye*, 4–6 (1924), 245–71.

—— 'Kult ciał niebieskich u starożytnych Hebrajczyków i szczątki tego kultu u współczesnego ludu żydowskiego' [The Cult Surrounding Celestial Bodies Among the Ancient Hebrews and the Vestiges of that Cult among Contemporary Jewry], *Archiwum Nauk Antropologicznych*, 1/6 (1921).

—— 'Kult wody u starożytnych Hebrajczyków i szczątki tego kultu u współczesnego ludu żydowskiego' [The Cult Surrounding Water Among the Ancient Hebrews and the Vestiges of that Cult among Contemporary Jewry], *Archiwum Nauk Antropologicznych*, 3/2 (1930).

—— 'Przesądy żydowskie' [Jewish Superstitions], *Wisła*, 12 (1898), 277–84; 14 (1900), 318–22, 639–44.

—— *Święta żydowskie w przeszłości i teraźniejszości* [Jewish Festivals in the Past and in the Present], 3 vols. (Kraków, 1908–19).

—— 'Wierzenia, przesądy i praktyki ludu żydowskiego' [Beliefs, Superstitions, and Practices of the Jewish Folk], *Wisła*, 18 (1904), 105–13; 19 (1905), 148–76.

—— 'Zjawiska przyrody w wyobrażeniu i praktyce ludu żydowskiego' [Natural Phenomena in the Imagination and Practice of the Jewish Folk], in Jan Kirszot (ed.), *Safrus, Książka zbiorowa poświącona sprawom żydostwa* [Safrus: A Collective Book Devoted to Jewish Matters] (Warsaw, 1905), 56–62.

—— 'Życie pozagrobowe i świat przyszły w wyobrażeniu ludu żydowskiego' [Life Beyond the Grave and the World to Come in the Imagination of the Jewish Folk', *Lud*, 8 (1902), 350–3.

LINDE, SAMUEL BOGUMIŁ, *Słownik języka polskiego* [A Polish Dictionary], 6 vols. (Lwów, 1859).

LINDEMANN, MARY, *Medicine and Society in Early Modern Europe* (Cambridge, 2010).

LINDENBERG, GABRIEL, 'Our Town as I Remember It' (Heb.), in Shimshon Meltser (ed.), *The Book of Horodenka* [Seyfer horodenke] (New York, 1963), 45–70.

LINETSKI, ISAAC JOEL, *The Hasidic Boy* [Dos khsidishe yingl] (Vilna, 1897).

LIPIETS, ISAAC, *Sefer matamim* (Warsaw, 1890).

LIPIETS, ISAAC, *Sefer matamim beḥadash* (Warsaw, 1893/4).

LOEWE, HEINRICH, 'Jüdische Volkserzählungen aus Polen', *Mitteilungen zur Jüdischen Volkskunde*, 3–4 (1915), 61–3.

LOEWENTHAL, NAFTALI, *Communicating the Infinite: The Emergence of the Habad School* (Chicago, 1990).

LUKIANOVSKI, SHALOM, *Yad shalom* (Piotrków, 1910).

MAGGID, DAVID, 'Inoyazichniye zagavori u ruskikh yevrieyev v XVIII i nachale XIX v.', *Yevreiskaya Starina*, 3 (1910), 580–91.

MAIMON, SALOMON, *An Autobiography*, trans. J. Clark Murray (Urbana, Ill., 2001).

MAIMONIDES, MOSES, *Moreh nevukhim* (Jerusalem, 1960).

MAJER, JÓZEF, and FRYDERYK K. SKOBEL, *Uwagi nad niektóremi wyrazami lekarskiemi* [Remarks on Certain Medical Expressions] (Kraków, 1835).

MARCUS, IVAN G., *The Jewish Life Cycle: Rites of Passage from Biblical to Modern Times* (Seattle, 2004).

MARGOSHES, YOSEF, *Memories from My Life* [Erinerungen fun mayn lebn] (New York, 1936).

MARK, YUDL, 'A Collection of Folk Comparisons' (Yid.), *Yidishe shprakh*, 5 (1945), 97–140.

——(ed.), *Great Dictionary of the Yiddish Language* [Groyser verterbukh fun der yidisher shprakh], 4 vols. (New York, 1980).

——'The Language of the Comedy *Di genarte velt*' (Yid.), *Yidishe shprakh*, 3 (1943), 75.

MARKUZE, MOSES, *Sefer refuot hanikra ezer yisra'el* [The Book of Medicaments; or, An Aid to Israel] (Poritsk, 1790).

MARMOR, KALMEN, *My Life Story* [Mayn lebns-geshikhte], 2 vols. (New York, 1959).

'Marriage', *Encyclopaedia Judaica* (Detroit, 2007), xiii. 563–76.

MATRAS, HAGIT, 'Books of Remedies and Medicaments in Hebrew: Contents and Sources' ['Sifrei segulot urefuot be'ivrit—tekhanim umekorot'], Ph.D. diss. (Hebrew University, 1997).

——'Jewish Folk Medicine in the 19th and 20th Centuries', in *Jews and Medicine: Religion, Culture, Science* (Tel Aviv, 1995), 113–35.

——'Wholeness and Holiness in Sifrei Segulot', *Koroth*, 9 (1988), 96–107.

MEISELS, AVRAHAM, *Vihyitem li segulah*, vol. i (Montreal, 2009).

MEKLER, DAVID LEIB, *Fun rebns hoyf: Fun Tshernobil biz Talne*, 2 vols. (New York, 1931).

*Mekor dimah: Shas tekhinah ḥadashah im ma'aseh alfes verav peninim* (Vilna, 1911/12).

*Mekor ḥayim*, in Isaac Arama, *Akedat yitshak* (Lemberg, 1868).

MELER, D., *Besorot tovot* (Biłgoraj, 1926/7); unpaginated.

MENDELE MOYKHER-SFORIM, *The Travels of Benjamin the Third: Collected Works* [Masoes binyomin hashlishi, geklibene verk], 5 vols. (New York, 1946).

MESLER, KATELYN, 'The Three Magi and Other Christian Motifs in Medieval Hebrew Medical Incantations: A Study in the Limits of Faithful Translation', in Resianne Fontaine and Gad Freudenthal (eds.), *Latin-into-Hebrew: Texts and Studies* (Leiden, 2013), i. 161–218.

METZLER, IRINA, *Disability in Medieval Europe: Thinking about Physical Impairment During the High Middle Ages, c.1100–1400* (London, 2006).

MICHALEWICZ, JERZY, *Żydowskie okręgi metrykalne i żydowskie gminy wyznaniowe w Galicji* [Jewish Public Records Districts and Jewish Religious Communities in Galicia] (Kraków, 1995).

MILKH, YANKEV, *Autobiographical Sketches* [Otobiografishe shkitsn] (New York, 1946).

MILLER, AVRAHAM, 'Once Upon a Time in Our Town' (Yid.), in Dov Rabin (ed.), *Krynki Memorial Book* [Pinkas krinki] (Tel Aviv, 1970), 205–11.

'Minor Collections of Folklore' (Yid.), *Yidishe filologye*, 2–3 (1924), 201–4.

MIZISH, MATISYAHU, 'Gentiles as Sorcerers' (Yid.), *YIVO bleter*, 13 (1938), 147–71.

M.L.G., 'Hresk' (Yid.), in *Slutsk Memorial Book* [Pinkas slutsk uvenoteiha] (Tel Aviv, 1962), 436.

MORGNSHTERN-SHIFMAN, ISRAEL, 'Budzanów as It Is' (Yid.), in Yitshak Siegelman (ed.), *The Book of Budzanów* [Sefer budzanov] (Haifa, 1970), 13–25.

MOSES BEN BENJAMIN WOLF, *Yarum mosheh* (Amsterdam, 1678/9).

MOSHKOVITSH, TSEVI (ed.), *Otsar hasipurim*, 20 vols. (Jerusalem, 1952/3).

MOSZYŃSKI, KAZIMIERZ, *Kultura ludowa Słowian, Cz. II: Kultura duchowa* [The Folk Culture of the Slavs, Part II: Spiritual Culture] (Kraków, 1934).

MOYSHELES, VELVL, 'Singer the Feldsher' (Yid.), in Zeev Tsurnamal (ed.), *Lask. Memorial Book* [Lask. Sefer zikaron] (Tel Aviv, 1968), 245–9.

M.P., 'Jüdische Sprichwörter und Redensarten aus Öst.-Ungarn', *Mitteilungen der Gesellschaft für Jüdische Volkskunde*, 1 (1899), 41–4.

NAGELBERG, AKIBA, 'Das Ipisch bei galizischen Juden', *Am Ur-Quell*, 3 (1892), 286.

—— 'Sagen galizischer Juden. Zwei Schytfym', *Am Ur-Quell*, 4 (1893), 257.

NAKHALIEL, A., 'A Town There Was' (Yid.), in Nakhmen Blumental (ed.), *The Memorial Book of Baranów* [Sefer yizkor Baranov] (Jerusalem, 1964), 58–62.

N.C., 'Places of Learning in Pruzhana in the Second Half of the Nineteenth Century' (Yid.), in Mordkhe W. Bernstein and Dovid Forer (eds.), *Memorial Book of Pruzhana, Bereze, Maltsh, Shershev, Selts: Their Foundation, History, and Destruction* [Pinkes pruzhene, bereze, maltsh, shershev, selts: zeyer oyfkum, geshikhte un umkum] (Buenos Aires, 1958), 104–10.

NEUMANN, BERL, 'Our Town' (Yid.), in Yitshak Idan (Zeldin) (ed.), *The Memorial Book of David-Horodok* [Sefer zikaron david-horodok] (Tel Aviv, 1957), 420–4.

NIGAL, GEDALIAH, *'Dybbuk' Stories in Jewish Literature* [Sipurei 'dibuk' besifrut yisra'el] (Jerusalem, 1994).
—— *The Hasidic Tale* (Oxford, 2008).
NÜSEL, L., 'Sprichwörter und Redensarten aus Posen', *Mitteilungen zur Jüdischen Volkskunde*, 2 (1906), 67–8.
OCHANA, RAPHAEL, *Mareh hayeladim* (Jerusalem, 1900).
'Omens and Remedies' (Yid.), in Yehudah Leib Kahan (ed.), *Jewish Folklore* [Yidisher folklor], Shriftn fun yidishn visnshaftlekher institut 9 (Vilna, 1938), 277–97.
OPATOSHU, YOSEF, *A Day in Regensburg* [A tog in regensburg] (New York, 1933).
—— 'From My Lexicon' (Yid.), *Yidishe shprakh*, 1 (1941), 118–20.
ORINSKI, G., 'A Document about Cholera in Pruzhana' (Yid.), in *Pinkas of the Town of Pruzhana* [Pinkes fun der shtot pruzhene] (Pruzhene, 1930), 39–42.
OSHEROVITSH, S., 'According to Rubiezhevich Custom' (Yid.), in David Shtokfish (ed.), *The Book of Rubiezhevich, Derevna, and the Area* [Sefer rubizhevitsh, derevne vehasevivah] (Tel Aviv, 1968), 61–81.
PALUCH, ADAM, 'Suchoty: przyczynek do ludowego pojęcia o chorobie, etiologii i terapii' [Consumption: A Contribution on the Folk Conception of the Disease, Its Aetiology, and Its Treatment], in Wojciech J. Burszta and Jerzy Damrosz (eds.), *Pożegnanie paradygmatu? Etnologia wobec współczesności* [Departing the Paradigm? Ethnology and Contemporaneity] (Warsaw, 1994), 192–201.
—— *Świat roślin w tradycyjnych praktykach leczniczych wsi polskiej* [The Plant World in Traditional Healing Practices in Rural Poland] (Wrocław, 1988).
*Passover Haggadah* [Hagadah shel pesaḥ], in Yom-Tov Levinski (ed.), *Sefer hamo'adim* (Tel Aviv, 1948), ii. 125–82.
PATAI, RAPHAEL, 'Jewish Folk-Cures for Barrenness', *Folklore*, 54 (1943), 117–24.
—— 'Jewish Folk-Cures for Barrenness, II', *Folklore*, 56/1 (1945), 208–18.
—— 'Lilith', *Journal of American Folklore*, 77/306 (1964), 295–314.
—— *On Jewish Folklore* (Detroit, 1983).
PELTO, PERTTI J., and GRETEL H. PELTO, 'Studying Knowledge, Culture, Behavior in Applied Medical Anthropology', *Medical Anthropology Quarterly*, NS 11/2 (1997), 147–63.
PENKALA-GAWĘCKA, DANUTA, 'Antropologia medyczna dzisiaj: kontynuacje, nowe nurty, perspektywy badawcze' [Medical Anthropology Today: Continuation, New Currents, Research Perspectives], *Socjologia i antropologia medycyny w działaniu* [The Sociology and Anthropology of Medicine in Action], Włodzimierz Piątkowski and Bożena Płonka-Syroka (eds.) (Wrocław, 2008), 219–42.
PERETS, ISAAC LEYBUSH, *One Does Not Die of Cholera if One Does Not Want To* [Az men vil nisht, shtarbt men nisht fun khole-ra] (Warsaw, 1893).
PERLES, JOSEPH, 'Die Berner Handschrift des kleinen Aruch', in *Jubelschrift zum siebezigsten Geburtstage des Prof. Dr. H. Graetz* (Breslau, 1887), 1–38.

PERLMAN, MOSHEH, *The Midrash of Medicine* [Midrash harefuah], 3 vols. (Tel Aviv, 1926).

PESAH, YA'AKOV, *Zevaḥ pesaḥ* (Zhovkva, 1722).

PETROVSKY-SHTERN, YOHANAN, *The Golden Age Shtetl: A New History of Jewish Life in East Europe* (Princeton, 2014).

—— 'Magic and Folk Remedy' (Heb.), in Israel Bartal, Alexander Kulik, and Ilia Lurie (eds.), *History of the Jews of Russia* [Toledot yehudei rusyah], 3 vols. (Jerusalem, 2010–15), 349–65.

—— 'The Master of an Evil Name: Hillel Ba'al Shem and his *Sefer ha-Heshek*', *AJS Review*, 28 (2004), 217–48.

—— '"You Will Find It in the Pharmacy". Practical Kabbalah and Natural Medicine in the Polish-Lithuanian Commonwealth, 1690–1750', in Glenn Dynner (ed.), *Holy Dissent* (Detroit, 2011), 13–53.

PIĄTKOWSKA, IGNACJA, 'Ludoznawstwo żydowskie' [Jewish Folk Studies], *Wisła*, 11/4 (1897), 803–10.

PINTSHEVSKI, DOVID, 'Opatów and the Rise of Hasidism' (Yid.), in Zvi Yashiv (ed.), *Opatów: Memorial Book of an Important Town that Once Existed but Is no More* [Apt (Opatów). Sefer zikaron le'ir ve'em beyisra'el asher haytah ve'einenah od] (Tel Aviv, 1966), 55–62.

PIROZHNIKOV, YITSHAK, *Jewish Proverbs* [Yidishe shprikhverter] (Vilna, 1908).

PLAUT, HEZEKIAH FAYVL, *Likutei ḥever ben ḥayim*, 5 vols. (Munkács, 1883).

PODBERESKI, ANDRZEJ, 'Materyały do demonologii ludu Ukraińskiego. Z opowiadań ludowych w powiecie Czehryńskim' [Material on Ukrainian Folk Demonology: From the Folk Tales of the District of Chekhryn], *Zbiór Wiadomości do Antropologii Krajowej*, 4 (1880), 3–82.

POLLAK, HAYIM YOSEF, *Mekor ḥayim* (n.p., n.d.).

POMERANTS, BUNTSHE, 'Reb Yankl the Ritual Slaughterer', in S. Kants (ed.), *The Book of Burshtin: Memorial Books of the Diaspora Communities* [Sefer Burshtin: sifrei zikaron likehilot hagolah] (Jerusalem, 1960), 215–20.

POTOCKA, ANNA, *Mój pamiętnik* [My Memoir] (Kraków, 1927).

POZNIAK, KHANE, and YETI LAUFER (eds.), *This Is How We Sang* [Azoy hobn mir gezungen] (Tel Aviv, 1974).

PRESMAN, ISROEL, *The Road We Have Travelled* [Der durkhgegangener veg] (New York, 1950).

PREUSS, JULIUS, *Biblical and Talmudic Medicine* (New York, 1978).

—— *Biblisch-talmudische Medizin* (Berlin, 1911).

PRILUTSKI, NOYEKH, and SHMUEL LEHMAN, 'Jewish Proverbs, Sayings, Expressions, and Insults about Lands, Regions, Towns and Shtetls' (Yid.), *Noyekh prilutskis zamlbikher far yidishn folklor, filologye un kulturgeshichte*, 1 (1912), 9–87.

PULNER, JOSIP, 'Obryady i povirya spolucheni z bagitnoyu, porodileyu i narozh-dentsem u Zhidiv' (Ukr.) [Rituals and Beliefs Connected to Pregnancy, Delivery, and Birth among the Jews], *Etnografichniy Visnik*, 8 (1929), 100–14.

PUŚ, WIESŁAW, *Żydzi w Łodzi w latach zaborów 1793–1914* [The Jews in Łódź in the Years of the Partition, 1793–1914] [Łódź, 1998].

'Rabbis and Tsadikim from Gliniany' (Yid.), in Henokh H. Halpern (ed.), *The Gliniany Scroll: Reminiscences and Experiences from an Annihilated Community* [Megiles gline: zikhroynes un iberlebungen fun a khorev gevorener kehile] (New York, 1950), 68–76.

RABINOVITSH, SOLOMON, *Tiferet shelomoh al hazemanim umo'adim* (Jerusalem, 1982).

RABOKH, BERL, 'Another Handful of Jewish Cares' (Yid.), *Yidishe shprakh*, 24 (1964), 61.

RAPOPORT-ALBERT, ADA, 'God and the Zaddik as the Two Focal Points of Hasidic Worship', *History of Religion*, 18 (1979), 296–325; repr. in a newly edited version in Ada Rapoport-Albert, *Hasidic Studies: Essays in History and Gender* (Liverpool, 2018), 124–60.

—— 'Hasidism', in *Jewish Women: A Comprehensive Historical Encyclopedia*, Jewish Women's Archive website (accessed 13 Feb. 2014).

RECHTMAN, AVROM, *Jewish Ethnography and Folklore* [Yidishe etnografye un folklor] (Buenos Aires, 1958).

—— 'Some Customs and Their Folk Explanations' (Yid.), *YIVO bleter*, 42 (1962), 249–64.

*Refuot ha'am im darkhei yesharim* (Slavita [Lwów], *c.*1870); unpaginated.

REISER, DANIEL, 'Idea nieuświadomionego (the unconscious) a chasydyzm w Galicji i Polsce' [The Idea of the Unconcscious and Hasidism in Galicia and Poland], trans. Małgorzata Lipska, *Cwisz: Żydowski Kwartalnik o Literaturze i Sztuce*, 1–2 (2014), 43–55.

'Reminiscences: A Little Bit of Everything' (Yid.), in Nakhmen Blumental (ed.), *The Book of Borshchiv* [Sefer borshtshiv] (Tel Aviv, 1960), 38–76.

REUBEN BEN ABRAHAM, *Sefer derekh yesharah* (Livorno, 1788).

REYMAN, BERL, 'Notes on Women's Professions' (Yid.), *Yidishe shprakh*, 19 (1959), 28–9.

'The River in Gliniany' (Yid.), in Henokh H. Halpern (ed.), *The Gliniany Scroll: Reminiscences and Experiences from an Annihilated Community* [Megiles gline: zikhroynes un iberlebungen fun a khorev gevorener kehile] (New York, 1950), 113.

RIVKIND, ITSHOK, *Jewish Money in Life, Culture, and Folklore* [Yidishe gelt in lebnshteyger, kultur-geshikhte un folklor] (New York, 1959).

—— 'Notes on Words' (Yid.), *Yidishe shprakh*, 17 (1957), 11–13.

ROBINSON, IRA, 'Literary Forgery and Hasidic Judaism: The Case of Rabbi Yudel Rosenberg', *Judaism*, 40 (1991), 61–78.

—— 'The Tarler *Rebbe* of Łódź and his Medical Practice: Towards a History of Hasidic Life in Pre-First World War Poland', in Antony Polonsky (ed.), *Focusing on Aspects and Experiences of Religion*, Polin: Studies in Polish Jewry 11 (1998), 53–61.

ROBINSOHN, IZAAK, 'An ajen-hore oder Güt Auge' (Ger.), *Am Ur-Quell*, 5 (1894), 19–20.

—— 'Tierglaube bei Juden Galiziens', *Der Urquell*, 1/1 (1897), 46–9.

ROBOTYCKI, CZESŁAW, and WIESŁAW BABIK (eds.), *Układ gniazdowy terminów i słownik słów kluczowych wybranych kategorii kultury: Medycyna ludowa* [The Group System of Terms and Dictionary of Keywords in Selected Categories of Culture: Folk Medicine] (Kraków, 2005).

ROKER, JOSHUA, *The Sanzer Tsadik* [Der sanzer tsadik] (New York, 1961).

—— *Toledot anshei shem* [A History of Renowned Personages] (Cleveland, 1938).

ROSENBERG, YEHUDAH YUDL, *Der malekh refo'el* (Przemyśl, 1913).

—— *Rafa'el hamalakh* (Piotrków, 1911).

—— *Segulot urefuot . . . ibergezetst oyf zhargon fun heyligen seyfer rafa'el hamalakh* [Remedies and Medicaments . . . Translated into Yiddish from the Holy Book Rafa'el Hamalakh] (Łódź, *c*.1920).

ROSENZWEIG-BLANDER, DVOYRE, 'Lifestyle, Customs, Remedies' (Yid.), in Berl Kahan (ed.), *The Szydłowiec Memorial Book* [Shidlovtser izker-bukh] (New York, 1974), 154–7.

ROSNER, FRED, *Medicine in the Bible and the Talmud* (New York, 1977).

—— 'Pigeons as a Remedy for Jaundice', in Fred Rosner and J. David Bleich (eds.), *Jewish Bioethics* (Hoboken, NJ, 2000), 59–68.

ROTHSTEIN, SHEMUEL, [S. NISNZOHN], *Dos malkhesdike khsides* (Warsaw, 1936).

—— *Nowy Sącz Hasidism* [Tsanzer khsides] (Warsaw, 1937).

—— *Tsadikim and Hasidim* [Tsadikim un khasidim] (New York, 1950).

ROTNER, BARUKH, *Sipurei nifla'ot* [Miracle Stories] (Zhitomir, 1901).

ROZEN, BER Y., 'A Collection of Idiomatic Expressions' (Yid.), *Yidishe shprakh*, 6 (1946), 49–84.

ROZEN, DAVID J., 'Biomedicine, Religion and Ethnicity: Healing in a Hasidic Jewish Community', *High Plains Applied Anthropologist*, 23 (2003), 112–24.

ROZENTAL, Z., 'Folk Songs' (Heb.), *Reshumot*, 2 (1927), 358–78.

ROZMUS, DARIUSZ, *De Judeorum arte sepulcrali: Motywy artystyczne w żydowskiej sztuce sepulkralnej* [De Judeorum arte sepulcrali: Artistic Motifs in Jewish Sepulchral Art] (Kraków, 2005).

ROZOVSKI, MORDKHE, *Collected Writings* [Geklibene shriftn] (Buenos Aires, 1947).

RUBINSTEIN, YEHOSHUA YONATAN, *Zikhron ya'akov yosef* (Jerusalem, *c*.1930).

RULIKOWSKI, EDWARD, 'Zapiski etnograficzne z Ukrainy' [Ethnographic Notes from the Ukraine], *Zbiór Wiadomości do Antropologii Krajowej*, 3 (1879), 62–166.

SADAN DOV, 'The Book of the Covenant' (Yid.), *Yerusholaimer almanakh*, 2–3 (1974), 187–94.

SAILLANT, FRANCINE, 'Home Care and Prevention', *Medical Anthropology Quarterly*, NS 12/2 (1998), 188–205.

SALZ, CHARLES (KHONE), 'My Town Pochayiv' (Yid.), in H. Gelernt (ed.), *The Pochayiv Memorial Book* [Pitshayever izker-bukh] (Philadelphia, 1960).

SAMUEL OF PRZEMYŚL, *Teshuvot haga'on rabi shemuel mipremesla* [Responsa of Rabbi Samuel of Przemyśl], in [Solomon ben Judah Leybush of Lublin, *Piskei veshe'elot uteshuvot maharash milublin* [The Rulings and Responsa of the Maharash of Lublin] (New York, 1988), 247–96.

SCHMID, DANIELA, 'Jüdische Amulette aus Osteuropa—Phänomene, Rituale, Formensprache', Ph.D. diss. (Vienna: Universität Wien, 2012).

SCHNEERSOHN, DOV BER, *Sefer refuot* [Book of Medicaments] (Lemberg, c.1850); unpaginated.

SCHOLEM, GERSHOM, *Gnosticism, Mysticism and Talmudic Tradition* (New York, 1965).

SCHREIBER, MOSES, *Ḥatam sofer*, 'Yoreh de'ah' [responsa] (New York, 1957/8).

SCHRIRE, THEODORE, *Hebrew Amulets* (New York, 1982).

SCHWARTZ, HOWARD, *Tree of Souls: The Mythology of Judaism* (New York, 2004).

SCHWARZ, YOSEF, 'Characters and Personalities' (Yid.), in S. Kants (ed.), *The Book of Burshtin* [Sefer burshtin] (Jerusalem, 1960), 264–72.

SCHWARZBAUM, CHAIM, *Studies in Jewish and World Folklore* (Berlin, 1968).

SCHWARZPUTTER, MOYSHE YECHIEL, 'From Years Gone By' (Yid.), in Berl Kahan (ed.), *The Szydłowiec Memorial Book* [Shidlovtser izker-bukh] (New York, 1974), 102–10.

SCHWEIZER, ISROEL, 'The Overgrown Path' (Yid.), in Isroel Schweizer (ed.), *Pinkas Szczekociny: The Szczekociny Memorial Book—The Life and Death of a Jewish Shtetl* [Pinkas shtshekotshin: shtshekotshiner izker-bukh—lebn un umkum fun a yidish shtetl] (Tel Aviv, 1959), 9–58.

*Sefer abudraham* (Warsaw, 1877).

*Sefer harefuot* [Book of Medicaments] (Vienna, 1926/7).

*Sefer hatsadik r. yosef zundl misalant verabotav* (Jerusalem, 1927).

*Sefer razi'el hamalakh* (Amsterdam, 1701).

SEGEL [SCHIFFER], BENJAMIN WOLF, 'Alltagglauben und volktümliche Heilkunde galizischer Juden', *Am Ur-Quell*, 4 (1893), 170–1, 272–3.

—— 'Chasydzi i chasydyzm' [The Hasidim and Hasidism], *Wisła*, 8 (1894), 677–90.

—— 'Eliah der Prophet', *Am Ur-Quell*, 4 (1893), 11–14, 42–5.

—— 'Materyały do etnografii Żydów wschodnio-galicyjskich' [Material for the Ethnography of the East Galician Jews], *Zbiór Wiadomości do Antropologii Krajowej*, 17 (1894), 261–332.

—— [Bar-Ami], 'Thekuphah', *Izraelita*, 35 (1902), 409–10, and 36 (1902), 421.

—— 'Wierzenia i lecznictwo ludowe Żydów' [Folk Beliefs and Remedies of the Jews], *Lud*, 3 (1897), 49–61.

*Sha'ar efrayim* (Fürth, 1726/7).

SHABAD, TSEMAKH, 'On Erysipelas' (Yid.), *Folksgezunt*, 4 (1927), 53–4.

—— 'On Favus (Ringworm)' (Yid.), *Folksgezunt*, 6 (1924), 159–60.

*Shemirot usegulot nifla'ot* [Amulets and Miraculous Remedies] (Warsaw, 1913).

SHIFMAN, L., 'Dangerous Beliefs about Measles' (Yid.), *Folksgezunt*, 4 (1923), 31–2.

SHLAFERMAN, S., 'The Folklore, Customs, and Stories of Kazimierz' (Yid.), in David Shtokfish (ed.), *Memorial Book of Kazimierz* [Pinkas kuzmir] (Tel Aviv, 1970), 167–75.

SHNEYER, NAFTALI, 'Fools' (Yid.), in Daniel Laybl (ed.), *The Book of Dębica* [Sefer dembits] (Tel Aviv, 1960), 53–4.

SHOLEM ALEICHEM, 'The Creature' (Yid.), in Sholem Aleichem, *The Complete Works* [Ale verk] (New York, 1918), i. 173–89.

—— *From the Fair: The Autobiography of Sholom Aleichem*, trans. and ed. Curt Leviant (New York, 1985).

SHOYS, CHAIM, *The Book of Jewish Festivals* [Dos yontev-bukh] (New York, 1933).

—— 'A Jewish Child is Born' (Yid.), *YIVO Bleter*, 17 (1941), 59.

SHULMAN, ELEAZAR, *The Ashkenazi Jewish Language* [Sefat yehudit-ashkenazit] (Riga, 1913).

SHUSTER, AARON, 'The Grandfather Healer' (Yid.), in Mosheh Silberman-Silon and Ya'akov Berger-Tamir (eds.), *The Community of Lipkany: A Memorial Book* [Kehilat lipkani: sefer zikaron] (Tel Aviv, 1963), 176–80.

*Siddur According to the Rite of Poland, Lithuania, Ruthenia, and Moravia* [Sidur keminhag polin, lita veraysn umern] (Ostroh, 1817).

SILVERMAN-WEINREICH, BEATRICE, 'Beliefs' (Yid.), *Yidisher folklor*, 2 (1955), 33.

—— (ed.), *Yiddish Folktales*, trans. Leonard Wolf (New York, 1997).

SIMNER, ZEKHARYAH, *Sefer zekhirah* (Heb.) (Johannisburg, c.1860).

SIMON, ANTONI ARNOLD, *Medycyna ludowa, czyli treściwy pogląd na środki ochronne, poznawanie i leczenie chorób* [Folk Medicine, or: a Substantial Overview of Protective Measures, Diagnosis, and Treatment of Diseases] (Warsaw, 1860).

SINGER, ISAAC BASHEVIS, 'The Gentleman from Cracow', in *Gimpel the Fool and Other Stories* (New York, 2006), 23–44

—— *The Magician of Lublin* (New York, 1965).

SIRAT, COLETTE, *A History of Jewish Philosophy in the Middle Ages* (Cambridge, 1996).

SLUTSKI, YEHUDA, 'Bobruysk (A Monograph)' (Yid.), in Yehuda Slutski (ed.), *Bobruysk: The Memorial Book of the Community in Bobruysk and the Surrounding Area* [Bobruysk: sefer zikaron likehilat bobruysk uvenoteiha], trans. Y. L. Pines (Tel Aviv, 1967), 113–220.

SOKOŁÓW, FLORIAN, *My Father* [Mayn foter], trans. Naftole Zilberberg (Tel Aviv, 1972).

SOSNOWIK, ELIOHU, 'Material on Jewish Folk Medicine in Belarus' (Yid.), *Yidishe filologye*, 2–3 (1924), 160–8.

SPERBER, DANIEL, 'Marriage', in Raphael Patai and Haya Bar-Itzhak (eds.), *Encyclopedia of Jewish Folklore and Traditions* (New York, 2013), 354–5.

SPERLING, ABRAHAM ISAAC, *Ta'amei haminhagim oyf ivri taytsh* [Reasons for the Customs in Yiddish], 2 vols. (Lemberg, 1909).

—— *Ta'amei haminhagim umekorei hadinim* [Reasons for the Customs and the Sources of Laws] (Jerusalem, 1957).

SPINNER, J., 'Zur Volkkunde galizischer Juden', *Am Ur-Quell*, 4 (1893), 95–6.

*Sposób domowy leczenia tak ludzi jak bydląt albo apteczka w domu przytomna zawsze* [The Domestic Method of Treating Both Humans and Livestock, or: the Ever-Ready Domestic Medicine Chest] (Kalisz, 1784).

'The Steam Bath' (Yid.), in Henokh H. Halpern (ed.), *The Gliniany Scroll: Reminiscences and Experiences from an Annihilated Community* [Megiles gline: zikhroynes un iberlebungen fun a khorev gevorener kehile] (New York, 1950), 113–14.

STEINBERG, ISRAEL, *From the Fount of the Wisdom of the Jewish People* [Mima'ayan haḥokhmah shel am yisra'el] (Tel Aviv, 1962).

STERN, YEKHIEL, 'A Translation School in Tyszowce' (Yid.), *Shriftn far psikhologye un pedagogik*, 2 (1940), 265–82.

STOL, MARTEN, *Epilepsy in Babylonia* (Groningen, 1993).

STOMMA, LUDWIK, *Antropologia kultury wsi polskiej XIX w.* [Cultural Anthropology of Nineteenth-Century Rural Poland] (Gdańsk, 2000).

STUTSHKOV, NOKHEM, *Thesaurus of the Yiddish Language* [Der oytser fun der yidisher shprakh] (New York, 1991).

SUKHER, SHLOYME, 'With the Hasidim of Vizhnits' (Yid.), in Shimshon Meltser (ed.), *The Book of Horodenka* [Seyfer horodenke] (New York, 1963), 249–51.

'Superstitions and Folk Sayings' (Yid.), in Elkhanan Erlikh (ed.), *The Book of Staszów* [Sefer stashov] (Tel Aviv, 1962), 327–8.

SZUBERT, WACŁAW, *Ubezpieczenie społeczne: Zarys system* [Social Security: An Overview of the System] (Warsaw, 1987).

SZUKIEWICZ, WANDALIN, 'Wierzenia i praktyki ludowe (zabobony, przesądy, wróżby i.t.d.), zebrane w gubernji wileńskiej' [Folk Beliefs and Practices (Superstitions, Omens, etc.) Gathered in the Vilno Guberniya], *Wisła*, 17 (1903), 432–44.

Szychowska-Boebel, Barbara, *Lecznictwo ludowe na Kujawach: materiały i rozważania* [Folk Healing in Cuiavia: Material and Musings] (Toruń, 1972).

Taglicht, J., 'Songs from Slovakia' (Yid.), *Mitteilungen zur Jüdischen Volkskunde*, 2 (1906), 58–62.

'Tales and Traditions' (Yid.), in Yehudah Leib Kahan (ed.), *Jewish Folklore* [Yidisher folklor], Shriftn fun yidishn visnshaftlekher institut 9 (Vilna, 1938), 167–73.

Talko-Hryncewicz, Julian, *Zarys lecznictwa ludowego na Rusi Południowej* [An Outline of Folk Treatments in Southern Rus] (Kraków, 1893).

Tarlau, J., 'Volksmedizinisches aus dem jüdischen Russland (Gouv. Mohilev)', *Mitteilungen der Gesellschaft für Jüdische Volkskunde*, 10 (1902), 144.

Ta-Shma, Israel, 'The Ban on Drinking Water at Tekufah and Its Origin' (Heb.), *Meḥkerei yerushalayim befolklor yehudi*, 17 (1995), 21–32.

——'Minhagim Books', in *Encyclopaedia Judaica* (Detroit, 2007), xiv. 278–9.

Taub, Yeshaya, 'The Appearance of a Jewish Home' (Yid.), *YIVO bleter*, 44 (1973), 277–81.

*Tehilim im sefer mishpat tsedek* (Vienna, 1856).

Temesváry, Rudolf, *Volksbräuche und Aberglauben in der Geburtshilfe und der Pflege des Neugeborenen in Ungarn* (Leipzig, 1900).

Tenenbaum, Shea, *Ayzik Ashmeday* (Yid.) (New York, 1965).

'The Town' (Yid.), in Henokh H. Halpern (ed.), *The Gliniany Scroll: Reminiscences and Experiences from an Annihilated Community* [Megiles gline: zikhroynes un iberlebungen fun a khorev gevorener kehile] (New York, 1950), 16–27.

Trachtenberg, Joshua, *Jewish Magic and Superstition* (New York, 1939).

Trayevitski, Yehuda, 'Personalities' (Yid.), in *The Community of Turzec and Yeremichi: A Memorial Book* [Kehilat turets veyeremits: sefer zikaron] (Tel Aviv, 1978), 203–5.

Trunk, Israel Yehoshua, *Poland: Memories and Images* [Poyln: zikhroynes un bilder], 7 vols. (New York, 1946).

Trzciński, Andrzej, *Symbole i obrazy: Treści symboliczne przedstawień na nagrobkach żydowskich w Polsce* [Symbols and Images: The Symbolic Content of Visual Imagery on Jewish Tombstones in Poland] (Lublin, 1997).

——'Zachowane wystroje malarskie bóżnic w Polsce' [Preserved Interior Painting in Synagogues in Poland], *Studia Judaica*, 4/1–2(7–8) (2001), 67–95.

Tsart, A., 'Superstitions and Beliefs in Our Region' (Yid.), *Folksgezunt*, 2–3 (1923), 51–2.

'Tsava'at rabi yehudah heḥasid', in Judah Hehasid, *Sefer ḥasidim* (Lwów, 1934/5), 5–16.

Tsherniak, F., 'Medical Assistance and Medical Institutions' (Yid.), in Benzion H. Ayalon (ed.) *Antopol (Antepolie) Yizkor Book* [Antopol. Sefer yizkor] (Tel Aviv, 1972), 527–36.

TSHERNIAK, YOSEF, 'Linguistic Folklore and Narrative Style' (Heb.), *Yeda am*, 10 (1964), 29–35.

—— 'Linguistic Folklore in Yiddish' (Heb.), *Yeda am*, 11 (1965), 96–104.

TUSZEWICKI, MAREK, 'Chasydzi w Galicji wobec współczesnej farmacji w świetle dzieła "Beerot ha-majim" (Przemyśl 1888)' [The Attitudes of Hasidim in Galicia towards Contemporary Pharmaceutics in Light of the Work *Be'erot hamayim* (Przemyśl, 1888)], *Medycyna Nowożytna*, 18 (2012), 49–83.

—— 'O pasożytach wywołujących suchoty. Na styku żydowskiej kultury ludowej i dawnej medycyny' [Regarding Parasites Causing Consumption: Where Folk Culture Meets Early Medicine], *Kwartalnik Historii Żydów*, 4(348) (2013), 613–34.

—— 'Żydowska medycyna ludowa: Pomiędzy swojskością a obcością' [Jewish Folk Medicine: Between the Familiar and the Alien], in Eugenia Prokop-Janiec (ed.), *Polacy—Żydzi: Kontakty kulturowe i literackie* [Poles—Jews: Cultural and Literary Contacts] (Kraków, 2014), 25–56.

UDZIELA, MARIAN, *Medycyna i przesądy lecznicze ludu polskiego* [Medicine and Treatment-Related Superstitions of the Polish Folk] (Warsaw, 1891).

UDZIELA, SEWERYN, 'Materiały etnograficzne zebrane z miasta Ropczyc i okolicy' [Ethnographic Material Gathered from the Town of Ropczyce and the Surrounding Region], *Zbiór Wiadomości do Antropologii Krajowej*, 10 (1886), 75–156.

UNGER, MENASHEH, *The Hasidic World* [Di khsidishe velt] (New York, 1955).

—— *Hasidism and the Jewish Festivals* [Khsides un yontev] (New York, 1958).

—— *Pshiskhe and Kotsk* [Pshiskhe un kotsk] (Buenos Aires, 1949).

'Useful Proverbs' (Yid.), *Yidishe shprakh*, 10 (1950), 59–62; 11 (1951), 55–8; 14 (1954), 61–2.

*Vade mecum medicum* (Częstochowa, 1721).

VARAD, MALKA, 'Every Jewish Festival with Its Own Atmosphere' (Yid.), in Yosef Kariv (ed.), *The Book of Horokhov* [Sefer Horokhov] (Tel Aviv, 1966), 47–8.

'Various Medicaments for Toothache', *Yidisher folklor*, 3 (1962), 70.

VARSHAVSKI, YITZHOK, 'Of the Old and New Homelands' (Yid.), *Forverts*, 1 Nov. 1963.

*Vayikra rabah* (New York, 1973/4).

VEYNIG, NAFTOLE, 'Doctors and Medicine in Jewish Sayings' (Yid.), *Sotsyale meditsin*, 11–12 (1936), 17–23.

—— 'Hygiene and Sanitation Services among Galician and Romanian Jews in the First Half of the Nineteenth Century' (Yid.), *Sotsyale meditsin*, 1–2 (1935), 22–6.

—— 'Mageyfe Weddings' (Yid.), *Sotsyale meditsin*, 9–10 (1937), 24–33.

—— 'Medicaments and Remedies among the Jews in Times of Epidemics' (Yid.), *Sotsyale meditsin*, 11–12 (1937), 25–31.

VIETUKHOV, ALEXEI, *Zagovory, zaklinaniya, obieregi i drugiye vidy narodnogo vrachevaniya* [Conjurations, Whispers, Amulets, and Other Folk Treatment Methods] (Warsaw, 1907).

VILNER, Y., 'People from the Shtetl' (Yid.), in Avraham Levita (ed.), *The Brzozów Memorial Book* [Sefer zikaron kehilat breziv (bzhozov)] (n.p., 1984), 155–7.

VIRSHUBSKI, AVRAHAM, 'The Dybbuk' (Yid.), *Folksgezunt*, 20 (1929), 319–20.

WASILEWSKI, JERZY S., 'Po śmierci wędrować. Szkic z zakresu etnologii świata znaczeń, cz. II' [Wandering after Death: A Sketch from the Field of the Ethnology of the Semantic World, Part II], *Teksty*, 4 (1979), 58–84.

—— 'Tabu, zakaz magiczny, nieczystość. Część II. Tabu a paradygmaty etnologii' [Taboo, Magical Interdiction, Uncleanness. Part II: Taboo and Ethnological Paradigms], *Etnografia Polska*, 34/1–2 (1990), 7–45.

WĘGRZYNEK, HANNA, 'The "Shvartze khasene": The Black Wedding among the Polish Jews', in Glenn Dynner (ed.), *Holy Dissent* (Detroit, 2011), 55–68.

WEINREICH, MAX, *Geschichte der jiddischen Sprachforshung* (Atlanta, 1993).

—— *History of the Yiddish Language*, trans. Shlomo Noble, 2 vols. (New York, 2008).

—— 'Lantukh: The History of a Jewish Demon' (Yid.), *Filologishe shriftn*, 1 (1926), 217–36.

WEINREICH, URIEL, 'Beliefs: Remedies for Warts' (Yid.), *Yidisher folklor*, 3 (1962), 62–3.

WEINSTEIN, BERISH, *Rzeszów: An Extended Poem* [Rayshe. Poeme] (New York, 1947).

WEINSTOCK, MOSES YA'IR, *Kodesh hilulim* (New York, 1949).

WEISSENBERG, SAMUEL, 'Beiträge zur Volkskunde der Juden', *Globus*, 77/21 (1900), 130–1, 339–41.

—— 'Das Feld- und das Kejwermessen', *Mitteilungen zur Jüdischen Volkskunde*, 1 (1906), 39–42.

—— 'Das neugeborene Kind bei den südrussischen Juden', *Globus*, 93/6 (1908), 85–8.

—— 'Eine jüdische Hochzeit in Südrussland', *Mitteilungen zur Jüdischen Volkskunde*, 1 (1905), 59–93.

—— 'Hygiene in Brauch und Sitte der Juden', in Max Grunwald (ed.), *Die Hygiene der Juden* (Dresden, 1911), 29–43.

—— 'Kinderfreud und -leid bei den südrussischen Juden', *Globus*, 83/20 (1903), 315–20.

—— 'Krankheit und Tod bei den südrussischen Juden', *Globus*, 91/23 (1907), 357–63.

—— 'Palästina in Brauch und Glauben der heutigen Juden', *Globus*, 92/17 (1907), 261–4.

—— 'Südrussische Amulette', *Verhandlungen der Berliner Gesellschaft für Anthropologie, Ethnologie und Urgeschichte*, 29 (1897), 367–9.

WEISSMAN, MOYSHE, *A Half-Century in America* [A halber yorhundert in amerike] (Tel Aviv, 1960).

WEISSMAN, MOYSHE, 'The Victory of the Jewish Doctor (Dr Goldberger)' (Yid.), in Eliezer Tash (Tur-Shalom) (ed.), *The Siemiatycze Community* [Kehilat Siemiatitsh] (Tel Aviv, 1965), 347–8.

WELLESZ, J., 'Volksmedizinisches aus dem jüdischen Mittelalter', *Mitteilungen zur Jüdischen Volkskunde*, 2 (1910), 117–20.

WEREŃKO, FRANCISZEK, 'Przyczynek do lecznictwa ludowego' [An Introduction to Folk Healing], *Materyały Antropologiczno-Archeologiczne i Etnograficzne*, 1 (1896), 99–228.

WERTHEIM, AARON, *Law and Custom in Hasidism* (New York, 1992).

WHITELEY, KATHLEEN, 'Hippocrates' *Diseases of Women* Book 1—Greek Text with English Translation and Footnotes', MA thesis (University of South Africa, Pretoria, 2003).

WIĘCKOWSKA, ELŻBIETA, *Lekarze jako grupa zawodowa w II Rzeczypospolitej* [Physicians as a Professional Group in the Second Polish Republic] (Wrocław, 2004).

WIENER, LEO, 'Aus der Russisch-Jüdischen Kinderstube', *Mitteilungen der Gesellschaft für Jüdische Volkskunde*, 2 (1898), 40–9.

—— 'Märchen und Schwänke in Amerika aus dem Munde russischer Juden aufgezeichnet', *Mitteilungen der Gesellschaft für Jüdische Volkskunde*, 2 (1902), 98–121.

WIENER-RAM, MALKA, 'Our Town and Its Jews' (Heb.), in David Yakubovitsh (ed.), *Memorial Book for the Communities of Vadovitse, Andrikhov, Kalvaria, Mishlenits, Sukha* [Sefer zikaron likehilot Vadovitse, Andrikhov, Kalvaria, Mishlenits, Sukha] (Ramat Gan, 1967), 53–9.

WILFF, SOLOMON, *Imrot shelomoh, vehu ḥupat ḥatanim heḥadash* (Kraków, 1906).

WINTER, SHEMUEL, 'Tatars and Witches' (Yid.), *Yidishe filologye*, 4–6 (1924), 394–6.

WODZIŃSKI, MARCIN, 'Dybuk. Z dokumentów Archiwum Głównego Akt Dawnych w Warszawie' [The Dybbuk: From Documents in the Central Archives of Historical Records in Warsaw], *Literatura Ludowa*, 6 (1992), 19–29.

WOLFSON, ELLIOT R., *Through a Speculum That Shines: Vision and Imagination in Medieval Jewish Mysticism* (Princeton, NJ, 1994).

WOLRAT, DOVID, 'The Rabbi's Funeral' (Yid.), in A. S. Shteyn and Gavriel Vaysman (eds.), *The Memorial Book of Sochaczew* [Pinkes Sokhatshev] (Jerusalem, 1962), 92–5.

WUTTKE, ADOLF, *Der deutsche Volksaberglauben der Gegenwart* (Berlin, 1900).

YARMUSH, ABEL, *Of Two Homes* [Fun tsvey heymen] (Buenos Aires, 1965).

YELIN, ABRAHAM, *Derekh tsadikim* (Piotrków, 1911/12).

YEUSHSOHN, B. [MOYSHE BUNEM YUSTMAN], *From Our Old Treasure* [Fun undzer altn oytser], 4 vols. (Warsaw, 1934).

YODER, DON, 'Folk medicine', in Richard M. Dorson (ed.), *Folklore and Folklife* (Chicago, 1982), 191–215.

YOFE, YUDA A., and YUDL MARK (eds.), *The Great Dictionary of the Yiddish Language* [Groyser verterbukh fun der yidisher shprakh], 4 vols. (New York, 1961).

YOFFIE, LEA RACHEL, 'Popular Beliefs and Customs among the Yiddish-Speaking Jews of St. Louis, Mo', *Journal of American Folklore*, 38 (1925), 375–99.

YUNIS, ZEV, 'The Old Homeland' (Yid.), in Yakov Shatski (ed.), *Mława Memorial Book* [Pinkes mlave] (New York, 1950), 27–130.

ZADOFF, MIRJAM, *Next Year in Marienbad: The Lost Worlds of Jewish Spa Culture* (Philadelphia, 2012).

ZALER, ISAAC, *Yalkut yitsḥak* (Warsaw, 1894/5).

ZAMLUNG, EZRIEL HAYIM, *Eser zekhiyot* (Benei Berak, 1973/4).

ZANDVAYS, SHLOYME, 'Sarny—Its Foundation, Existence, and Decline' (Yid.), in Yosef Kariv (ed.), *The Sarny Community Memorial Book* [Sefer yizkor likehilat sarni] (Tel Aviv, 1961), 82–154.

ZAWADSKI, WŁADYSŁAW, *Obrazy Rusi Czerwonej* [Images from Red Ruthenia] (Poznań, 1869).

ZAWILIŃSKI, ROMAN, 'Przesądy i zabobony z ust ludu w różnych okolicach zebrane' [Superstitions and Old Wives' Tales Gathered from the Mouths of the People in Various Circumstances], *Zbiór Wiadomości do Antropologii Krajowej*, 16 (1892), 252–67.

ZELKOVITSH, YOSEF, 'Death and Its Accompanying Moments in Jewish Ethnography and Folklore' (Yid.), *Lodzer visnshaftlekhe shriftn*, 1 (1938), 149–90.

*Zemirot leshabat kodesh veyom tov, nusaḥ vizhnits* [Songs for the Sabbath and Festivals: The Vizhnits Rite] (Kiryat Vizhnits, 2008).

ZEVIN, Y. Y., *All the Stories of the Talmud and the Ein Ya'akov* [Ale agodes fun talmud un ein ya'akov], 3 vols. (New York, 1922).

ZEYERMAN, SHRAGA, 'Medical Care' (Yid.), in Dov Shuval (ed.), *The Sarnaki Community Memorial Book* [Sefer yizkor likehilat sarnaki] (Haifa, 1968), 125–7.

ZIMMELS, HIRSCH JACOB, *Magicians, Theologians and Doctors: Studies in Folk Medicine and Folklore as Reflected in the Rabbinical Responsa 12th–19th Centuries* (London, 1952).

ZINBERG, ISRAEL, *A History of Jewish Literature* [Di geshikhte fun der literatur bay yidn], 8 vols. (New York, 1943).

ZŁOTNIK, YEHUDAH LEIB [YEHUDAH AVIDA], 'Incantations and Remedies in Arabic and Yiddish' (Heb.), *Yeda am*, 5 (1958), 3–7.

—— [Elzet], 'Some Jewish Customs' (Heb.), *Reshumot*, 1 (1918), 335–77.

ZOLLER, I., 'Lilith' (Yid.), *Filologishe shriftn*, 3 (1929), 121–42.

ZUKER, MORDKHE, 'A Dybbuk' (Yid.), in Yitshak Perlov and Alfred Lipson
    (eds.), *The Book of Radom* [Sefer radom] (Tel Aviv, 1961–3), 273.

ZUKER, YEHUDAH LEIB, 'Ritual Slaughterers' (Yid.), in Yitshak Perlov and
    Alfred Lipson (eds.), *The Book of Radom* [Sefer radom] (Tel Aviv, 1961–3),
    59–62.

# INDEX OF PLACES

# INDEX OF SUBJECTS

Printed and bound by CPI Group (UK) Ltd, Croydon, CR0 4YY

09/06/2025

14685961-0003

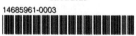